Telemedicine: A Practical Approach

Telemedicine: A Practical Approach

Editor: Brittany McGrath

FOSTER
ACADEMICS
www.fosteracademics.com

www.fosteracademics.com

FOSTER
ACADEMICS

Cataloging-in-Publication Data

Telemedicine : a practical approach / edited by Brittany McGrath.
p. cm.
Includes bibliographical references and index.
ISBN 978-1-63242-841-7
1. Telecommunication in medicine. 2. Medical telematics. 3. Medicine. I. McGrath, Brittany.
R119.9 .T45 2019
610.285--dc23

Foster Academics,
118-35 Queens Blvd., Suite 400,
Forest Hills, NY 11375, USA

ISBN 978-1-63242-841-7 (Hardback)

Printed and bound in China.

Contents

Preface

Telemedicine refers to the health care provided from a distance with the help of telecommunication and information technology. It is helpful in improving access to medical services in distant rural areas. It plays a significant role in saving lives in critical and emergency cases. Teleconferencing and videotelephony are the most common forms of telemedicine. Telepharmacy is a sub-field of telemedicine. It involves the delivery of pharmaceutical care to patients through information technology and telecommunications. Patient counseling, drug therapy monitoring along with prior and refill authorization for prescription drugs are some of the telepharmacy services. This book is a compilation of chapters that discuss the most vital concepts and emerging trends in the field of telemedicine. Some of the diverse topics covered herein address the varied branches that fall under this field. It aims to serve as a resource guide for students and experts alike and contribute to the growth of the discipline.

This book has been the outcome of endless efforts put in by authors and researchers on various issues and topics within the field. The book is a comprehensive collection of significant researches that are addressed in a variety of chapters. It will surely enhance the knowledge of the field among readers across the globe.

It gives us an immense pleasure to thank our researchers and authors for their efforts to submit their piece of writing before the deadlines. Finally in the end, I would like to thank my family and colleagues who have been a great source of inspiration and support.

Editor

1

Willingness to Adopt Telemedicine in Major Iraqi Hospitals

Mohd Khanapi Abd Ghani and Mustafa Musa Jaber

Biomedical Computing and Engineering Technologies (BIOCORE) Applied Research Group, Faculty of Information and Communication Technology, Universiti Teknikal Malaysia Melaka, Durian Tunggal, 75450 Ayer Keroh, Malacca, Malaysia

Correspondence should be addressed to Mustafa Musa Jaber; mustafamusajaber@yahoo.com

Academic Editor: Malcolm Clarke

The Iraqi healthcare services are struggling to regain their lost momentum. Many physicians and nurses left Iraq because of the current situation in the country. Despite plans of calling back the skilled health workforce, they are still worried by the disadvantages of their return. Hence, technology plays a central role in taking advantage of their profession through the use of telemedicine. Studying the factors that affect the implementation of telemedicine is necessary. Telemedicine covers network services, policy makers, and patient understanding. A framework that includes the influencing factors in adopting telemedicine in Iraq was developed in this study. A questionnaire was distributed among physicians in Baghdad Medical City to examine the hypothesis on each factor. The Statistical Package for the Social Sciences was utilized to verify the reliability of the questionnaire and Cronbach's alpha test shows that the factors have values more than 0.7, which are standard.

1. Introduction

Developing countries are using telemedicine to link health centers, tertiary centers, and referral hospitals. Several e-health applications, such as telemedicine, can be found with different degrees of success in majority of developing countries [1, 2]. According to [3], the following two factors explain the wide use of telemedicine: the lack of alternatives such as building hospitals in each village which is costly and (2) the apparent geographical superiority of telemedicine over traditional medicine. Despite high expectations from the technology, configuring its use into a certain routine is impossible [4].

The framework of adopting telemedicine in Iraq was categorized into four characteristics, namely, technological, organizational, environmental, and individual. Fourteen influencing factors were explicated, and each was included in its appropriate characteristic. This framework can enhance the quality of the healthcare sector in Iraq. Thus, the influencing factors are enablers in the decision-making and e-participation of hospitals [5]. This study illustrates a suitable design of the questionnaire on willingness to adopt telemedicine of telemedicine in Iraq to evaluate the framework. A pilot study was conducted to improve the reliability of the questionnaire.

Several benefits can be expected from the use of telemedicine. These benefits can affect not only the health providers and the patients, but also the entire healthcare organization. For example, a study on physicians and health managers in the Quebec health region in Canada by [6] found that the benefits and usefulness of the telemedicine system were seen on three levels: (1) clinical/patient, (2) professional/educational, and (3) organizational.

2. Limitations of the Research

This study aims to examine the feasibility and acceptance level telemedicine framework in Iraq. However, a number of limitations should be considered. First, studies regarding telemedicine in Iraq are limited, with few studies conducted by the Ministry of Health of Iraq. This situation caused some difficulties in designing the questionnaire. Second, the physicians' level of understanding of telemedicine is limited because telemedicine is a new technology in Iraq [5, 7]. Third, only a handful of physicians practice electronic consultation (e-consultation). Fourth, physicians have limited grasp and knowledge of data warehouse because it is viewed and considered as a new tool in telemedicine. Fifth, the number of respondents was 35 only. Finally, the unstable political climate and strife in Iraq added challenges to the scope and limitations of this study.

3. The Framework

The technology-organization-environment (TOE) framework, which was developed by [8], is chosen and applied as the framework of this study. [1, 2], These studies have demonstrated consistent support for TOE's ability to provide a comprehensive perspective on innovation adoption, while facilitating the flexibility to identify and categorize unique factors that may emerge in particular situations [9]. Moreover, the main reason for selecting this framework is that this approach has the potential to address issues of this study. On the subject of appropriate framework selection, [10] advocates a framework that has been adapted and adopted and requires further development and fine-tuning in its application for contextual matching.

This study adapted the TOE framework to improve its suitability in the field of telemedicine. This adaption considers technological, organizational, environmental, and individual characteristics. In addition, social exchange theory, diffusion of innovation theory, TOE adoption framework, and previous studies are employed to investigate the factors that influence telemedicine in Iraq. These theories have been applied in electronic information sharing studies [11, 12]. Social exchange theory refers to shared information in the public sector [13]. This theory is based on power and trust. Thus, factors such as top management support of upper-level leadership are employed. The focus of this theory is to help organizations and individuals in deciding whether to adopt or reject a new innovation and to estimate the duration of acceptance and use of a new technology. In reality, the theory has been used to clarify and evaluate a wide range of IT adoption, such as that of the Internet [14], database machine [15], software engineering techniques [16], and IT in general [17].

The remaining factors have been adopted from researches done in Middle Eastern countries such as Kuwait and Jordan. Each characteristic has numerous influencing factors. The influencing factors of the current research are privacy, culture, attitude to telemedicine, benefit, connectivity, IT capability, compatibility, data warehouse concept, technical support, top management support, cost, approach, and upper-level leadership. This study also introduces 13 hypotheses. One hypothesis is formulated for every factor. Figure 1 shows the framework of this study.

The factors that can promote engagement in the willingness to accept telemedicine have been identified. The pilot study is performed to evaluate the questionnaire items and to determine the appropriate questions for the survey.

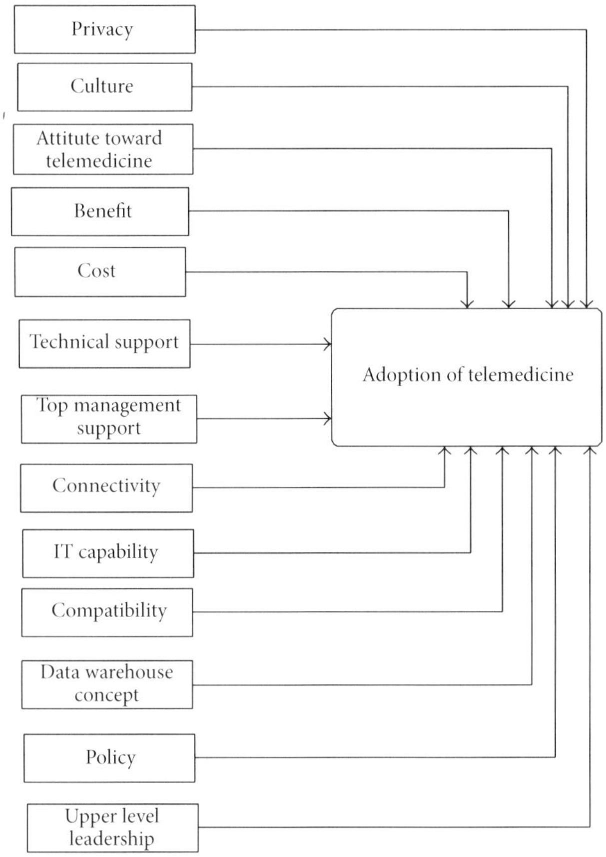

FIGURE 1: Framework of willingness to adopt telemedicine in Iraq.

The questionnaires were distributed among physicians. The succeeding section explains the questionnaire design.

4. Research Methods

The survey method is employed in this study because surveys are prevalently used to begin reports and it is a suitable method for examining factors and hypotheses. The questionnaire methodology is used for data collection. Paper [18] shows that the questionnaire design relies on three criteria, namely, the manner by which the questions are written, planning for the classification of variables, and the appearance of the questionnaire. This study uses a six-part questionnaire. Part 1 includes the questions related to demographic factors. Part 2 relates to the state of telemedicine. Part 3 relates to the characteristics of telemedicine. Part 4 relates to organizational characteristics. Part 5 includes questions related to technological characteristics. Part 6 relates to environmental characteristics. Please refer to the Appendix.

The questionnaire is designed based on the content of each factor. Suggestions and advice from colleagues and supervisors are considered in improving the design of the questionnaire, as well as in developing the questionnaire. The questionnaire is written in English and then translated into Arabic, which is the official language in Iraq. Table 1 shows the operationalization of the factors and items.

Table 1: Operationalization of the factors and items.

Factor	Items	References
Privacy	3 items	[17, 19]
Culture	3 items	[19–21]
Attitude toward telemedicine	3 items	[22, 23]
Benefit	5 items	[20, 21, 24]
Connectivity	3 items	[25, 26]
IT capability	3 items	[20, 21, 24, 27]
Compatibility	3 items	[5, 13, 28]
Data warehouse	3 items	[29–31]
Technical support	3 items	[21, 32]
Top management support	3 items	[5, 13, 28, 33]
Cost	4 items	[20, 24, 34]
Policy	3 items	[5, 13, 20, 21, 28]
Upper-level leadership	3 items	[5, 13, 35]

Table 2: Demographic characteristics.

	% of participants	
	Pilot study 1	Pilot study 1
Variable		
Male	24	80.0%
Female	6	20.0%
Less than 30	3	10.0%
From 30 to 40	21	70.0%
From 41 to 50	5	16.7%
More than 50	1	3.3%
Bachelor	21	70.0%
Master's	8	26.7%
Ph.D.	1	3.3%
Experience in years		
From 1 to 5	6	20.0%
From 6 to 10	14	46.7%
From 11 to 15	8	26.7%
More than 15	2	6.7%
Type of position		
Administrator	12	40.0%
Nonadministrator	18	60.0%

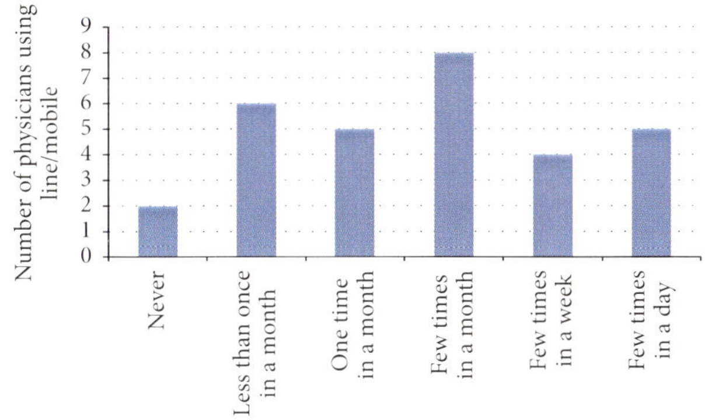

Figure 2: Line/mobile usage.

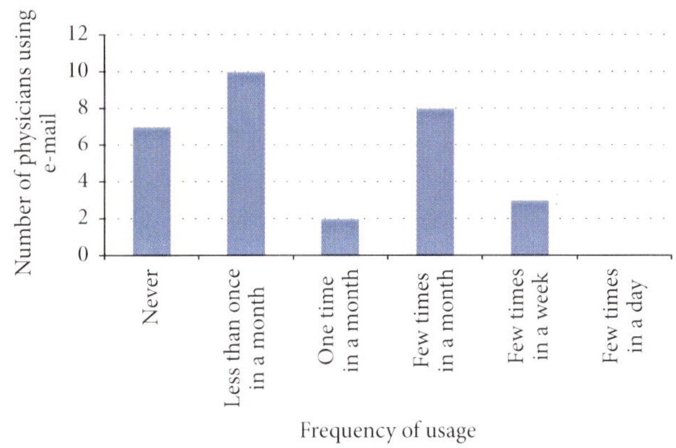

Figure 3: E-mail usage.

5. Pilot Study

Questionnaires were distributed among physicians who are working in Baghdad Medical City. Among the 35 questionnaires collected, only 5 were not correctly answered. Table 2 illustrates the demographic characteristics of the pilot study.

5.1. Usage of Devices. Queries on the method of how physicians conduct electronic consultation in inputting patient information were conducted in this study. Five methods were mentioned in the questionnaire, but the participants were provided an option to add another method that they have used. However, no other method of information sharing was added by the participants. Thus, each study reveals different percentages related to the five methods used. Figures 2, 3, 4, and 5 illustrate the percentages of the most used method of electronic consultation. The data collected reveal that e-mail is the most used method in electronic consultation.

The database was not utilized by the participants to access the ministry's information. The results from the two pilot studies reveal that the most used means of electronic consultation between physicians and patients are phone, e-mail, and website. The findings also show that the use of webcam is limited. The use of database was mentioned only once in both studies.

5.2. Percentage and Initiation Time of Sharing Information. The electronic information sharing practice in the Iraqi healthcare sector was measured in terms of the percentage of electronic consultation used and the time information consultation was initiated. Thus, based on the findings, the participants of the pilot studies illustrated the percentage of electronic consultation used. Most of the participants revealed that the percentage of consultation is 63.3% from 1% to 20% of their work. Most of the participants mentioned that electronic consultation was initiated between 1 year and 3 years ago. Table 3 shows the consultation percentage per year was initiated.

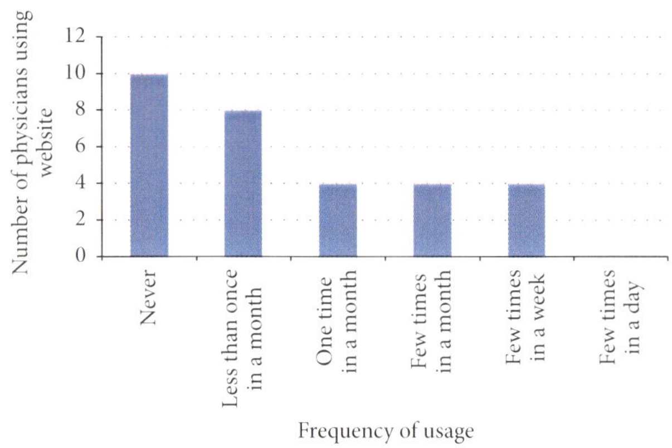

FIGURE 4: Website usage.

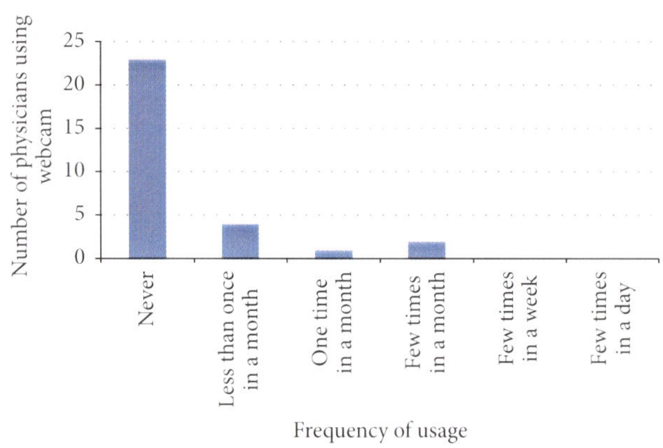

FIGURE 5: Webcam usage.

TABLE 3: Percentage and start/initiation time of consultation.

Variables	Number of participants	% of participants
Percentage of consultation		
Zero	5	16.7%
From 1% to 20%	19	63.3%
From 21% to 40%	5	16.7%
From 41% to 60%	1	3.3%
From 61% to 80%	0	0.0%
From 81% to 100%	0	0.0%
Years of consultation		
Zero	1	3.3%
Less than a year	9	30.0%
From 1 to 3 years	18	60.0%
From 4 to 6 years	2	6.7%
From 7 to 9 years	0	0.0%
10 years or more	0	0.0%

6. Results of Data Analysis

The most commonly used test in reliability measurement of any pilot study questionnaire is Cronbach's alpha [18, 36]. According to [37], Cronbach's alpha test possesses values within the range of 0 to 1; a higher level of range indicates greater value of reliability. Values of 0.9 and above are excellent, 0.8 and above are good, 0.7 and above are acceptable, 0.6 and above are questionable, and less than 0.6 are poor [37, 38].

TABLE 4: Cronbach's alpha and number of items.

Factor	Cronbach's alpha	Number of items
Privacy	.756	3
Culture	.926	3
Attitude toward telemedicine	.755	3
Benefit	.729	5
Connectivity	.794	3
IT capability	.706	3
Compatibility	.763	3
Data warehouse	.749	3
Technical support	.787	3
Top management support	.706	3
Cost	.728	4
Policy	.815	3
Upper-level leadership	.818	3

The data collected from the two pilot studies have been analyzed using Statistical Package for the Social Sciences 20 to identify the values of each factor in Cronbach's alpha. Based on the pilot study, no change should be made in the items of the pilot study. These items were rewritten to create a clear and easy-to-understand questionnaire. The items of the factors were also reduced. Thus, all factors have values of more than 0.7, which are acceptable. Table 4 shows Cronbach's alpha and number of items for each factor.

7. Conclusion and Future Work

This study was proposed to examine the influencing factors in the willingness to adopt and practice telemedicine in Iraq. This study was prompted by a real need to examine the requirements, challenges, and gaps in adopting this new technology. A set of items of questionnaires was designed based on previous studies on the adoption of telemedicine in the Middle Eastern countries, such as Kuwait, Saudi Arabia, Jordan, and Syria. The pilot studies were conducted to examine each influencing factor in the hypotheses and to test the reliability of the questionnaire. The pilot study was required to verify the items. Cronbach's alpha test in the pilot study reveals that the factors have values more than 0.7, which are acceptable. The pilot study was conducted using questionnaires that were disseminated to physicians in Iraq. A research paper will follow this study to illustrate the results of the data analysis of the survey. Future research will then test the hypotheses and validate the framework. The results of the tests are expected to contribute to furthering the understanding and grasp of electronic information sharing in the healthcare sector. In addition, research of willingness to adopt telemedicine needs to be examined in rural area since it has different factors to measure.

Table 5: Part 3: individual characteristic.

	Strongly disagree	Disagree	Neutral	Agree	Strongly agree
Pri1: being concerned about patient privacy is important.					
Pri2: we have to keep the privacy of patients.					
Pri3: telemedicine is not private and confidential.					
Cul1: applying telemedicine will be negatively affected by culture and religion issues.					
Cul2: social issues (culture and religion) have a potential effect on applying telemedicine.					
Cul3: our culture and social norms refuse the use of telemedicine.					
ATT1: I trust technology to work.					
ATT2: I am happy using ICT/the Internet for patient care.					
ATT3: general comfort exists in using ICT/Internet to store, retrieve, and communicate patient information with other health institutions.					
Ben1: telemedicine enhances collaboration in the public sector.					
Ben2: telemedicine improves the healthcare service quality in Iraq.					
Ben3: telemedicine reduces cost in overall healthcare expenses.					
Ben4: telemedicine improves efficiency and resource utilization.					
Ben5: telemedicine improves access to healthcare services and care delivery, especially for people in rural and remote communities.					

Table 6: Part 4: technological characteristic.

	Strongly disagree	Disagree	Neutral	Agree	Strongly agree
Con1: the connectivity is important for healthcare delivery.					
Con2: physicians have to be connected to the Internet.					
Con3: physicians have to be connected to patients.					
ITc1: our healthcare requires information system applications.					
ITc2: our healthcare requires good ICT infrastructure.					
ITc3: telemedicine requires basic IT skills.					
Compat1: physician ICT is different from patient ICT.					
Compat2: telemedicine does not contrast with healthcare needs.					
Compat3: different telemedicine applications will not affect the efficiency.					
DWc1: we should keep patient health record perpetually.					
DWc2: there are needs of patient health record to have statistic.					
DWc3: we should store our patient's record in a common database to make them accessible.					

Table 7: Part 5: organization characteristic.

	Strongly disagree	Disagree	Neutral	Agree	Strongly agree
TS1: telemedicine requires good technical support.					
TS2: a specific focus on long-term sustainability is a common trait among successful programs.					
TS3: technical support provides measurement and feedback to physicians.					
TMS1: our top managers are interested in applying telemedicine.					
TMS2: our top managers have properly identified telemedicine needs.					
TMS3: our top managers have prioritized telemedicine needs.					
Cost 1: high cost of equipment might be the cause of not adopting telemedicine.					
Cost 2: telemedicine is less costly than traditional healthcare delivery.					
Cost 3: staff training is costly.					
Cost 4: software and hardware maintenance is costly.					

Table 8: Part 6: environmental characteristic.

	Strongly disagree	Disagree	Neutral	Agree	Strongly agree
Policy 1: the government should amend policies to support the telemedicine project.					
Policy 2: our hospitals require legislations and policies to apply the telemedicine project.					
Policy 3: legislations and policies build good relationship and trust among our staff.					
Upper 1: the Ministry of Health recommends the application of telemedicine.					
Upper 2: the Ministry of Health requests the application of telemedicine.					
Upper 3: the Ministry of Health provides the requirements to implement telemedicine.					

Appendix

Factors and Items

See Tables 5, 6, 7, and 8 and Figures 2 and 3.

References

[1] J. A. Blaya, H. S. F. Fraser, and B. Holt, "E-health technologies show promise in developing countries," *Health Affairs*, vol. 29, no. 2, pp. 244–251, 2010.

[2] M. M. Jaber, M. K. A. Ghani, and N. S. Herman, "A review of adoption of telemedicine in Middle East countries: toward building Iraqi telemedicine framework," *Science International*, vol. 26, no. 5, pp. 1795–1800, 2014.

[3] K. Schlein, A. Y. De La Cruz, T. Gopalakrishnan, and D. Montagu, "Private sector delivery of health services in developing countries: a mixed-methods study on quality assurance in social franchises," *BMC Health Services Research*, vol. 13, article 4, 2013.

[4] S.-H. Hsieh, S.-L. Hsieh, P.-H. Cheng, and F. Lai, "E-health and healthcare enterprise information system leveraging service-oriented architecture," *Telemedicine and e-Health*, vol. 18, no. 3, pp. 205–212, 2012.

[5] M. K. A. Ghani, M. M. Jaber, and N. Suryana, "Telemedicine supported by data warehouse architecture," *ARPN Journal of Engineering and Applied Sciences*, vol. 10, no. 2, pp. 415–417, 2015.

[6] M.-P. Gagnon, G. Godin, C. Gagné et al., "An adaptation of the theory of interpersonal behaviour to the study of telemedicine adoption by physicians," *International Journal of Medical Informatics*, vol. 71, no. 2-3, pp. 103–115, 2003.

[7] M. A. Mohammed, M. H. Kadhim, A. Fuad, and M. M. Jaber, "Follow up system for directorate of scholarship and cultural relations in Iraq," in *Proceedings of the International Conference on Computer, Communications, and Control Technology (I4CT '14)*, pp. 182–187, Langkawi, Malaysia, September 2014.

[8] L. G. Tornatzky, M. Fleischer, and A. K. Chakrabarti, *Processes of Technological Innovation*, Lexington Books, 1990.

[9] K. Zhu, K. Kraemer, and S. Xu, "Electronic business adoption by European firms: a cross-country assessment of the facilitators and inhibitors," *European Journal of Information Systems*, vol. 12, no. 4, pp. 251–268, 2003.

[10] S. Kurnia and R. B. Johnston, "The need for a processual view of inter-organizational systems adoption," *The Journal of Strategic Information Systems*, vol. 9, no. 4, pp. 295–319, 2000.

[11] A. Y. Akbulut, *An investigation of the factors that influence electronic information sharing between state and local agencies [Ph.D. thesis]*, Louisiana State University, Baton Rouge, La, USA, 2003.

[12] A. Ziaee Bigdeli, M. M. Kamal, and S. de Cesare, "Electronic information sharing in local government: the decision-making process," in *Proceedings of the 20th European Conference on Information Systems (ECIS '12)*, Barcelona, Spain, June 2012.

[13] R. M. Emerson, "Social exchange theory," *Annual Review of Sociology*, vol. 2, no. 1, pp. 335–362, 1976.

[14] N. Prammanee, "A critical analysis of the adoption and utilization of the internet in Thailand for education purposes," *First Monday*, vol. 8, no. 1, 2003.

[15] J. A. Hoffer and M. B. Alexander, "The diffusion of database machines," *ACM SIGMIS Database*, vol. 23, no. 2, pp. 13–19, 1992.

[16] J. Bayer and N. Melone, "A critique of diffusion theory as a managerial framework for understanding adoption of software engineering innovations," in *Proceedings of the 21st Annual Hawaii International Conference on System Sciences, Volume II. Software Track*, pp. 311–316, Kailua-Kona, Hawaii, USA, January1988.

[17] G. C. Moore and I. Benbasat, "Development of an instrument to measure the perceptions of adopting an information technology innovation," *Information Systems Research*, vol. 2, no. 3, pp. 192–222, 1991.

[18] U. Sekaran and R. Bougie, *Research Methods for Business: A Skill Building Approach*, Wiley, London, UK, 2010.

[19] D. Ludwick and J. Doucette, "Primary care physicians' experience with electronic medical records: barriers to implementation in a fee-for-service environment," *International Journal of Telemedicine and Applications*, vol. 2009, Article ID 853524, 2009.

[20] A. Buabbas, *Investigation of the adoption of telemedicine technology in the Kuwaiti health system: strategy and policy of implementation for overseas referral patients [Ph.D. thesis]*, School of Information Systems, Computing and Mathematics, Brunel University, Uxbridge, UK, 2013.

[21] M. Alajlani and M. Clarke, "Effect of culture on acceptance of telemedicine in middle eastern countries: case study of Jordan and Syria," *Telemedicine and e-Health*, vol. 19, no. 4, pp. 305–311, 2013.

[22] C. S. Gadd and L. E. Penrod, "Assessing physician attitudes regarding use of an outpatient EMR: a longitudinal, multi-practice study," in *Proceedings of the AMIA Annual Symposium*, p. 194, Washington, DC, USA, November 2001.

[23] K. D. Kleiner, R. Akers, B. L. Burke, and E. J. Werner, "Parent and physician attitudes regarding electronic communication in pediatric practices," *Pediatrics*, vol. 109, no. 5, pp. 740–744, 2002.

[24] N. Almotiri, *Teleconsultation perspective for cardiovascular patients in Saudi Arabia [Ph.D. thesis]*, Brunel University, School of Information Systems, Computing and Mathematics, 2012.

[25] M. K. A. Ghani, M. M. Jaber, and N. Suryana, "Barriers faces telemedicine implementation in the developing countries: toward building Iraqi telemedicine framework," *Journal of Engineering and Applied Sciences*, vol. 10, no. 4, pp. 1562–1567, 2015.

[26] A. A. Abera, G. H. Mengesha, and P. F. Musa, "Assessment of Ethiopian health facilities readiness for implementation of telemedicine," *Communications of the Association for Information Systems*, vol. 34, article 67, 2014.

[27] R. M. Baroud, "How ready are the stakeholders in the Palestinian healthcare system in the Gaza strip to adopt e-health?" *Dissertation Abstracts International Section B: The Sciences & Engineering*, vol. 69, no. 4, 2008.

[28] F. Jing and Z. Pengzhu, "A field study of G2G information sharing in Chinese context based on the Layered behavioral model," in *Proceedings of the 42nd Annual Hawaii International Conference on System Sciences (HICSS '09)*, pp. 1–13, Big Island, Hawaii, USA, January 2009.

[29] T. Ariyachandra and H. Watson, "Key organizational factors in data warehouse architecture selection," *Decision Support Systems*, vol. 49, no. 2, pp. 200–212, 2010.

[30] X. Lu, F. Liu, and R. Pei, "E-government implementation performance and information sharing: an analysis among multi-level departments," in *Proceedings of the International Conference on Network Computing and Information Security (NCIS '11)*, vol. 1, pp. 279–283, Guilin, China, May 2011.

[31] M. A. Mohammed, A. R. Hasson, A. R. Shawkat, and N. J. Al-Khafaji, "E-government architecture uses data warehouse techniques to increase information sharing in Iraqi universities," in *Proceedings of the IEEE Symposium on E-Learning, E-Management and E-Services (IS3e '12)*, pp. 1–5, IEEE Explore, Kuala Lumpur, Malaysia, October 2012.

[32] R. Latifi, "Ten critical steps for a successful telemedicine program," in *Establishing Telemedicine in Developing Countries: From Inception to Implementation*, vol. 104 of *Studies in Health Technology and Informatics*, pp. 60–68, IOS Press, Amsterdam, The Netherlands, 2004.

[33] S. Khoja, H. Durrani, and A. Fahim, "Scope of policy issues for eHealth: results from a structured review," in *Proceedings of the Making the eHealth Connection*, Bellagio, Italy, July-August 2008.

[34] N. S. Wickramasinghe, A. M. A. Fadlalla, E. Geisler, and J. L. Schaffer, "A framework for assessing e-health preparedness," *International Journal of Electronic Healthcare*, vol. 1, no. 3, pp. 316–334, 2005.

[35] S. Al Hasnawi, "Physicians' shortage in Iraq: impact and proposed solutions," *Iraqi Journal of Community Medicine*, vol. 3, pp. 214–218, 2013.

[36] L. J. Cronbach, "Response sets and test validity," *Educational and Psychological Measurement*, vol. 6, pp. 475–494, 1946.

[37] D. George and M. Mallery, *Using SPSS for Windows Step by Step: A Simple Guide and Reference*, Allyn y Bacon, Boston, Mass, USA, 2003.

[38] J. F. Hair, A. H. Money, P. Samouel, and M. Page, "Research methods for business," *Education + Training*, vol. 49, pp. 336–337, 2007.

2

Robust Sounds of Activities of Daily Living Classification in Two-Channel Audio-Based Telemonitoring

David Maunder, Julien Epps, Eliathamby Ambikairajah, and Branko Celler

School of Electrical Engineering and Telecommunications, The University of New South Wales, Sydney, NSW 2052, Australia

Correspondence should be addressed to Julien Epps; j.epps@unsw.edu.au

Academic Editor: Sotiris A. Pavlopoulos

Despite recent advances in the area of home telemonitoring, the challenge of automatically detecting the sound signatures of activities of daily living of an elderly patient using nonintrusive and reliable methods remains. This paper investigates the classification of eight typical sounds of daily life from arbitrarily positioned two-microphone sensors under realistic noisy conditions. In particular, the role of several source separation and sound activity detection methods is considered. Evaluations on a new four-microphone database collected under four realistic noise conditions reveal that effective sound activity detection can produce significant gains in classification accuracy and that further gains can be made using source separation methods based on independent component analysis. Encouragingly, the results show that recognition accuracies in the range 70%–100% can be consistently obtained using different microphone-pair positions, under all but the most severe noise conditions.

1. Introduction

1.1. Home Telemonitoring. The devotion to one's parents has been displayed in various cultures throughout time and, as such, has usually included the care of one's parents in old age. In colonial times, the care of frail aged persons was primarily the responsibility of the family. Today in the West, elderly people are primarily cared for in hospitals, nursing homes, or by their families.

The United Nations predicts that by 2100, 28.1% of the world population will be aged 65 years or older, compared with 10.0% in 2000 and 6.9% in 1990 [1]. The resulting increased demand on the health system, coupled with decreasing taxpayer support and fewer younger people to care for the elderly, will introduce significant pressure on aged care services. The main needs of these services are monitoring and supporting elderly people. For example, the fifth highest cause of death for elderly people is falls [2], and while the falls themselves may not be easily preventable, in many circumstances the deaths following them are, with appropriate monitoring and support. Consequently, significant research interest has been focused towards home-telecare solutions allowing elderly people to live safely and independently in their homes.

In recent years, it has been suggested that sound "signatures" are well suited to automated telemonitoring of elderly people and superior to video cameras from the perspective of privacy [3]. Telemonitoring using sound signatures is a relatively less explored area in the literature, in comparison with other techniques such as gait parameters and posture and motion information.

The main methods for monitoring elderly people are the "Health Smart Home," wearable devices, or a combination of the two. The first Health Smart Home [4] used magnetic switches between doors, infrared sensors, and sound sensors to monitor which room or part of a room the person was in and the activity they were undertaking. In [5], infrared sensors and magnetic switches were used to monitor the activities of the subject and compare them with expected behaviour. The main shortcomings of the Health Smart Home are the restriction to monitoring only nonbiomechanical parameters, its inability to monitor elderly subjects outside their home, and the need to distinguish the elderly person from others in the home.

Wearable devices are designed to measure biomechanical/physiological parameters and can be attached to clothing, worn either as jewellery or as a separate device [6]. Pedometers, foot-switches, and heart rate measurements can monitor the level of a person's daily activity and energy expenditure. Accelerometers measure the acceleration along the x, y, and z axes and can measure dynamic and static activities over a short or long period of time. Gyroscopes measure the Coriolis acceleration from rotational angular velocity and can therefore measure changes in the wearer's posture. The major disadvantage of wearable devices is that they are not able to be used by people who are incapable, physically or mentally, of operating and maintaining them.

Investigations into telemonitoring using sound sensors have been performed by a French consortium of the CLIPS and TIMC laboratories, who developed a five-microphone system [3, 7, 8]. The main shortcoming of this work is the specialised wiring in the dedicated test apartment [9]. In addition, sound files in their database were recorded in a controlled environment and the noise sources mixed in artificially. Nevertheless, this group has demonstrated the feasibility of classifying a range of different household sounds [6, 8–10].

Source separation is a problem in which a sound sensor receives a number of component sources, and the goal is to determine the original component sources. One technique for single-microphone source separation is to express each separated source as a weighted sum of subbands (refiltering) [11]. A newer algorithm, which uses sub-band independent component analysis, has been proposed where each of the frequency bins is composed of a linear combination of the corresponding frequency bins. This technique is combined with a beamformer which estimates the direction of arrival [12]. In [13], an acoustic event classification system is described which applies temporal ICA on a single-microphone audio signal to determine the temporal window during which features should be extracted, resulting in improved system performance. In this context, ICA was used as a method segmenting different sound sources rather than for separating them in an acoustic sense using multiple microphones.

A variant of the bionic wavelet transform, an adaptive wavelet transform derived from a nonlinear auditory model of the cochlear, has been applied to the task of single-microphone speech enhancement [14]. A novel prefilter has also been developed and uses temporal and simultaneous masking thresholds to shape the speech spectrum in order to obtain a better estimate of the autoregressive coefficients that characterize the speech spectrum [15].

1.2. Robust Sounds of Daily Life Classification from Two-Channel Audio. In many instances, the objective of telemonitoring is to form a model of the "activities of daily life" [6], so that deviations from this model can be used to automatically prompt for help. In sound-based telemonitoring, the aim is similar: to distinguish between different "sounds of daily life" (SDLs), which may correspond to some or all of the activities of daily life.

Figure 1 depicts a generic sound signature classification system. Extraction of sound signature parameters occurs at the "front-end," where information putatively useful for differentiating between sound signatures is obtained from the microphone signal. As a precursor to the front-end, clearly it would be desirable to detect the presence or absence of a relevant SDL. Similar approaches have been adopted in [3, 7, 8, 16] where the energy of the most discriminating bands from the discrete wavelet transform (DWT) were used to distinguish between an event and noise. For example, to distinguish between a kettle sound and a door slap, energy may be a useful parameter, as the energy in the kettle sound would be significantly lower than that of the door slap (assuming the microphones were equidistant from each sound source). Sound modelling and classification are then conducted in the back-end. Since both microphones will normally contain both signal and noise components, a two-stage system is proposed, with the first stage attempting to determine estimates for the signal and noise.

1.3. Source Separation. In general, multimicrophone sensing of sounds of daily life in realistic environments is likely to produce individual microphone signals comprising the superposition of the sound of daily life and other background noises. A related problem is known as the "cocktail party effect," in which a number of people are speaking and a listener desires to listen exclusively to one of them. In a telemonitoring application, the objective is somewhat different: to separate the sound source from the background noise source, in order to classify it more accurately. Suppose that we define each microphone signal $x_i[n]$, $i = 1, 2, \ldots, M$, as a linear combination of the unknown sources $s_j[n]$, $j = 1, 2, \ldots, N$,

$$\begin{bmatrix} x_1[n] \\ x_2[n] \\ \vdots \\ x_m[n] \end{bmatrix} = \begin{bmatrix} a_{11} & a_{12} & \cdots & a_{1p} \\ a_{21} & a_{22} & \cdots & a_{2p} \\ \vdots & \vdots & \ddots & \vdots \\ a_{m1} & a_{m2} & \cdots & a_{mp} \end{bmatrix} \begin{bmatrix} s_1[n] \\ s_2[n] \\ \vdots \\ s_p[n] \end{bmatrix}. \quad (1)$$

Independent component analysis (ICA) assumes that the input source distributions are non-Gaussian and independent. ICA estimates a matrix $\mathbf{B}$, which is the inverse of $\mathbf{A} = (a_{ij})_{M\times N}$ (in the case $M = N$) from (1), to separate the sources [17].

ICA uses the central limit theorem result, which states that a linear combination of non-Gaussian independent sources will converge to a Gaussian distribution. Therefore, the distributions of the sensor signals $x_i[n]$ will be more Gaussian than those of the sources $s_i[n]$. ICA estimates the matrix $\mathbf{B}$, which when applied to the sensors $x_i[n]$ attempts to minimise the Gaussianness of the estimated separated sources. This leads to $\hat{s}_i[n]$, $i = 1, 2, \ldots, N$ estimated separated sources. Various metrics are available for measuring a source's Gaussianness, including kurtosis and negentropy [17].

In the context of this work, the sensor signals are recorded by $N = 2$ microphones $m_1[n]$ and $m_2[n]$. Each microphone is composed of a linear combination of the sound of daily life source $s_{\mathrm{SDL}}[n]$ and noise source $s_{\mathrm{noise}}[n]$:

$$\begin{bmatrix} m_1[n] \\ m_2[n] \end{bmatrix} = \begin{bmatrix} a_{11} & a_{12} \\ a_{21} & a_{22} \end{bmatrix} \begin{bmatrix} s_{\mathrm{SDL}}[n] \\ s_{\mathrm{noise}}[n] \end{bmatrix}. \quad (2)$$

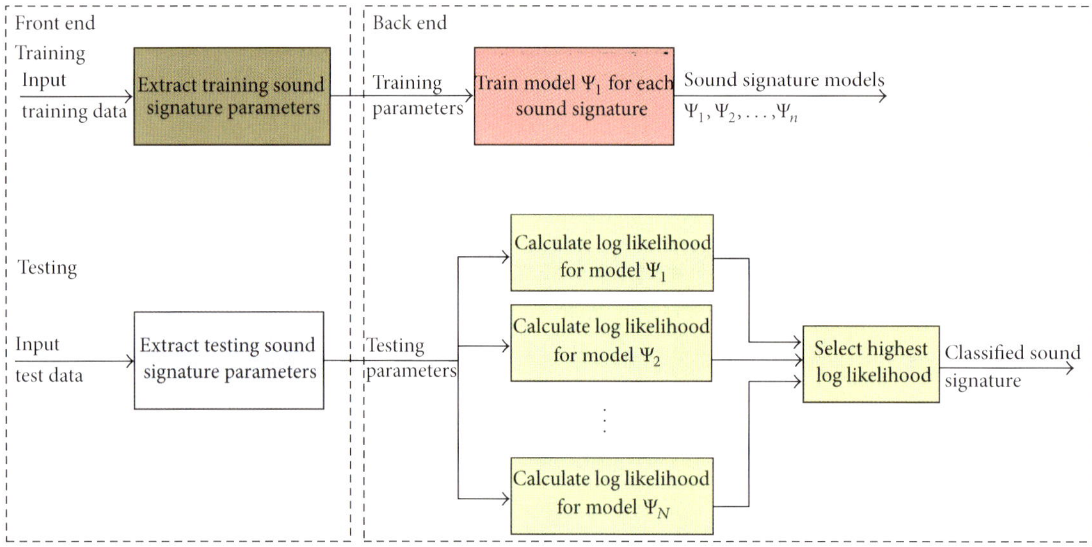

FIGURE 1: Typical configuration for a "sounds of daily life" classification system, which we refer to herein as the baseline system. Classified sound signatures can then be modelled for telemonitoring purposes.

ICA estimates the matrix **B**, which minimizes the Gaussianness of $s_{\text{sep1}}[n]$ and $s_{\text{sep2}}[n]$ and determines estimates for the separated sources:

$$\begin{bmatrix} s_{\text{sep1}}[n] \\ s_{\text{sep2}}[n] \end{bmatrix} = \begin{bmatrix} b_{11} & b_{12} \\ b_{21} & b_{22} \end{bmatrix} \begin{bmatrix} m_1[n] \\ m_2[n] \end{bmatrix}. \quad (3)$$

There are two problems encountered using ICA:

(1) ICA only determines the separated sources up to a scaling factor. The matrix **B** could be multiplied by a scaling factor without changing the Gaussianness of $s_{\text{sep1}}[n]$ and $s_{\text{sep2}}[n]$;

(2) ICA separates the sources, but does not identify which is the SDL and which is the noise source.

The focus of this paper is the classification of sounds of daily life (SDLs) from multiple microphones of unknown location, in the presence of noise. If a range of SDLs can be detected, a distress situation such as a thud, which could correspond to a fall or a cry for help, could be discovered and appropriate medical care sent to the house. In addition, a model of elderly people's daily activities can be developed from which important information about their functional health status derived. This work is more portable than previously reported systems that employ fixed microphones [3, 6–10], employing two microphones which can be easily installed in a private residence, and data has been recorded in realistic scenarios in the presence of typical background noises.

In particular, we develop methods for addressing the problems of identifying the $s_{\text{SDL}}[n]$ signal following source separation and sound activity detection, as shown in Figure 2, and evaluate these on a large and realistic new multi-microphone database. The work builds on and substantially extends earlier work on sound activity detection for robust sounds of daily life classification [18].

2. Proposed Source Selection Methods

Due to the prevalence of independent component analysis among source separation problems, we also adopt this method. To overcome the problem of ICA determining the sources only up to a scaling factor, the separated sounds of daily life are herein normalized to have a maximum value of 1. This makes the data consistent. There are a number of ways to overcome the problem of identifying the $s_{\text{SDL}}[n]$ signal following source separation, each with its advantages. The main approach adopted herein is to determine which separated source has the least noise; however, it may not always be straightforward to identify which signal components are sounds of daily life and which are noise. Five possible solutions to this problem are proposed as follows.

2.1. Source Selection with a Priori SNR. If prior knowledge is available about which microphone has the best SNR, the separation matrix can be analysed to determine which separated source has the superior SNR. Without loss of generality, assume that $m_1[n]$ has the best SNR. If it does not, it can be swapped with $m_2[n]$ to ensure it does. If $|b_{11}|^2 > |b_{12}|^2$, the first separated source contains more data from the microphone with the best SNR and therefore has the least noise in it. Alternatively, if $|b_{11}|^2 < |b_{12}|^2$, the second separated source has the smaller amount of noise:

$$\hat{s}_{\text{SDL\_Apriori}}[n] = \begin{cases} s_{\text{sep1}}[n] & \text{if } |b_{11}|^2 > |b_{12}|^2 \\ s_{\text{sep2}}[n] & \text{if } |b_{11}|^2 < |b_{12}|^2. \end{cases} \quad (4)$$

The main shortcoming of this algorithm is that it requires prior information as to which microphone has the best SNR. This requirement is addressed by the three methods given in the ensuing subsections.

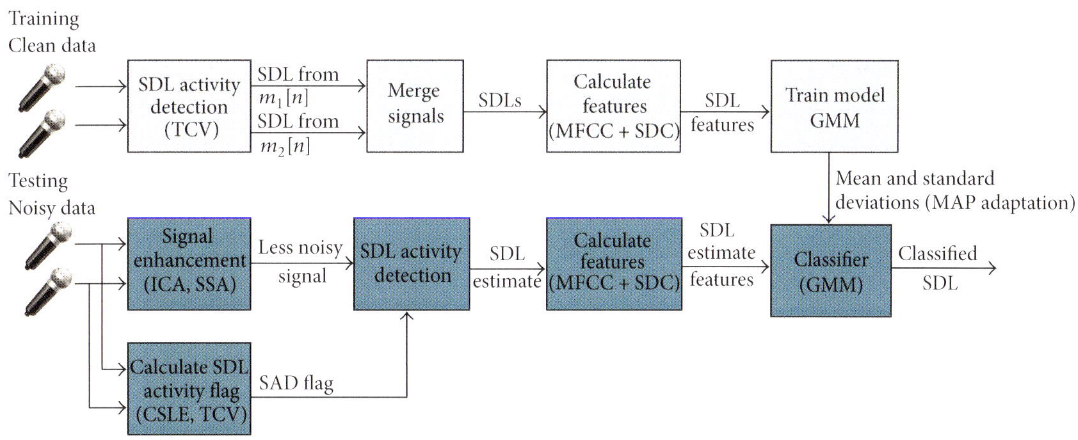

Figure 2: Proposed configuration for a robust "sounds of daily life" classification system, based on multiple microphones.

2.2. SNR Estimation Source Selection Using Microphone with Best SNR. This method extends the first method and automates the process of determining which microphone has the least amount of noise. A related problem is the determination of whether a sound is present or not, which we term sound activity detection (SAD). For each of the microphone signals, the SAD algorithm is applied (see Section 3), the SDL and noise segments are found using a reliable SAD algorithm—we used CSLE—and an estimate of the SNR determined using the following formula:

$$\widehat{\mathrm{SNR}}_{\mathrm{BestMic}} = \frac{\sigma^2_{\mathrm{SDL}+w}}{\sigma^2_w}, \quad (5)$$

where $\sigma^2_{\mathrm{SDL}+w}$ is the average SDL (signal plus noise) power and σ^2_w is the average noise power, estimated from segments of the signals suspected to contain SDLs and noise, respectively.

The microphone with the largest SNR is found and (5) is applied. This method has the advantage of not requiring prior information. In addition, due to the varying microphones, noise and SDL locations, the microphone with the least noise may change. However, the main shortcoming is that if the SAD is not sufficiently accurate, the microphone with the least amount of noise could be incorrectly selected which will result in not choosing the SDL correctly.

A variant of this method is

$$\widehat{\mathrm{SNR}}_{\mathrm{LeastNoise}} = \frac{1}{\sigma^2_w}, \quad (6)$$

where σ^2_n is the average noise power. This means that the SAD algorithm only needs to classify noise frames correctly (its performance is unaffected by noise frames which are classified as SDL frames).

2.3. Source Selection Using Separated SDL with Best SNR. The SNR estimates from the previous subsection extract information from the input microphone signals to determine which separated source has the best SNR. The methods detailed in this section use information from the separated sources to determine which has the least amount of noise. This approach obtains an SNR estimate by applying (8) to each separated source and determines which has the best SNR:

$$\hat{s}_{\mathrm{SDL\_BestSNR}}[n] = \begin{cases} s_{\mathrm{sep1}}[n] & \text{if } \mathrm{SNR}\left(s_{\mathrm{sep1}}[n]\right) > \mathrm{SNR}\left(s_{\mathrm{sep2}}[n]\right) \\ s_{\mathrm{sep2}}[n] & \text{if } \mathrm{SNR}\left(s_{\mathrm{sep1}}[n]\right) < \mathrm{SNR}\left(s_{\mathrm{sep2}}[n]\right). \end{cases} \quad (7)$$

2.4. Source Selection Using Separated SDL with Least Noise. This method is similar to that of Section 2.3, however only the noise segments are used. The SNR estimate is determined using $\widehat{\mathrm{SNR}}_{\mathrm{LeastNoise}}$, which is then used as the SNR estimate in (7), to produce a separated source $\hat{s}_{\mathrm{SDL\_LeastNoise}}[n]$. As with the calculation of $\widehat{\mathrm{SNR}}_{\mathrm{LeastNoise}}$, this technique means the SAD classification does not need to be as stringent.

2.5. SNR Steepest Ascent (SSA) for Improvement of the Unmixing Matrix. As discussed in Section 2.1, in some situations it is possible to use sound activity detection to identify regions of the signal for which there is noise only or sound and noise together. For the special case of two-source separation, this information can be used to estimate improved estimates of the unmixing matrix entries. Consider the separated SDL from (7) and without loss of generality, assume that $s_{\mathrm{sep1}}[n]$ is the separated SDL following source selection. We define the SNR of the separated SDL as follows:

$$\widehat{\mathrm{SNR}}_{\mathrm{SDL\_SA}}(b_{11}, b_{12}) = \frac{\left(1/\left|\{n_K, n_{K+1}, \ldots, n_G\}\right|\right)\sum_{n\in\{n_K,n_{K+1},\ldots,n_G\}}\left(b_{11}m_1[n] + b_{12}m_2[n]\right)^2}{\left(1/\left|\{n_L, n_{L+1}, \ldots, n_H\}\right|\right)\sum_{n\in\{n_L,n_{L+1},\ldots,n_H\}}\left(b_{11}m_1[n] + b_{12}m_2[n]\right)^2}, \quad (8)$$

where $\{n_K, n_{K+1}, \ldots, n_G\}$ are the SDL and noisy sample indices, and $\{n_L, n_{L+1}, \ldots, n_H\}$ are the noisy sample indices.

As b_{11} and b_{12} are varied, the SNR varies. The SNR space may exhibit an arbitrary number of peaks if both parameters

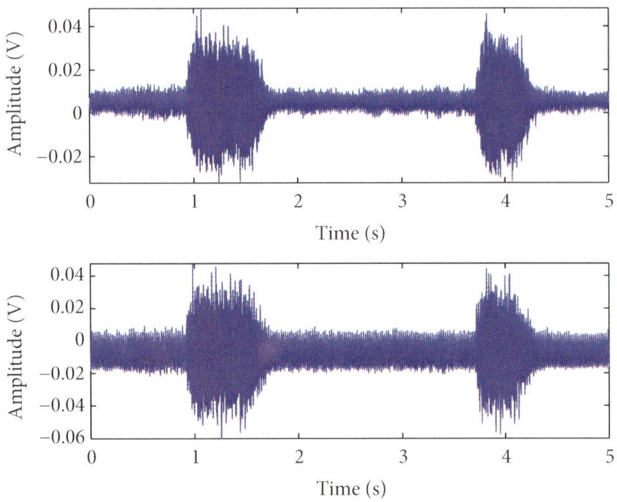

FIGURE 3: Example microphone signals for a phone ringing (sound of daily life—higher energy segments) with the radio on (background noise—lower energy segments).

are varied. If one of the parameters is constant and the other is varied, only one peak should exist.

Figure 4 depicts the variation in SNR for the two microphone signals in Figure 3 as a function of b_{12}. The first plot shows $m_1[n]$ set as the primary and $m_2[n]$ set as the secondary microphone. The second swaps $m_1[n]$ and $m_2[n]$ (which is equivalent to not swapping the microphones, but holding b_{12} constant and varying b_{11}). Both plots yield the same peak SNR, suggesting that the algorithm only needs to be performed for one combination of the microphone signals.

Attempting to find the SNR over an entire range of suitable b_{12} values is computationally burdensome. Therefore, a steepest ascent approach is proposed. Let $m_{\text{best}}[n]$ and $m_{\text{worst}}[n]$ be the microphone signals with the best and worst SNRs, respectively. If $b_{11} = 1$ and $b_{12} = 0$ then

$$s_{\text{SDL}}[n] = b_{11} m_{\text{best}}[n] + b_{12} m_{\text{worst}}[n]. \tag{9}$$

The algorithm can be initialized by $b_{11} = 1$ and $b_{12} = 0$, that is, the initial separated SDL will have the same SNR as that of the microphone with the best SNR. The approach adopted is to vary the separated source by adding or subtracting a scaled version of the microphone with the worst SNR for the purpose of improving the SNR of the separated source,

$$b_{12} = b_{12} + \mu \frac{\partial \text{SNR}_{\text{SDL}}}{\partial b_{12}}, \tag{10}$$

where

$$\begin{aligned}
\frac{\partial \text{SNR}_{\text{SDL}}}{\partial b_{12}} &= \frac{\partial}{\partial b_{12}} \frac{(1/N)\sum_{n\in S}\left(b_{11} m_{\text{best}}[n] + b_{12} m_{\text{worst}}[n]\right)^2}{(1/M)\sum_{n\in N}\left(b_{11} m_{\text{best}}[n] + b_{12} m_{\text{worst}}[n]\right)^2} \\
&= \frac{Q - R}{\left((1/M)\sum_{n\in N}\left(b_{11} m_{\text{best}}[n] + b_{12} m_{\text{worst}}[n]\right)^2\right)^2}, \\
Q &= \frac{1}{M}\sum_{n\in N}\left(b_{11} m_{\text{best}}[n] + b_{12} m_{\text{worst}}[n]\right)^2 \\
&\quad \times 2\frac{1}{N}\sum_{n\in S}\left(b_{11} m_{\text{best}}[n] + b_{12} m_{\text{worst}}[n]\right) m_{\text{worst}}[n], \\
R &= \frac{1}{N}\sum_{n\in S}\left(b_{11} m_{\text{best}}[n] + b_{12} m_{\text{worst}}[n]\right)^2 \\
&\quad \times 2\frac{1}{M}\sum_{n\in N}\left(b_{11} m_{\text{best}}[n] + b_{12} m_{\text{worst}}[n]\right) m_{\text{worst}}[n].
\end{aligned} \tag{11}$$

Since the vector $(1, \partial \text{SNR}_{\text{SDL}}/\partial b_{12})$ "points" in the direction of steepest ascent in the (b_{11}, b_{12}) space, adapting the parameter b_{12} in this direction will increase the SNR of the separated source.

In (10), the adaptation parameter μ is constant and determines the convergence of the algorithm. If $\mu < 0$, b_{12} approaches a value that yields the smallest SNR. If $\mu > 0$, b_{12} approaches a value yielding the largest SNR. Additionally, if μ is small, the rate of convergence will be slow. If μ is large, there is possible instability in the result—although both issues are mitigated through adapting μ, as outlined below.

The SNRs in the database of SDLs are very diverse. As a result, for some values of μ, the algorithm will converge quickly, some will converge slowly, and others will overshoot and miss the peak completely. To overcome this, an adaptive μ is implemented. The value of μ begins with a high value and when overshoot is detected (which is found by a negative change in SNR), the algorithm backtracks by one iteration and μ is decreased. A suitable method for achieving this, determined empirically, is multiplying μ by a factor of 0.1 each time an overshoot is detected. Figure 5 shows how the SNR evolves in each iteration of the algorithm for the example recorded in Figure 3.

It was investigated whether the algorithm would converge in less time than if the optimum SNR was found through an exhaustive search. Recordings from the databases for different SDLs with radio noise were used. Two recordings were chosen at random, for each of the eight SDLs from the radio at pleasant listening level and male speaker databases, using microphones 1 and 3. Figure 6 shows a plot of the difference between the best SNR (which was determined by an exhaustive search across $b_{12} \in [-10, 10]$ and the SNR) which evolves in the algorithm. Figure 7 shows the difference between the value of b_{12}, corresponding to the best SNR value, and the evolved value of b_{12}. In both cases, all SDLs converge in under 30 iterations. To obtain the same SNR maximum using an exhaustive search over the region $b_{12} \in [-10, 10)$

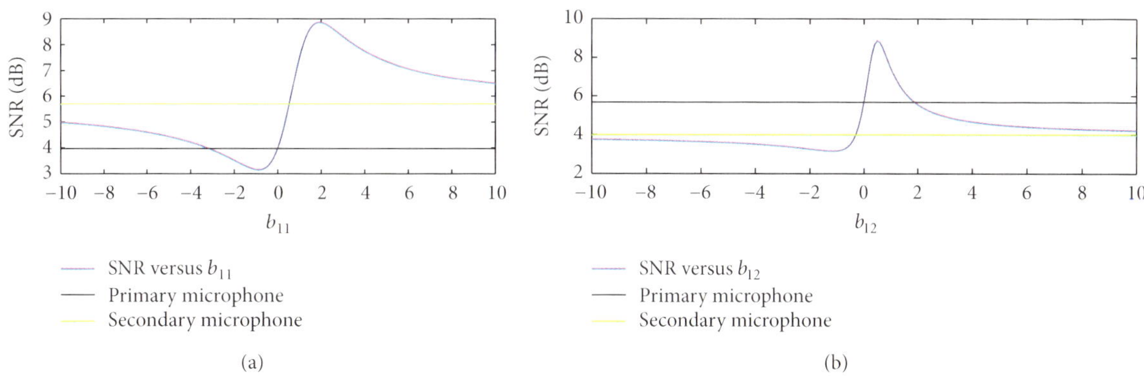

FIGURE 4: Plot of SNR as the unmixing matrix coefficient b_{12} is varied, for the two channels shown in Figure 3. The first (a) fixes the primary microphone as constant and adds the secondary microphone scaled by b_{12}. The second (b) fixes the secondary microphone as constant and adds the primary microphone scaled by b_{12}. Both yield approximately the same peak.

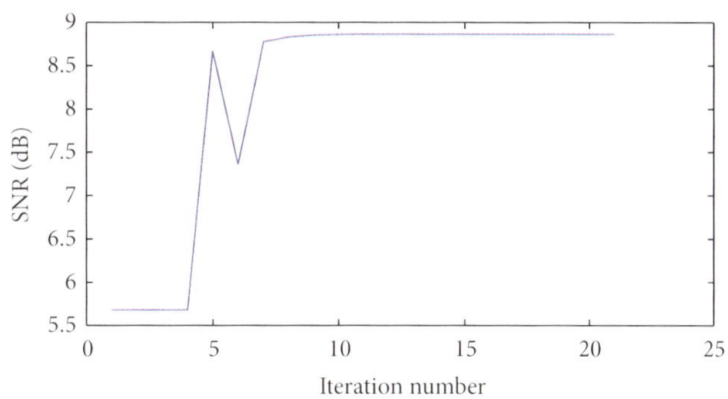

FIGURE 5: Example SNR versus iteration number for the SNR steepest ascent method. Overshoot is detected at iteration 6, at which point the value of μ is decreased to minimise the likelihood of the algorithm overshooting again.

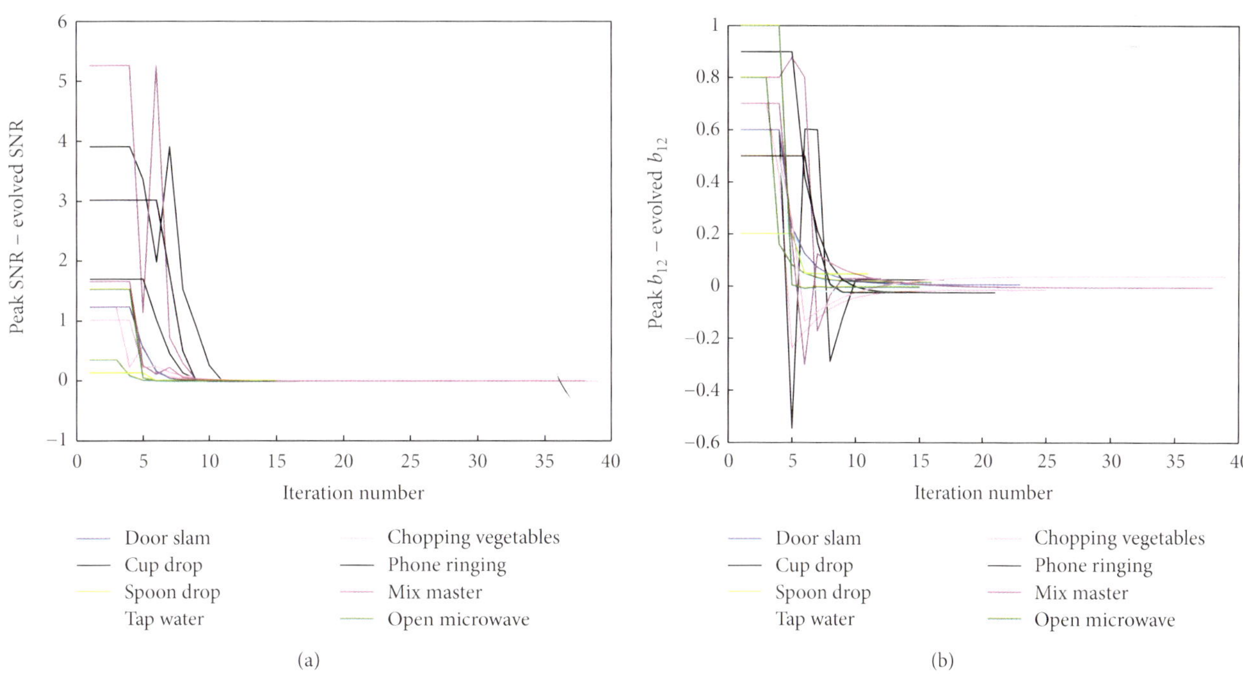

FIGURE 6: Convergence behaviour of the SSA algorithm: differences between the optimum SNR and evolved SNR (a) and optimum b_{12} value minus evolved b_{12} (b), for various example sounds of daily life (as indicated) with background radio noise at pleasant listening level, using microphones 1 and 3. Two SDLs from each sound class were chosen at random.

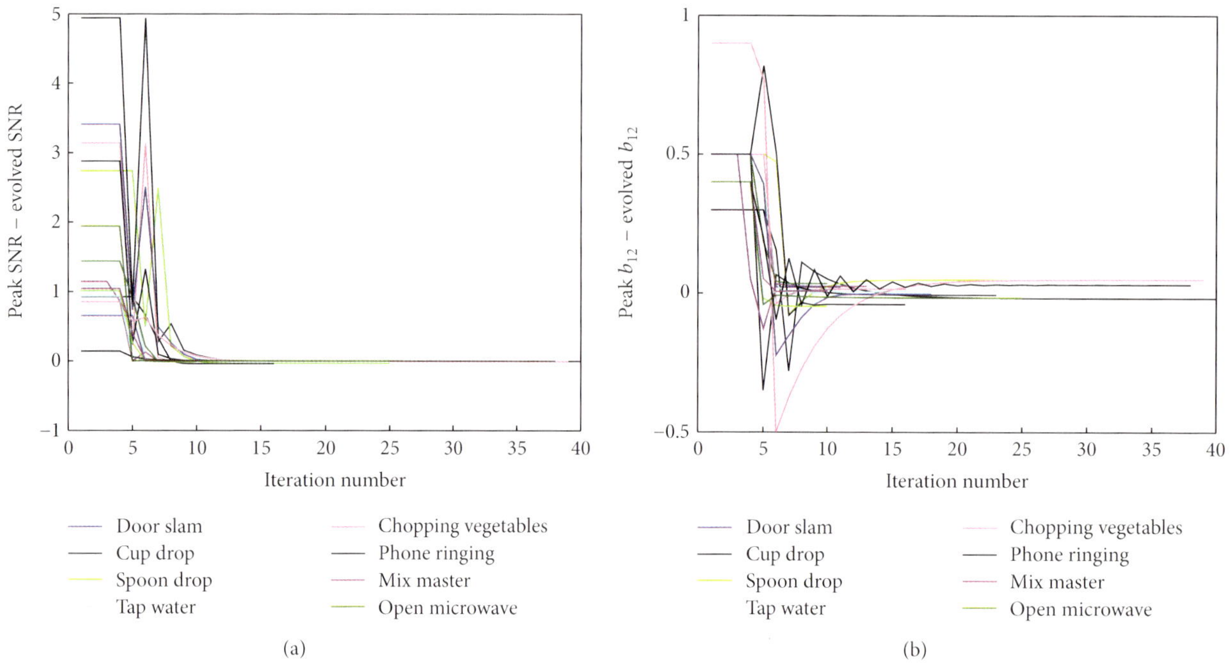

FIGURE 7: Difference between best SNR and evolved SNR (a) and best b_{12} value minus evolved b_{12} (b), for the database with a male speaker in the background, using microphones 1 and 3.

(assuming we knew which region to select) with a resolution of 0.01, the number of iterations needed would be 2000.

2.6. Noise Inverse Steepest Ascent (NISA) for Improvement of the Unmixing Matrix. This method is identical to the SSA method described in Section 2.4, except that here the goal is to minimize the noise power in the pure noise segments. This means that the SAD algorithm only needs to accurately classify the noise frames.

3. Sound Activity Detection

The purpose of sound activity detection (SAD) is to identify the location of the SDL in the audio signal (either a raw microphone signal or separated signal) and attempts to remove silence or pure noise components that produce unwanted variability during classification. SAD requires the extraction of features that can distinguish between signal and noise, followed by a classification rule. In these respects, SAD is analogous to voice activity detection in speech processing, and indeed some methods discussed below can be traced to speech processing research.

The spatial separation of the multiple microphones suggests that differences in the relative energies of the sound and background noise in each microphone signal can be exploited to detect the presence or absence of the sound. In array processing, where sensors are placed in a known spatial pattern, eigenvalue methods have been used with success to estimate the bearing of a signal of interest [19]. In the current problem, the spatial pattern of microphone sensors is unknown; however, changes in the composition of the microphone signals due to the presence or absence of a particular source (i.e., the sound of daily life) can still be detected using similar techniques. Motivated by similar considerations, we define the cross-spectral matrix as [18]:

$$\mathbf{C}[k] = \begin{bmatrix} |M_1[k]|^2 & |M_1[k]|\,|M_2[k]| \\ |M_2[k]|\,|M_1[k]| & |M_2[k]|^2 \end{bmatrix}, \qquad (12)$$

where $M_1[k]$ and $M_2[k]$ are the discrete Fourier transforms (DFTs) of the respective microphone signals $m_1[n]$ and $m_2[n]$. Under the assumption that the noise is uncorrelated with the signal of interest, it has been shown that the largest eigenvalue of $\mathbf{C}[k]$ comprises signal variance and noise variance terms, while the remaining eigenvalues comprise only noise variance terms [19].

Since $\mathbf{C}[k]$ is a rank one matrix, we consider instead a cross-spectral matrix

$$\overline{\mathbf{C}}[k] = \sum_{m=1}^{M} \mathbf{C}_m[k] \qquad (13)$$

that has been averaged over M consecutive frames, where $\mathbf{C}_m[k]$ is the cross-spectral matrix at the mth frame calculated using (13), as suggested in [20]. The eigenvalues of this matrix are now [18]

$$\lambda_{1,2} = \frac{1}{2}\left(\overline{|M_1[k]|^2} + \overline{|M_2[k]|^2}\right) \pm \frac{1}{2}\sqrt{4\overline{|M_1[k]\,M_2[k]|^2} + \left(\overline{|M_1[k]|^2} - \overline{|M_2[k]|^2}\right)^2}. \qquad (14)$$

In the problem at hand, assumptions of uncorrelated signal and noise cannot be made (typical sounds of daily life and noises are discussed in Section 4); however, the choice of frequency or frequency range over which $\mathbf{C}[k]$ is computed can be chosen empirically to minimize the correlation, by selecting frequencies in which the signal and noise are likely to have maximally different spectral characteristics.

The eigenvalues of the rank one matrix $\mathbf{C}[k]$ are

$$\lambda_{1,2} = \left\{0, \left|M_1[k]\right|^2 + \left|M_2[k]\right|^2\right\}, \tag{15}$$

which can be trivially determined from the DFTs of the microphone signals.

When only the noise source is active, $s_{\text{kitchen}}[k] = 0$. Therefore [18],

$$\lambda_2 = \begin{cases} \left(\left|a_{21}\right|^2 + \left|a_{22}\right|^2\right)\left|s_{\text{noise}}[k]\right|^2 \\ \quad \text{if only noise source is active} \\ \left(\left|a_{21}\right|^2 + \left|a_{22}\right|^2\right)\left|s_{\text{noise}}[k]\right|^2 \\ \quad + \left(\left|a_{11}\right|^2 + \left|a_{12}\right|^2\right)\left|s_{\text{kitchen}}[k]\right|^2 \\ \quad + 2\left(\left|a_{11}a_{12}\right| + \left|a_{21}a_{22}\right|\right)\left|s_{\text{kitchen}}[k]\right|\left|s_{\text{noise}}[k]\right| \\ \quad \text{if SDL is occurring.} \end{cases} \tag{16}$$

Therefore, one would expect a significant change in λ_2 when the SDL is occurring. Since $\lambda_2 \geq 0$, λ_2 is the largest eigenvalue and the smallest eigenvalue is $\lambda_1 = 0$ (in practice $\lambda_1 \neq 0$ but $\lambda_1 \ll \lambda_2$).

Therefore, a significant change in the largest eigenvalue is expected when an SDL is occurring, in comparison to during the pure noise segments. As the cross-spectral matrix has rank one, it is averaged across several Hamming windowed frames, making it have rank two, allowing the eigen decomposition to be performed. The largest eigenvalues are calculated for each windowed frame average for $k = 0, 1, \ldots, (N/2) - 1$ where N is the length of the DFT.

The quantities $(1/2)(\overline{|M_1[k]|^2} + \overline{|M_2[k]|^2})$, $\overline{4|M_1[k]M_2[k]|^2}$, and $\overline{(|M_1[k]|^2 - |M_2[k]|^2)^2}$, representing terms of (14), were also investigated; however, none of them in isolation matched the performance of λ_2 as a method for sound activity detection.

Figure 8 shows a time-frequency plot of the largest eigenvalues for a recording when a spoon was dropped. It was determined empirically that in the 3-4 kHz band, the eigenvalues are approximately zero when only the noise source is active and nonzero when the SDL is occurring for all SDLs in the databases. An example of the 3-4 kHz band is shown for the spoon dropping recording in the presence of radio noise in Figure 9.

An average of the eigenvalues is calculated across the 3-4 kHz band, then converted to a dB scale and normalized to the range $[-1, 0]$ dB. This yields an indicator which is small during the pure noise segments and much higher when the SDL is occurring. A threshold was then applied to this largest eigenvalue-based indicator, a method we refer to as baseline SAD.

An example result of the CSLE algorithm, showing where the SDL was found for a dropping spoon recording, is given in Figure 10. The estimated endpoints are within ±6% of the true endpoints. In the sound files checked across the entire database described in Section 4, similar deviations from the true endpoints were found.

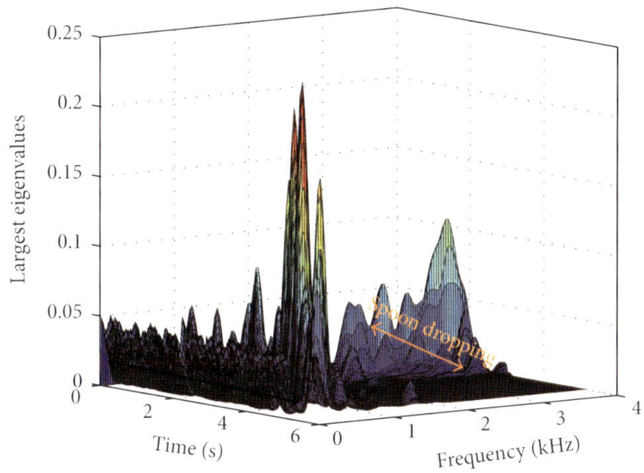

FIGURE 8: Time-frequency plot of the largest eigenvalues of the averaged cross spectral matrices for a dropping spoon sound in radio noise.

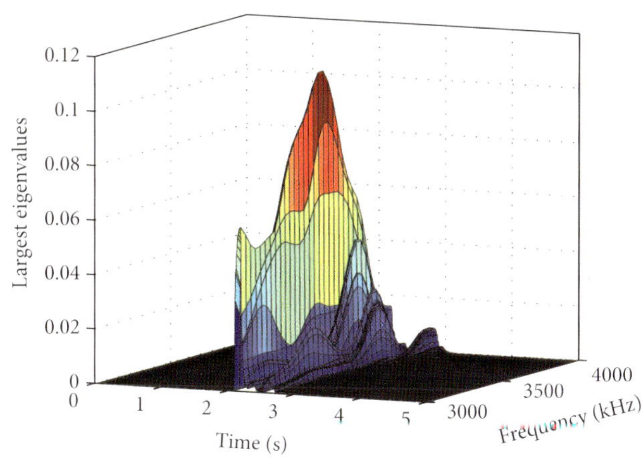

FIGURE 9: Close-up view of the 3-4 kHz region from the time-frequency plot in Figure 8. This shows a significant non-zero component when the SDL is occurring.

4. Evaluation

4.1. Noisy Sounds of Daily Life Database. In previous work by the authors [18], a database of seven sounds of daily life was constructed, in which a single radio was located close to one microphone in the recording environment. While many noise reduction applications have a sound sensor almost completely dedicated to recording the noise, this is not realistic in a general practical environment, as the sound sensors and noise source might be located anywhere. Further, very high accuracies were produced using the database in [18]. Consequently, we decided to investigate more difficult microphone configurations and noises.

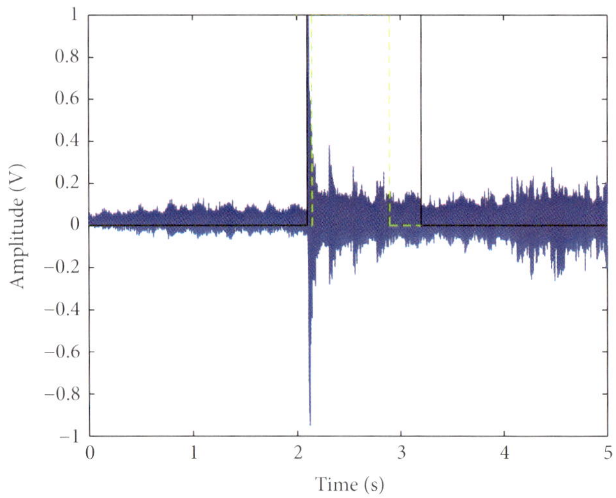

FIGURE 10: Time-domain waveform comparing an example segmentation (red) with the actual endpoints (green).

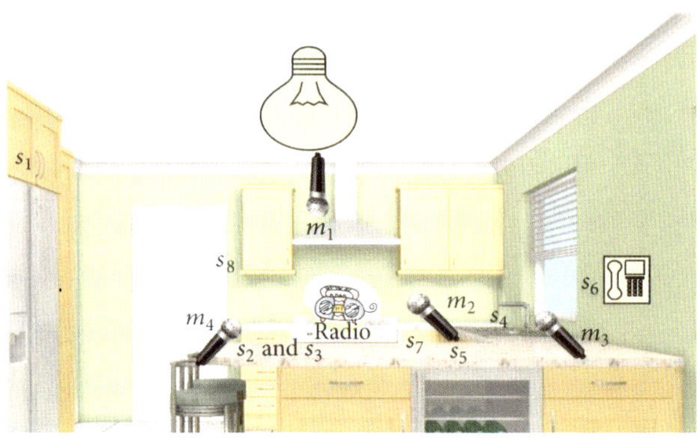

(1) Slamming cupboard door
(2) Dropping a cup
(3) Dropping a spoon
(4) Tap water
(5) Chopping vegetables
(6) Phone ringing
(7) Mixmaster
(8) Open microwave

FIGURE 11: Kitchen configured for data collection to investigate more difficult microphone configurations.

The microphone positions in the database described herein were carefully chosen with neither microphone as close to the radio as in [18]. In addition, the microphones were chosen, where possible, to be near either a power outlet, or the mains electricity (e.g, a light), to realistically evaluate the system's performance, as the microphones would be attached to the mains power if this were to become a commercial product. Microphone 1 was attached to a light, microphones 2 and 3 were mounted near power outlets and microphone 4 was placed diagonally and horizontally opposite microphones 2 and 3, respectively, as there were no more suitable positions near a possible entry to the mains electricity. The configuration for the noisy SDL recordings is depicted in Figure 11.

The eight SDLs recorded comprised a cupboard door slamming (s_1), a cup dropping (s_2), a spoon dropping (s_3), running tap water (s_4), chopping vegetables (s_5), a phone ringing (s_6), a mixmaster operating (s_7), and a microwave door opening (s_8).

TABLE 1: Estimated SNR ranges (dB) for the noisy sounds of daily life database, comprising various sounds recorded in the presence of radio noise (two volume levels), speech noise, and rain noise.

	Mic 1	Mic 2	Mic 3	Mic 4
Slamming cupboard door	19–25	23–32	15–18	18–23
Dropping a cup	15–19	12–20	1.0–1.5	3.5–5.0
Dropping a spoon	3.6–4.4	3.3–5.8	0.9–1.6	3.5–4.9
Tap water	1.2–1.7	2.6–5.2	1.4–2.0	2.6–3.2
Chopping vegetables	9–15	8–18	11–14	12–17
Phone ringing	4.5–6.1	5.8–8.7	4.3–5.7	4.3–6.3
Mixmaster	3.6–4.5	6.8–9.7	17–20	9.5–12
Open microwave	2.9–7.0	3.8–9.1	1.4–2.3	2.9–6.8

In each instance four channels were recorded to compare system performance in the same conditions for different microphone placements, but a maximum of two microphones were used in any evaluations reported herein.

Each recording had a duration of 5 seconds, and the total duration of the database across all conditions was 2.78 hours (90 training samples × 8 SDLs × 5 seconds = 1 hour. 40 training samples × 8 SDLs × 5 seconds × 4 noise degradations = 1.78 hours).

System performance in the presence of different noise types is of particular interest. In addition to the radio at pleasant listening level (as in [18]), other noise types recorded were the radio at a very loud volume, a male speaker talking in the background, and data recorded in the presence of rain (note that rain cannot be considered a point source, so does not satisfy the assumptions of CSLE). The estimated SNR ranges, across all conditions, are shown in Table 1.

4.2. System Description. The overall system is shown in Figure 2. The noise-corrupted testing data was preprocessed before feature extraction, using either signal enhancement, sound activity detection, or both. Features were then extracted and maximum a posteriori (MAP) adaptation was applied before using the adapted Gaussian mixture model (GMM) to determine the most likely SDL.

Feature extraction was performed using Mel frequency cepstral coefficients (MFCCs), following earlier work showing that importance of magnitude spectrum information in distinguishing between the SDLs [21]. Shifted delta cepstral (SDC) features were also employed, to allow some modelling of the temporal variation of the magnitude spectrum, and based on previous results [21, 22].

A GMM classifier with six mixture components was employed, following successes in related applications [21, 23, 24]. This was trained using 10 iterations of the EM algorithm. MAP adaptation of the GMM mean vectors was conducted, to enhance the discrimination between the different sounds of daily life classes over the simpler alternative configuration comprising GMMs trained separately on data from each class. Since, during GMM training, random initialization of

GMM parameters was employed, the results reported are the averages across 10 different initializations.

Classifier training was performed using clean sounds of daily life data. If it is trained using a noisy set, it will be unrealistically optimized for a specific spectral and spatial configuration. In any case, mismatch between the training data and real test data is to be expected. The system was trained using data from two microphones. If only one microphone is used, the classifier is biased towards data from that microphone (as it has a unique frequency response and additive noise characteristics). A noise-reduced signal will contain data from two microphones, as suggested by (2). Consequently, even though the SNR of the signal is improved by training using the microphone with the best SNR, the classification performance may not be improved because the unmixed signal passed to the classifier will contain data from both microphones.

TABLE 2: Classification accuracy of seven ICA-based methods for source separation for data comprising clean sounds of daily life data in which noise was artificially mixed, to ensure that noise components were perfectly correlated between channels.

	Mic 1, 20 dB, Mic 2, 15 dB Accuracy	Mic 1, 25 dB, Mic 2, 20 dB Accuracy
$ICA_{SDL\_Apriori}$	61.33%	62.83%
$ICA_{BestMic}$	61.72%	62.94%
$ICA_{LeastNoise}$	61.61%	63.94%
$ICA_{SDL\_BestSNR}$	58.11%	59.79%
$ICA_{SDL\_LeastNoise}$	59.56%	60.72%
ICA_{SSA}	65.61%	65.94%
ICA_{NISA}	**66.06%**	**66.17%**

4.3. Experiments. All experiments were performed in MATLAB and focused on the eight-class classification accuracy of various components of the proposed system.

(1) A comparison of the seven ICA-based methods for source separation among the microphone sources was made in which noise was artificially mixed into clean sounds of daily life data. The objective of this experiment was to eliminate delay between microphones, due to sound propagation, as a source of uncertainty in the results.

(2) Combinations of the source separation and sound activity detection methods were tested for one of the microphone configurations of the noisy SDL database, for four different noise configurations. In these experiments, CSLE was selected as the sound activity detection method of choice in most configurations, based on previous work [18].

(3) Three of the most promising source separation methods were combined with CSLE and tested for all microphone configurations of the noisy SDL database across all four different noise configurations.

In all tests, the GMM was trained with 30 recordings per sound class (with samples chosen uniformly across the database), and the system was tested using 40 noisy recordings per sound class across the different types of noise. The duration of each recording was 5 seconds.

5. Results and Discussion

5.1. Source Separation under Controlled Conditions. As seen in Table 2, under conditions where the noise was artificially mixed into the sounds of daily life, there was a clear advantage to using the steepest descent methods, with the noise inverse steepest ascent method of improving the unmixing coefficients producing the highest accuracies for both conditions tested. This suggests that the SSA and NISA methods may have often been able to find the optimum unmixing coefficients as occurred during the example of Figure 4.

5.2. Source Separation and SAD under Noisy Conditions. The advantage of steepest ascent methods over other source separation methods did not seem to be preserved for experiments on the noisy SDL database, in which noises were acoustically mixed in a realistic manner. As seen in Table 3, although the SNR steepest ascent method with CSLE performed best on the Mics 1 and 2 loud radio noise condition, this was by a narrow margin, and various other configurations proved slightly better for other noise conditions. In general, the results of Table 3 primarily demonstrate the importance and effectiveness of sound activity detection for the problem of multichannel SDL classification in noise.

5.3. Source Separation and SAD for Different Microphone Configurations under Noisy Conditions. Finally, in Table 4, the accuracies from a selection of the most promising configurations from all conditions are reported, with a view to recommending a good system configuration across all conditions tested. From Table 4, it is clear that sound activity detection using CSLE is the major single contributor to classification accuracy. However, further gains might be achieved using CSLE and ICA based on *a priori* SNR (Section 2.1), whose accuracy either improved on or was roughly comparable with that of CSLE alone.

6. Conclusion

This paper has reported the application of source separation and sound activity detection methods to the problem of classifying sounds of daily life for home telemonitoring under realistic noisy conditions using multiple arbitrarily positioned microphones. Overwhelmingly, the experimental evidence shows that the inclusion of an effective sound activity detection method, such as the cross-spectral largest eigenvalue (CSLE) method, in an "activities of daily life" classification system produces large and consistent gains in accuracy, up to 90% in terms of relative reduction in error rate under a range of noisy conditions. Source separation methods, including the ICA variants considered

Table 3: Classification accuracies of various combinations of source separation and sound activity detection methods for one of the microphone configurations of the noisy SDL database, across four different noise configurations. Despite this, source separation methods do provide relative reductions in error rate of up to 7%, 48%, and 2% compared with CSLE alone for the radio normal, rain, and radio loud conditions, respectively.

Method	Radio normal (Mic 1 and Mic 2)	Rain (Mic 1 and Mic 2)	Radio loud (Mic 1 and Mic 2)	Talking (Mic 1 and Mic 2)
Baseline (channel with best SNR + Baseline SAD)	44.04%	61.39%	28.58%	39.54%
SAD alone: baseline SAD	56.33%	77.78%	32.92%	46.96%
SAD alone: CSLE	71.96%	97.18%	40.25%	**69.45%**
$ICA_{SDL\_Apriori}$	44.54%	61.06%	29.71%	48.75%
$ICA_{SDL\_Apriori}$ + CSLE	71.63%	98.01%	41.04%	66.95%
$ICA_{BestMic}$	43.83%	61.30%	29.71%	41.54%
$ICA_{BestMic}$ + CSLE	72.13%	97.08%	41.38%	67.12%
$ICA_{LeastNoise}$	43.04%	60.88%	30.46%	44.83%
$ICA_{LeastNoise}$ + CSLE	72.00%	**98.10%**	41.50%	68.25%
$ICA_{SDL\_BestSNR}$	44.46%	60.88%	29.50%	41.63%
$ICA_{SDL\_BestSNR}$ + CSLE	73.04%	97.50%	41.08%	67.75%
$ICA_{SDL\_LeastNoise}$	43.83%	60.56%	30.42%	45.75%
$ICA_{SDL\_LeastNoise}$ + CSLE	**73.79%**	96.81%	40.88%	68.75%
ICA_{SSA}	44.08%	61.90%	29.83%	40.92%
ICA_{SSA} + CSLE	71.04%	97.04%	**41.58%**	68.21%

Table 4: Classification accuracy of promising system configurations, for all three microphone configurations of the noisy SDL database, across four different noise configurations.

Method	Radio normal (Mic 1 and Mic 2) (Mic 1 and Mic 3) (Mic 1 and Mic 4)	Rain (Mic 1 and Mic 2) (Mic 1 and Mic 3) (Mic 1 and Mic 4)	Radio loud (Mic 1 and Mic 2) (Mic 1 and Mic 3) (Mic 1 and Mic 4)	Talking (Mic 1 and Mic 2) (Mic 1 and Mic 3) (Mic 1 and Mic 4)	Average
	44.04%	61.39%	28.58%	39.54%	43.39%
Baseline (channel with best SNR)	51.25%	61.71%	28.75%	44.61%	46.58%
	49.38%	64.91%	33.17%	44.42%	47.97%
	71.95%	97.18%	40.25%	**69.46%**	69.71%
SAD alone: CSLE	**84.08%**	99.77%	55.21%	79.67%	79.68%
	79.21%	**98.66%**	**50.63%**	**73.13%**	**75.41%**
	71.63%	**98.01%**	41.04%	66.96%	69.41%
$ICA_{SDL\_Apriori}$ + CSLE	83.46%	**100%**	55.88%	**81.67%**	**80.25%**
	77.88%	98.24%	48.71%	44.79%	67.41%
	73.04%	97.50%	41.08%	67.75%	**69.84%**
$ICA_{SDL\_BestSNR}$ + CSLE	82.79%	99.07%	**57.17%**	76.94%	78.99%
	76.63%	98.24%	49.00%	69.96%	73.46%
	71.04%	97.04%	**41.58%**	68.21%	69.47%
ICA_{SSA} + CSLE	82.50%	99.07%	55.29%	79.00%	78.97%
	75.00%	97.13%	47.29%	67.46%	71.72%

herein, provided at best modest gains. Among these, the $ICA_{SDL\_Apriori}$ method, which identifies the two unmixed signals using estimates of their SNRs, seems to perform well, providing relative reductions in error rates of up to 10% in the best case. The overall classification performance on an eight-class task provided accuracies between 70%–100% across three different microphone-pair conditions and three noise conditions, while the most challenging low-SNR loud radio noise condition resulted in accuracies in 40%–50% range, still well above chance level. Future work will examine the long-term performance of this system in the homes of elderly subjects, detecting a range of sounds that are found to commonly occur, and will begin correlating their occurrence with clinical indicators.

References

[1] United Nations, *Long-Range World Population Projections: Based on the 1998 Revision. The Population Division*, Department of Economic and Social Affairs; United Nations Secretariat, 2003.

[2] D. Trewin, *Australian Bureau of Statistics*, Causes of Death in Australia, Canberra, Australia, 1996.

[3] D. Istrate, E. Castelli, M. Vacher, L. Besacier, and J. F. Serignat, "Information extraction from sound for medical telemonitoring," *IEEE Transactions on Information Technology in Biomedicine*, vol. 10, no. 2, pp. 264–274, 2006.

[4] B. G. Celler, T. Hesketh, W. Earnshaw, and E. Ilsar, "Instrumentation system for the remote monitoring of changes in functional health status of the elderly at home," in *Proceedings of the 16th Annual International Conference of the IEEE Engineering in Medicine and Biology Society*, pp. 908–909, November 1994.

[5] N. Noury, T. Herve, V. Rialle et al., "Monitoring behaviour in the home using a smart fall sensor and position sensors," in *Proceedings of the 1st Annual International Conference on Microtechnologies in Medicine and Biology*, pp. 607–610, 2000.

[6] A. Fleury, M. Vacher, and N. Noury, "SVM-based multimodal classification of activities of daily living in health smart homes: sensors, algorithms, and first experimental results," *IEEE Transactions on Information Technology in Biomedicine*, vol. 14, no. 2, pp. 274–283, 2010.

[7] M. Vacher, D. Istrate, L. Besacier, J. F. Serignat, and E. Castelli, "Sound detection and classification for medical telesurvey," in *Proceedings of the IASTED International Conference on Biomedical Engineering*, pp. 395–399, ACTA Press, Innsbruck, Austria, February 2004.

[8] G. Virone, D. Istrate, M. Vacher, N. Noury, J. F. Serignat, and J. Demongeot, "First steps in data fusion between a multichannel audio acquisition and an information system for home healthcare," in *Proceddings of the 25th Annual International Conference of the IEEE Engineering in Medicine and Biology Society*, pp. 1364–1367, September 2003.

[9] E. Castelli, M. Vacher, D. Istrate, L. Besacier, and J. F. Serignat, "Habitat telemonitoring system based on the sound surveillance," in *Proceedings of the International Conference on Information Communication Technologies in Health*, 2003.

[10] M. Vacher, D. Istrate, F. Portet et al., "The sweet-home project: audio technology in smart homes to improve well-being and reliance," in *Proceedings of the IEEE International Conference on Engineering in Medicine and Biology*, pp. 5291–5294, August 2011.

[11] S. T. Roweis, "One microphone source separation," in *Advances in Neural Information Processing Systems*, pp. 793–799, 2001.

[12] H. Saruwatari, S. Kurita, K. Takeda, F. Itakura, T. Nishikawa, and K. Shikano, "Blind source separation combining independent component analysis and beamforming," *Eurasip Journal on Applied Signal Processing*, vol. 2003, no. 11, pp. 1135–1146, 2003.

[13] F. Kraft, R. Malkin, T. Schaaf, and A. Waibel, "Temporal ICA for classification of acoustic events in kitchen environment," in *Proceedings of the International Conference on Speech and Language Processing*, pp. 2689–2692, 2005.

[14] M. T. Johnson, X. Yuan, and Y. Ren, "Speech signal enhancement through adaptive wavelet thresholding," *Speech Communication*, vol. 49, no. 2, pp. 123–133, 2007.

[15] Y. Wang, J. An, V. Sethu, and E. Ambikairajah, "Perceptually motivated pre-filter for speech enhancement using Kalman filtering," in *Proceedings of the 6th International Conference on Information, Communications and Signal Processing (ICICS '07)*, pp. 1–4, Singapore, December 2007.

[16] B. S. Atal and L. R. Rabiner, "Pattern recognition approach to voiced-unvoiced-silence classification with applications to speech recognition," *IEEE Transactions on Acoustics, Speech, and Signal Processing*, vol. 24, no. 3, pp. 201–212, 1976.

[17] A. Hyvärinen and E. Oja, "Independent component analysis: algorithms and applications," *Neural Networks*, vol. 13, no. 4-5, pp. 411–430, 2000.

[18] D. Maunder, E. Ambikairajah, J. Epps, and B. Celler, "Dual-microphone sounds of daily Life classification for telemonitoring in a noisy environment," *Proceedings of the Annual International Conference of the IEEE Engineering in Medicine and Biology Society*, vol. 2008, pp. 4636–4639, 2008.

[19] D. H. Johnson and S. R. DeGraaf, "Improving the resolution of bearing in passive sonar arrays by eigenvalue analysis," *IEEE Transactions on Acoustics, Speech, and Signal Processing*, vol. 30, no. 4, pp. 638–647, 1982.

[20] W. Wang and D. H. Johnson, "Computing linear transforms of symbolic signals," *IEEE Transactions on Signal Processing*, vol. 50, no. 3, pp. 628–634, 2002.

[21] N. C. Laydrus, E. Ambikairajah, and B. Celler, "Automated sound analysis system for home telemonitoring using shifted delta cepstral features," in *Proceedings of the 15th International Conference on Digital Signal Processing (DSP '07)*, pp. 135–138, Cardiff, UK, July 2007.

[22] P. A. Torres-Carrasquillo, E. Singer, M. A. Kohler, R. J. Greene, D. A. Reynolds, and J. R. Deller, "Approaches to language identification using Gaussian mixture models and shifted delta cepstral features," in *Proceedings of the International Conference of Spoken Language Processing*, pp. 89–92, 2002.

[23] D. A. Reynolds and R. C. Rose, "Robust text-independent speaker identification using Gaussian mixture speaker models," *IEEE Transactions on Speech and Audio Processing*, vol. 3, no. 1, pp. 72–83, 1995.

[24] F. Allen, E. Ambikairajah, and J. Epps, "Language identification using warping and the shifted delta cepstrum," in *Proceedings of the IEEE 7th Workshop on Multimedia Signal Processing (MMSP '05)*, pp. 1–4, Shanghai, China, November 2005.

3

Using Action Research and Peer Perspectives to Develop Technology That Facilitates Behavioral Change and Self-Management in COPD

Catherine McCabe,[1] John Dinsmore,[1] Anne Marie Brady,[1] Gabrielle Mckee,[1] Sharon O'Donnell,[1] and David Prendergast[2]

[1] *School of Nursing & Midwifery, Trinity College Dublin, 24 D'Olier Street, Dublin 2, Ireland*
[2] *Intel Ireland Ltd., Collinstown Industrial Park, Leixlip, County Kildare, Ireland*

Correspondence should be addressed to Catherine McCabe; camccabe@tcd.ie

Academic Editor: Frank Tost

Background. Behavioural change and self-management in patients with chronic illness may help to control symptoms, avoid rehospitalization, enhance quality of life, and decrease mortality and morbidity. *Objective*. Guided by action research principles and using mixed methods, the aim of this project was to develop peer based educational, motivational, and health-promoting peer based videos, using behavioural change principles, to support self-management in patients with COPD. *Methods*. Individuals ($n = 32$) living with COPD at home and involved in two community based COPD support groups were invited to participate in this project. Focus group/individual interviews and a demographic questionnaire were used to collect data. *Results*. Analysis revealed 6 categories relevant to behavioural change which included self-management, support, symptoms, knowledge, rehabilitation, and technology. Participants commented that content needed to be specific, and videos needed to be shorter, to be tailored to severity of condition, to demonstrate "normal" activities, to be positive, and to ensure that content is culturally relevant. *Conclusions*. This study demonstrated that detailed analysis of patient perspectives and needs for self-management is essential and should underpin the development of any framework, materials, and technology. The action research design principles provided an effective framework for eliciting the data and applying it to technology and testing its relevance to the user.

1. Introduction

Chronic obstructive pulmonary disease (COPD) is the 4th leading cause of death worldwide [1]. The pattern of care for patients with COPD often involves lengthy hospital admissions, followed by a return to the home environment with little follow-up support for the management of disease symptoms. This inevitably leads to the hospital readmission with acute symptom onset which is unsatisfactory for the individual and financially unsustainable for increasingly stretched health services.

Behavioral change and self-management in people with chronic illness may help to control symptoms, avoid unnecessary rehospitalization, enhance quality of life, and decrease overall mortality and morbidity [2]. Behavioral change techniques influence change by using motivating techniques, education, problem definition, collaborative goal setting/problem-solving, contract for change, continuing support, and evaluation [3].

Recent studies highlight the role that video and multimedia based information communication technologies (ICT) can play in COPD self-management. A comparative study revealed that individuals using a 19-minute video outlining the benefits of exercise followed by a 30-minute video exercise programme 4 days a week for 6 weeks had significantly improved physical and emotional functional capabilities [4]. This is important as the British Lung Foundation Survey revealed that less than 2% of COPD patients in the UK had access to a rehabilitation exercise programme [4].

A study on the use of video technology to provide motivation for exercise concluded that individuals with COPD showed improved quality of life (QoL), coping skills, and diminished fatigue when using a videotape series focused on motivation and exercise [5]. Two hundred fourteen COPD patients took part in this 3-tiered RCT (video intervention versus standard video versus control). Groups using the video intervention were twice as likely to change from sedentary states to moderate exercise compared to the control groups. The video intervention group saw an improvement in activities of daily living and was particularly effective at prompting exercise with 84% of patients reporting routine exercise at 9-month follow-up. This study shows a distinct correlation between improved health benefits, motivation, and behavioral change with video intervention, suggesting that videos provide an effective medium to disseminate knowledge and encourage self-management. A randomized controlled trial that measured the effects of an animated diagram and video-based online breathing programme for dyspnea in patients with stable COPD concluded that a video based online training programme resulted in improved pulmonary function, exercise capacity, and health status in the treatment group only [6].

The theory of innovation diffusion states that individuals are more likely to consider technology use when relevant to them [7]. Therefore it is important to design new technologies including content from a patient centric perspective with reference to the health condition and cultural context of the individual. Studies related to behavioral change and COPD show significant positive effects for self-efficacy and behavioral change on administration of a behavioral change programme [8]. This paper discusses findings from a project guided by action research principles that explored patient based self-management and technology based programmes for people living at home with COPD and concludes that action research principles can be an effective framework design for behavioral change video and multimedia content development.

The main aim of this project was to develop peer based educational, motivational, and health-promoting peer based videos, using behavioral change principles, to support self-management in patients with COPD.

An objective of the project was to explore the needs, sources of support, and experiences of people living at home in relation to their knowledge, ability, and readiness to self-manage their care needs in relation to COPD.

2. Method

Action research principles and a cross-sectional descriptive methodology were chosen as a suitable method of enquiry for the aim of this study. Action research is a process by which new knowledge is generated and used to achieve change [9]. The strength of this process of inquiry lies in its ability to generate solutions to practical problems. In this study the action research took place over 4 phases (Figure 3).

Ethical approval was provided by the relevant institutional ethics committee (Faculty of Health Sciences).

3. Action Research Process

Phase 1. The project began with a review of the literature to identify the main self-management needs and resources relevant to COPD in an ICT context. This was followed with completion of the demographic questionnaire and focus group/individual interviews to ascertain the knowledge, readiness for self-care, sources of support, and perceived care needs of people with COPD. Focus group and individual interviews were video recorded and content was used for development of self-management videos in Phase 2.

Phase 2. In conjunction with the data from the interviews and video recordings, existing educational resources currently accessed by the client group or available to meet their identified needs were reviewed. This data guided and informed the development of new educational, motivational, and health-promoting peer related videos specific to COPD. Eighteen videos representing the 6 key themes of knowledge, symptoms (prevention), self-management (practices), rehabilitation, support (including carers), and "Real Time Health" were produced. The theme of "Real time Health" was constructed to highlight the role of psychology and the constant need for individuals to manage their condition in a "real time" home environment.

Phase 3. Participants were invited to participate in follow-up focus group interviews to explore user views and satisfaction with the video material produced. They were shown a series of five, 3–5-minute videos representing areas of self-management based on data gathered in Phase 1. Participants were asked to discuss any perceived positive and negative aspects to each video as well as discuss any improvements they would like to be considered as part of the Phase 4 iteration process. The key issues that the participants commented on were that some content needed to be more specific and focused and videos needed to be shorter, to be tailored to level of severity of condition, to demonstrate "normal" day-to-day activities, to be positive, and to ensure that content is relevant to the Irish Health service.

Phase 4. Using feedback from Phase 3, a second and final stage of video development was conducted.

4. Participants

Treatment of COPD in Ireland is managed mainly through primary health care settings by general practitioners (GP) and community nurses. Admission to acute care facilities only occurs for exacerbations of symptoms and discharge is usually followed by attendance at a local rehabilitation programme which may last up to 6 weeks and GP visits as required. Until recently only informal local support groups provided information and social support to people with COPD; however, recently a national support organization has been established. For the purposes of this study, individuals living with COPD at home and involved in community based COPD support groups were invited to participate in this project. Study information sheets with contact details were distributed at community based COPD support group events. Eligibility criteria included a diagnosis of COPD, member of COPD support group, over 18, and English speaking. When eligible participants contacted the researcher specific sessions were organized for those who were interested in attending.

5. Instruments

Participants completed a brief questionnaire comprising 25 items which documented some sociodemographic characteristics of the participants. These included age, gender, medical insurance, medical/social history, comorbidities, BMI, perceived health status, independence rating, carer support, where COPD advice was obtained, confidence in self-management, and ICT use.

Focus group interviews were conducted at community locations convenient to the participants, with a researcher as a facilitator. There were 10 focus groups in total (5 in Phase 2 and 5 in Phase 3), with an average of 6 participants in each. The final total of focus group participants was 32 as participants in Phase 2 focus groups were the same as Phase 3. The themes explored in the interviews included experience, knowledge, self-management, social support, health professional support, social and personal life, quality of life, perceptions, cognitions, and confidence. Twelve individuals who participated in a focus group interview also completed an individual participant perspective interview, four of whom completed a second individual interview as part of the project's prolonged engagement methodology to gather in-depth information.

6. Data Analysis

Descriptive statistics, using SPSS version 19, were used to describe the demographic data and included means, standard deviations, percentages, and ranges. Descriptive statistics were also used to describe the exploratory questions of the second part of the questionnaire. All recordings from the interviews were transcribed and transferred into NVivo version 9 for analysis. A constant comparative methodology facilitated the identification of patterns in participant responses and unifying concepts facilitating initial coding and development of core categories, which were revisited and consolidated, in line with the steps in the textural content analysis of [10]. Analysis continued until theoretical saturation was obtained and the number of references for each theme was calculated. Data from the individual interviews was analysed with the focus groups to triangulate findings at Phases 1 and 3, respectively (Figure 1). The content from these interviews was also used to construct the peer-perspective videos.

In order to ensure consistency in coded findings research team members used NVivo to manage and review transcribed data from the focus group interviews. Several COPD patients that gave important insights within an interview after coding were interviewed for a second time (prolonged engagement). This is in line with guidelines for ensuring trustworthiness in qualitative interviewing [11].

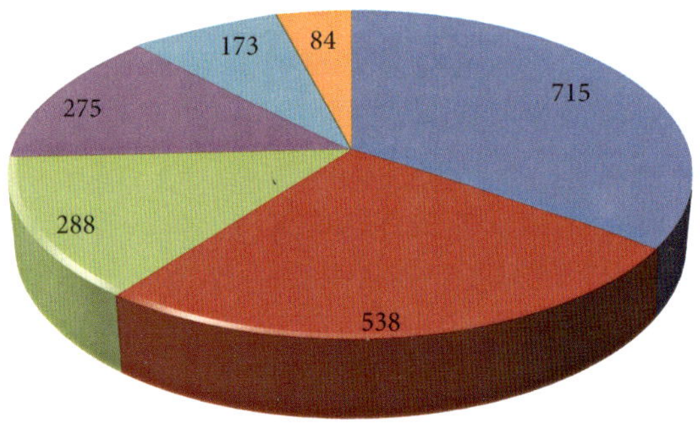

FIGURE 1: Core themes and reference totals extracted after coding analysis at Phase 1.

7. Results

Recruitment occurred from July to December 2011. Sociodemographic characteristics are outlined in Table 1. Thirty-two individuals participated in the initial focus groups at Phase 1 and again at Phase 2.

Coding of the transcripts from Phase 1 revealed 6 core categories relevant to COPD behavioral change. These included self-management, support, symptoms, knowledge, rehabilitation, and technology. Figure 1 outlines the number and portion of references attributed to each core theme across the focus groups and interviews.

Self-management was the main core theme discussed by participants followed by support. Management of symptoms and overall knowledge to the condition were almost equally referred to with rehabilitation methods the second last most talked about area. Each of these categories was further refined into various subthemes as outlined in Table 2.

7.1. Knowledge of the Condition. Participants distinguished between early stage knowledge immediately after diagnosis and knowledge obtained from years of living with the condition.

> *FG: "In the beginning you would just have got it from a consultant or the doctor—probably looked up the net after that."*

A distinct lack of online information related specifically to the Irish context was reported and also information was scattered across various sites rather than one site covering all areas of the condition effectively.

> *I've been on the British Lung Foundation and different sites on the Internet but they do not give a proper breakdown of things. And most of it is American, which is different to us, they have different facilities to use and they call things a different name and you know it makes life a bit*

Table 1: Focus group participant profile.

Participants (32)			
Gender breakdown	47% male, 53% female		
	Mean	Standard deviation	Range
Average age	67	8.44	46–78
BMI	25.8	4.64	20.40–38.52
Medical coverage	Have complete medical cards (84%) Covered by medical card for GP consultations (75%) Covered for medications and prescriptions (47%) Covered by private health insurance in their own name (34%) Covered through a family member (6%)		
Past medical history breakdown (%)	TIA/stroke (3%) Heart disease (16%) Hypertension (38%) Diabetes (6%) High cholesterol (22%) Anxiety and depression (31%) Other (47%)		
Accommodation support (%)	Lived alone (38%); lived with nondependents (56%); lived with dependents (6%)		
Smoking cessation (%)	Did smoke but have quit (78%); still smoke (9%); nonresponders (13%)		
Perceived health status (%)	Fair (41%); average (41%); poor (13%); good (13%)		
Independence rating (%)	Required some assistance (63%); fully independent (31%); nonresponders (3%)		
Carer support (%)	Spouse (47%); children (9.4%); friend (3.1%); partner (3.1%); other (12.5%); remainder—nonrespondents		
Obtaining information (%)	Books/newspapers/magazines (21%); Internet (12.5%); Digital Recordings (6%); health professionals (69%); alternative sources (25%)		
Confidence in self-management (%)	Yes (72%); no (29%)		
ICT use (%)	Standard mobile phone (91%); smart phone (25%); desktop home computer (25%); laptop (25%)		
Internet connectivity (%)	Have access to Internet based resources (50%); have access to an Internet connection (53%); use Internet daily (25%); use Internet a few times a week (9%); use Internet a few times per month (6%)		
Confidence in ICT use (%)	Fully confident (50%); partially confident (16%); neutral (12.5%); not confident (6%); nonrespondents (16%)		

more difficult. You cannot do the same things as they do because we haven't got it, we might not understand the jargon you know, they talk a lot about medi-care which we haven't got. (DE)

7.2. Symptoms. Participants reported 5 key subthemes in relation to the symptoms which were psychological symptoms, breathing difficulties, infections, symptom triggers, and relationship of symptoms with existing comorbidities. Psychological symptoms were broken down into 5 key branches: depression, isolation, frustration, embarrassment, and anger.

FG: "You do feel isolated, when your first given, told the news I mean I just wouldn't accept it at all... and that just led to depression, just couldn't cope."

Patients who commented that they did not feel depressed also commented on "feeling fed up," "worthless," "thinking of euthanasia," "disappointed," "browned off," "being vexed at why they got this," "having a lack of motivation," and little "joyfulness."

Participants remarked that when breathing was good participants were optimistic, calm, and positive. If breathing was poor participants reported being conscious of the condition, struggling, panicking, gasping for air, and being frustrated.

FG: "The shortness of breath in everything you do, just normal things like showering can be very frustrating."

7.2.1. Self-Management. Self-management was the most referenced topic of conversation amongst both the focus groups and interviewees. Results produced a four-way interlogical model to patient's views of COPD self-management; if one area was positively affected, then all other areas replicated a positive outcome. The areas of breathing, functional, social,

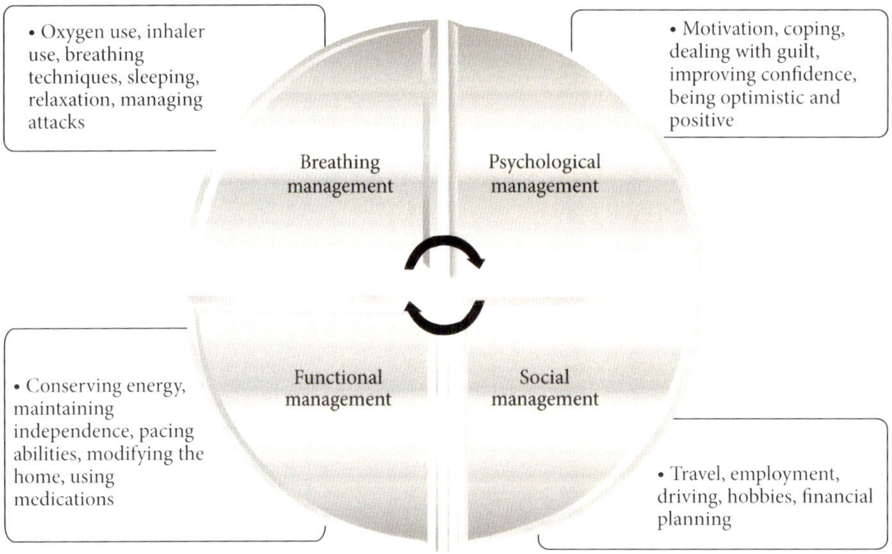

Figure 2: Four-way interactive structure for self-management.

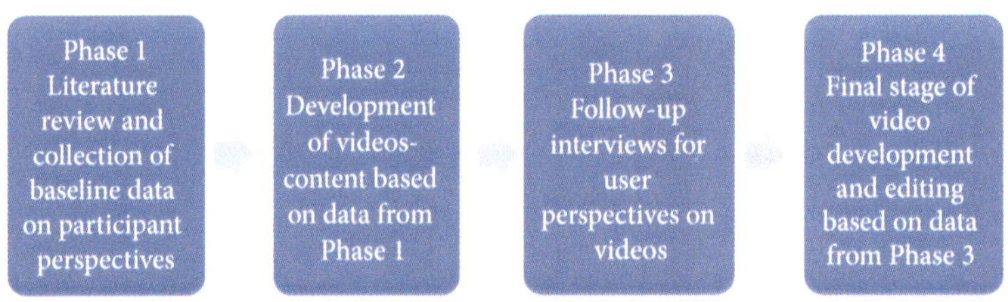

Figure 3: Action research process.

Table 2: Six core categories and subthemes.

Core theme	
Knowledge	Knowledge of the condition; knowledge of diagnosis; knowledge of the cause; awareness of COPD; stigma
Symptoms	Psychological; breathing related; infections; associated comorbidities and symptom triggers
Rehabilitation	Exercise; diet; smoking cessation; medical rehabilitation (including pulmonary)
Self-management (practice and strategies)	Breathing related; functional management; psychological; social management
Support	Health professional; peer support; friends and family; community and social support
Technology use	Internet; computers; videos; mobile phones; tablets

and psychological management (Figure 2) were seen as necessary to holistically self-manage in a primary care context.

> *BS: "The first time I was told when I was doing the rehab program, that I needed to go on oxygen I was absolutely devastated because I thought how in the name of God am I going to live my life on oxygen. And I was really down in the dumps about it until I kind of got used to the idea. And then I said you know well if it helps, if it makes life easier, now it does not stop me getting out of breath but it helps me recover my breath quicker."*

Functional management practices amongst participants in this study focused on the dispensation, conservation, and regulation of energy levels in order to maintain independence, which was referenced in relation to the ability to perform activities of daily living and social activities such as going to the local shop or cooking a meal.

> *FG: "If I do decide to cut the grass myself and its only a small bit of grass I'd only do half of it and I'd have to leave it and come in and go out maybe in an hour later to finish it. I wouldn't have the energy to do it all in the one."*

Tiredness and weakness associated with a lack of energy increased negative psychological responses to self-management.

> *FG: "It affects your social end of it, because you just do not have the energy, you know if there's something going on and you are not feeling great well you just have to pass on it, you know."*

The psychological processes behind COPD self-management revealed 5 core areas of importance for participants. These areas were patient motivation, coping ability/response, optimism or positivity, overcoming guilt, and confidence in self-management. Motivation was the most commented on area of importance referenced by participants followed closely by development of "coping" responses. Participants felt daily motivation to self-manage was difficult when they were feeling low or depressed, especially for those who were more socially isolated. Motivation was particularly difficult with regard to developing an exercise routine.

> *Also very important and others have said it too, is to motivate yourself to do things. That can be difficult at times especially if you are feeling a bit sorry for yourself which you can be from time to time. (FG)*

Peer and family support appeared to be important in improving motivational drives to self-management.

> *I set up a support group and from meeting those people at the support groups and I helped with a few support groups now and that gives me a sense of purpose or reason to do things. (ML)*

Learning to accept and live with the condition was referenced as key to participant's ability to cope; participants comment regularly that dwelling on their condition had an extremely negative impact on their motivation and confidence to self-manage.

> *We all adjust to a different quality of life, even with age, its amazing ... and my quality of life compared to what it used to be is what most people consider to be pretty awful but I do not, I'm happy with what I am able to do and I do it. (MA)*

The final subbranch to the psychological component of self-management was overcoming guilt. Participants almost exclusively felt guilt for their diagnosis and development of the condition. The foundation of this guilt was linked to regrets about previous behaviors such as smoking, which have been reported as a key to COPD onset. A consensus did emerge that their condition did not warrant sympathy due to the perception that the cause was self-inflicted.

> *I felt guilt and feel slightly that my condition is my own fault. And I have a huge guilt trip about that. (FG)*

Confidence appeared linked to perceived independence as a key determinate of successful self-management.

> *That's all part and parcel of your confidence so if you are independent you are going to have the confidence to go out and do exercises or whatever. (FG)*

Participants discussed 5 major areas of concern in relation to social activities; these include ability to drive, employment, hobbies, financial issues, and travel. Overall participant's felt that compared to prediagnosis their travel was now restricted and nonspontaneous particularly for those who required continuous oxygen therapy and needed to carry an oxygen tank.

> *DE: "If I go away I've got to have the c-pap machine, the nebulizer and the portable oxygen concentrator. I mean that takes up a suitcase, you get all that lot together. So I cannot travel light anymore. That was my first gut reaction was oh no I'm going to be on this for the rest of my life now."*

Additional problems associated with participant engagement in short-term travel included financial costs to fuel or public transport and the psychological feeling that they were restricting others' enjoyment.

Personal hobbies play an important role in maintaining confidence and independence as part of a social based self-management framework in COPD.

> *Some nights I go and I might not get up and dance at all ... if they are fast there's no way I could do them. But even if I do not do a dance I'm still keeping in touch with the friends that I made at the dancing over the years. (BE)*

Compensating for activities no longer possible is also central to participant coping strategies. Due to physical limitations several participants optimized current abilities and substituted new hobbies and practices.

> *I just sit back and relax, no good getting annoyed about it, just take it, sit back and read the paper, turn on my wireless and listen to a bit of music, you know. (JO)*

The loss of employment was devastating for younger participants in this study and contributed to decreased confidence in self-managing. Participants commented on wishing to go back to work, while simultaneously acknowledging that the physical limitations and uncertainty of their illness progression would not allow them to do so.

> *I would love to go back to work, I would love the purposefulness of it and the freedom of being able to earn your own money. I mean that's always been, I've always been to work up until I got the severity of this ... after that I did not feel like I could go to work after that, kind of knocked my confidence a bit I suppose. (DE)*

All participants received fixed income benefits and/or a pension as their primary income and commented on the difficulty of living on a minimal budget that does not provide flexibility to support areas of change for the participant outside of daily living essentials.

> *I'm fortunate my limited income just about covers what I have to do but it does not leave anything for holidays or anything out of the ordinary ... I must admit I would like a holiday, that is one thing I really miss. (DE)*

Rehabilitation was referenced 173 times compared to self-management at 715. Four areas of rehabilitation, exercise, smoking cessation, medical rehabilitation (including pulmonary rehabilitation clinics), and diet, were referenced by participants in this study.

> *I keep active. It can be tough at times but it has to be done. And the more you push yourself the better you feel anyway . . . I can see the difference; I'm that little bit more free. I can walk that little bit better. (ML)*

All participants consented that smoking contributed to the development of their condition and cessation of smoking was essential to rehabilitation and self-management strategies.

> *I should have stopped, I did not, I kept smoking . . . even when I was on the inhalers, even on that I used to smoke. I smoked until I couldn't smoke. (JO)*

7.2.2. Support. Support was the second most referenced area of concern for participants in this study (538 references) with health professional support, peer support, friends and family, and community/social support referenced in descending order.

> *FG: "When you're in the system, in the hospital with the doctors and that and the nurses, they're brilliant."*

> *FG: "On the rehab course you get not just the proper exercises for your lungs but you also get a lot of education and a lot of information on the condition and also about the medication and all that sort of thing which you wouldn't pick up really."*

> *FG: "Once they understand it, once they accept you know that this is it and this is you for the rest of your life. I find my family is great now with me, I go everywhere with them."*

7.2.3. Technology. Technologies used by participants as part of their current self-management practices included the Internet (most commonly referenced), desktop/laptop computer, videos, and mobile phone. The Internet was labeled separately from computers due to its availability on multiple devices and platforms. Fluency and usage levels varied amongst participants with 50% of individuals having access to Internet based facilities. Internet usage focused on e-mail, resourcing knowledge, and using Skype, particularly for individuals isolated or with distant relations.

> *DE: "Another thing about people on the internet you know at least if you look up what other people are going through you think oh I'm not that bad or you know it can make life a bit more bearable because during winter months I'm more or less indoors."*

8. Discussion

International published trials on COPD self-management (including ICT use) suggest that self-management is linked to improved health status, reduced emergency visits to health professionals, and reduced hospitalizations [12–14]. A Cochrane systematic review of 14 controlled trials on self-management education in patients with COPD stipulated that it is not clear what influence self-management education has on COPD patients. While self-management reduces hospitalization, data is insufficient to formulate clear recommendations regarding what should comprise content in a self-management educational programme, to integrate skills into everyday patient life (e.g., diet, exercise, smoking cessation, and sleep habits) and how best this should be disseminated using new technology [13].

Developing a model to promote healthy lifestyle change after diagnosis of COPD is an extremely detailed task. Core to the development of this model is the integration of structures for increased engagement, improved patient motivation, and self-efficacy. This study demonstrates that detailed analysis of patient perspectives on their condition and needs for self-management is essential and should underpin the development of any framework, materials, and technology. Inclusion of users in the process of design, development, and usability of a technology based self-management programme ensures a more positive user experience. According to NICE guidelines the three key requirements for high quality care include effectiveness, safety, and user experience. Involvement of users in the design of a service or product opens up opportunities for design, function, and safety issues that may have been otherwise unapparent [15]. The action research design principles that guided this project provided an effective framework for eliciting user perspective data, applying it to technology in a patient centric manner and testing its relevance to the user. This type of approach may result in increased and sustained user compliance.

Knowledge of COPD at diagnosis appears critical to the outlook and coping responses invoked by patients. Time should be taken by health professionals to ensure patients are confident in their knowledge of COPD as soon as possible following diagnosis and commencement of treatment. Sites or dissemination material should be tailored to various severity groups in COPD; for example, those with mild/moderate disease appear not to engage with web sites showing the severe aspects of the condition. Peer support and learning should be ideally constructed within the cultural and health system in which a patient resides. Participants in this study expressed frustration that available online peer resources were developed outside of the Irish context, particularly in the United States, referencing services and situations unfamiliar to their self-management situation in Ireland.

Psychological related symptoms to living with COPD were commonly referenced areas in this study, supporting previous research suggesting that emotional status determines health status to a greater extent than lung function or exercise tests in COPD patients [16]. Participants in this study perceived social and peer support as central to alleviating negative psychological symptoms such as depression. Future research into improving the social support structure of individuals with COPD is recommended. In assessing psychological symptoms of COPD it is important to also review their level of social and peer support. Participant responses in this study suggest that depression amongst individuals in Ireland with COPD may be a "silent" or underreported phenomenon. Future research is recommended into this potential phenomenon as positive psychological perceptions are key to successful behavioral change and self-management.

Overall participants in this study believe that self-management is a unique and subjective process that one learns based on their personal experience of COPD. Key actions participants used in self-management focused around conserving energy, seeking support, avoiding triggers, and being motivated to change their lifestyle. Uncertainty amongst participants in relation to the progression of their condition means planning on a day-to-day basis only with key motivational drives to maintaining health orientated around family/social life and maintaining independence. Bartlett et al. [3] had similar findings in relation to the importance of planning daily goals for successful self-management. In dealing with "triggers" to symptom exacerbations participants revealed a willingness to modify behavior and sustain daily techniques to anticipate and deal with changes in their condition. Similar to Dinesen et al. this project recommends that designing a framework to allow individuals to share these techniques via peer learning online would be off benefit in potential behavioral change and self-management on a daily basis [17].

Participant responses in this study revealed a potential logical interrelated self-management model based on function, breathing, psychological, and social management, which requires further detailed research (Figure 2). In order to support and facilitate effective self-management and behavioral change in patients with COPD, all 4 areas of this model need to be addressed when developing programmes.

Combining educational learning materials on the use of assistive breathing technologies with correct relaxation and breathing techniques appears crucial to the foundation of an effective breathing management behavioral change programme. Exercise is essential to patient rehabilitation and behavioral change and when constructing an exercise based behavioral change programme two key elements need to be incorporated. Firstly, an extensive educational and illustrative component is required to facilitate effective learning of required exercises. Secondly, a motivational component needs to be included based on learning via social contact with peers, family, and friends to encourage and support behavioral change, for example, face to face contact, e-mails, or phone call. Programmes that provide both elements for patients with COPD are very effective but limited [17].

Participants who reported guilt feelings were less inclined to seek support when needed. This may hamper effective rehabilitation and self-management and is an issue that needs to be addressed as part of the patient rehabilitation process as patients who do not seek adequate support due to a "guilt complex" may have their recovery stifled and experience decreased quality of life. Methods to overcome feelings of guilt should be incorporated in all behavioral change or psychoeducational self-management programmes as these feelings may prevent patients seeking support. This continued subtheme of social support avoidance due to feelings of guilt needs to be examined and treated within the wider COPD patient population.

The symbolism of oxygen use with loss of independence is a major worry for individuals with COPD. Addressing this with patients at an early stage in diagnosis is important as part of a lifestyle change process that facilitates successful self-management behaviors. Practical advice on issues like travelling long and short distances with portable oxygen can help patients adapt more easily to living with COPD. Any behavioral change program to improve breathing apparatus use needs to address individuals issues of using apparatus in public, teach appropriate breathing techniques to supplement apparatus use and breathing regulation, and also teach relaxation techniques to effectively regulate breathing techniques and apparatus use especially in stressful or panic situations.

When developing and recommending self-management programmes, financial costs also need to be taken into consideration as most patients will be on fixed income health benefits and/or pension supports which may not be sufficient to finance lifestyle/home modifications. Self-management programmes should include information on all potential financial and health assistance subsidies available.

Augmenting self-efficacy is important in determining which tasks an individual will perform or avoid based on level of knowledge. This process of knowledge empowerment has been seen to assist in developing patient self-efficacy to make relevant decisions in self-management [18]. Self-efficacy plays a major role in explaining health related behaviors [19] and thus it is essential that it is factored into any outputs from a self-management or behavioral change programme. Available studies show significant positive effects for self-efficacy and behavioral change following a structured educational programme [8, 20] with improved self-efficacy noted to improve and increase engagement with particular tasks [21]. A recent pilot RCT has demonstrated that compliance with behavior change programmes using technology was found to be high which resulted in increased benefits in terms of self-management [22].

Commonly adopted behavioral change models used in COPD self-management based programmes include the Transtheoretical Model (TTM) which concentrates on processes of change and support required to adopt a healthier lifestyle [23]. Other social cognition and health belief models used in the study of health related behaviors in COPD include the Theory of Planned Behavior; the Theory of Reasoned Action; the Health Belief Model, the Attitude-Social Influence-Efficacy Model [24] and the Self-Efficacy Model [25]. These models focus primarily on patient self-efficacy, giving the patient confidence to carry out a behavior necessary to reach a desired goal. Key to achieving self-efficacy is the modeling of patient beliefs and perceptions around their condition and potential recovery. The use of action research as a framework in this project demonstrates its feasibility and effectiveness in ensuring patient beliefs/perceptions form the basis for a technological approach to facilitate self-management in COPD.

The authors of this study recommend further investigation into relationships between perceived psychological self-management of those with COPD and the functional based selection, optimization, and compensation theory of successful ageing. In-depth knowledge of these processes with the COPD population may be of benefit when tailoring a self-management program to this group.

A key strength of this study is its demonstration in the feasibility and importance of codevelopment/design of technology based programmes for people with COPD, in order to ensure that content is relevant, easy to use, and needs based. This will improve compliance and ultimately increase behavioural change and self-management.

9. Limitations

Recruitment of participants was solely from COPD support groups. Individuals in these groups were more proactive in researching and promoting COPD knowledge, lifestyle changes, and societal awareness.

Acknowledgments

The authors wish to thank the following for their funding, support, and contribution: the TRIL Consortium (Technology Research for Independent Living), Intel Ireland Ltd., and COPD support groups in Bray and Sligo.

References

[1] World Health Report, World Health Organisation, Geneva, Switzerland, http://www.who.int/whr/2000/en/whr00_en.pdf.

[2] N. Henschke, R. W. Ostelo, M. W. van Tulder, and J. W. Vlaeyen, "Behavioural treatment for chronic low-back pain," *Cochrane Database of Systematic Reviews*, vol. 7, Article ID CD002014, 2010.

[3] K. Bartlett, P. Sheeran, and M. S. Hawley, "Effective behaviour change techniques in smoking cessation interventions for people with chronic obstructive pulmonary disease: a meta-analysis," *British Journal of Health Psychology*, vol. 19, pp. 181–203, 2014.

[4] J. Moore, H. Fiddler, J. Seymour et al., "Effect of a home exercise video programme in patients with chronic obstructive pulmonary disease," *Journal of Rehabilitation Medicine*, vol. 41, no. 3, pp. 195–200, 2009.

[5] Rose Biomedical, "Chronic obstructive pulmonary disease; NIH funded study identifies new tool to help individuals with COPD," Obesity, Fitness & Wellness Week, NewsRX, Atlanta, Ga, USA, 2004.

[6] F. Liu, F. Cai, Q. Tang et al., "Effects of an animated diagram and video-based online breathing program for dyspnea in patients with stable COPD," *Patient Prefer Adherence*, vol. 7, pp. 905–913, 2013.

[7] E. M. Rogers, *Diffusion of Innovations*, The Free Press, New York, NY, USA, 5th edition, 2003.

[8] Y. K. Scherer and L. E. Shmieder, "The effect of a pulmonary rehabilitation program on self-efficacy, perception of Dyspnea, and physical endurance," *Heart Lung*, vol. 26, pp. 15–22, 1997.

[9] G. Williamson, L. Bellman, and J. Webster, *Action Research in Nursing and Healthcare*, Sage, London, UK, 2012.

[10] S. M. Kolb, "Grounded theory and the constant comparative method: valid research strategies for educators," *Journal of Emerging Trends in Educational Research and Policy Studies (JETERAPS)*, vol. 3, pp. 83–86, 2012.

[11] R. M. Tappan, *Advanced Nursing Research; From Theory to Practice*, Jones and Bartlet Learning, Ontario, Canada, 2011.

[12] F. Gallefoss and P. S. Bakke, "Impact of patient education and self-management on morbidity in asthmatics and patients with chronic obstructive pulmonary disease," *Respiratory Medicine*, vol. 94, no. 3, pp. 279–287, 2000.

[13] T. Effing, E. M. Monninkhof, P. D. van der Valk et al., "Self-management education for patients with chronic obstructive pulmonary disease," *Cochrane Database of Systematic Reviews*, vol. 17, no. 4, Article ID CD002990, 2007.

[14] A. J. Krus, O. van Schayck, J. Veen, T. van der Malen, and N. H. Chavennes, "Successful patient self-management of COPD requires hands-on guidance," *The Lancet Respiratory Medicine*, vol. 1, pp. 670–672, 2013.

[15] National Institute for Health and Clinical Excellence (NICE), "Service user experience in adult mental health: improving the experience of care for people using adult: NHS mental health services NICE clinical guideline," no. 136, 2011, http://guidance.nice.org.uk/cg136.

[16] H. F. S. Kim, M. E. Kunik, V. A. Molinari et al., "Functional impairment in COPD patients: the impact of anxiety and depression," *Psychosomatics*, vol. 41, no. 6, pp. 465–471, 2000.

[17] B. Dinesen, L. Huniche, and E. Toft, "Attitudes of COPD Patients towards tele-rehabilitation: a cross-sector case study," *International Journal of Environmental Research and Public Health*, vol. 10, pp. 6184–6198, 2013.

[18] T. Bodenheimer, E. H. Wagner, and K. Grumbach, "Improving primary care for patients with chronic illness: the chronic care model—part 2," *Journal of the American Medical Association*, vol. 288, no. 15, pp. 1909–1914, 2002.

[19] R. M. Kaplan, A. L. Ries, L. M. Prewitt, and E. Eakin, "Self-efficacy expectations predict survival for patients with chronic obstructive pulmonary disease," *Health Psychology*, vol. 13, no. 4, pp. 366–368, 1994.

[20] M. K. Kaşikçi, "Using self-efficacy theory to educate a patient with chronic obstructive pulmonary disease: a case study of 1-year follow-up," *International Journal of Nursing Practice*, vol. 17, no. 1, pp. 1–8, 2011.

[21] A. Bandura, "The self system in reciprocal determinism," *The American Psychologist*, vol. 33, no. 4, pp. 344–358, 1978.

[22] M. Tabak, M. Vollenbroek-Hutten, P. van der Valk, J. van der Palen, and H. Hermens, "Telerehabilitation intervention for patients with chronic obstructive pulmonary disease: a randomized controlled pilot trial," *Clinical Rehabilitation*, 2013, http://cre.sagepub.com/content/early/2013/11/27/0269215513512495.

[23] J. O. Prochaska, C. A. Reeding, and K. E. Evers, "The transtheorectical model and stages of change," in *Health Behaviour and Health Education: Theory, Research and Practice*, K. Glanz and B. K. Rimer, Eds., Jossey-Bass, San Francisco, Calif, USA, 3rd edition, 2002.

[24] J. Brug and P. van Assema, "Beliefs about fat," in *Food, People and Society*, L. J. Frewer, E. Risvik, and H. Schifferstein, Eds., pp. 39–54, Springer, Berlin, Germany, 2001.

[25] I. Mesters, T. L. Creer, and F. Gerards, "Self-management and respiratory disorders: guiding patients from health and self-management perspectives," in *Respiratory Disorders and Behavioural Medicine*, A. A. Kaptein and L. Creer, Eds., pp. 139–174, Martin Dunitz Ltd., London, UK, 2002.

Web-Based Depression Screening and Psychiatric Consultation for College Students

Aya Williams,[1] Rachel LaRocca,[1] Trina Chang,[1] Nhi-Ha Trinh,[1] Maurizio Fava,[1] Joseph Kvedar,[2] and Albert Yeung[1]

[1] *Massachusetts General Hospital Depression Clinical and Research Program, One Bowdoin Square 6th floor, Boston, MA 02114, USA*
[2] *Massachusetts General Hospital Center for Connected Health, 25 New Chardon Street, Suite 300, Boston, MA 02114, USA*

Correspondence should be addressed to Albert Yeung; ayeung@partners.org

Academic Editor: Trevor Russell

Background. A steady rise in the prevalence of depression among college students has negatively affected student quality of life. This study investigates the feasibility and acceptability of a Web-based model, including Skype, to screen and provide psychiatric consultation to depressed college students. *Methods.* Students completed the 9-item Patient Health Questionnaire (PHQ-9) online; those who screened positive (PHQ-9 $\geq$ 10) or endorsed any level of suicidal ideation were offered Web-based psychiatric consultation using Skype. After the consultation, students filled out a 7-item satisfaction questionnaire to report on the acceptability of this Web-based method. *Results.* A total of 972 students consented to the online depression screening and 285 screened positive. Of those, 69 students consented and 17 students successfully completed the psychiatric consultation via Skype. Thirteen (76.4%) students found the interview useful in helping them understand their depression. Fifteen (88.2%) students thought that psychologists and psychiatrists could successfully see patients via videoconferencing. *Conclusions.* Current online technologies can provide depression screening and psychiatric consultation to college students; those who participated reported a positive experience. Future studies will need to address the low levels of participation among college students and attract students who are underserved, as well as use a videoconferencing platform that adequately protects data confidentiality.

1. Introduction

Major depressive disorder (MDD) is a highly prevalent illness affecting 2% to 3% of men and 5% to 9% of women in the United States at any particular point in time, with a lifetime risk of 5% to 12% in men and 10% to 25% in women [1]. A steady rise in the prevalence of depression among college students [2, 3] has negatively affected students' quality of life. According to the 2007 national survey across 39 university campuses, 43.2% of students reported "feeling so depressed it was difficult to function" and 10.3% admitted to "seriously considering attempting suicide" in the past year [4]. MDD among college students is associated with diminished academic performance [5, 6], increased alcohol consumption [7], increased maladaptive eating [8], compromised physical health [9], and increased suicidal ideation [10]. A depression diagnosis made during college is associated with twice the increased risk of discontinuation of the student's college career [11]. A systematic review of depression prevalence studies in university students suggests that these figures may underestimate the actual prevalence [12]. Thus, identification and management of depression in university settings are necessary.

Several studies have used Web-based surveys of depression and anxiety [13] to screen successfully for mood problems among college students [10, 14, 15]. However, online screening alone does not connect students with necessary resources for treatment. Up to 85% of students with positive screens for mental disorders do not receive any treatment from professionals [16]. Reasons include lack of problem recognition and need, delayed time to appointment, lack of time, financial constraints, and privacy concerns [14]. There is a need to address these barriers that exist between receiving a positive screen result and accessing professional treatment.

Kim et al. [13] argue that screening must be integrated with accessing professional services, so when a mental health need is identified via screening, a student can act on the need in the same session. Hass et al. [17] suggested that clinician-student dialogue and personalized assessment, unlike computer-generated feedback, could identify and help students resolve their resistance to treatment. Mailey et al. [18] similarly emphasized the need for a more interactive model of Internet interventions with live clinician instead of text-heavy communications to keep students socially engaged. A review of technology-assisted self-help and minimal contact therapies confirmed that therapist-assisted treatments remain optimal in the treatment of clinical depression [19].

Given these findings, researchers and clinicians have turned to videoconferencing, which allows real-time interaction between the student and the clinician while obviating the cost of logistical barriers such as transportation and the potential stigma surrounding visiting an on-campus mental health clinic. The clinician can gauge the student's appearance, including the choice of clothing and attire, facial expression, and bodily movement and use these visual cues to inform clinical diagnosis and treatment recommendations [20]. Many online counseling services have recently emerged [21–23]. Yet there are few studies assessing the effectiveness and safety of such therapies for mental health in the university setting [24]. Khasanshina et al. [25] developed a model of psychiatric services that connected students experiencing high distress with clinicians via videoconferencing. The model successfully supplemented mental health care for college students in the rural university setting, although the services could be delivered only at a clinic connected by a virtual private network.

Studies have examined the feasibility and acceptability of Skype to deliver psychotherapy to clinical populations, with positive results [26–28]. In a study measuring the feasibility and efficacy of exposure therapy for social anxiety disorder using Skype, 83% of the therapists rated delivering treatment through Skype as fairly or very feasible, and 95% of the patients reported that receiving treatment through Skype was fairly or very easy [26]. Two studies investigating the efficacy of cognitive behavioral therapy [27] and problem-solving therapy [28] through Skype for patients with depression demonstrated clinically significant improvement in depressive symptoms. Technical difficulties, such as sound quality (e.g., choppiness, softness, echoing, and delay) and video quality (e.g., blurriness, frozen picture, and delay), still remained in these studies. Skype was run on desktop computers or laptops from home or primary care offices. Moreover, telephone screening or in-person setup of the technology occurred prior to the initiation of Skype psychotherapy.

This study investigated the feasibility and acceptability of a Web-based model that reached out to college students for online depression screening immediately followed by scheduling of an online psychiatric consultation if the student screened positive. The entire procedure from recruitment to consultation was carried out online, with no in-person screening or setup. The consultations were offered by licensed off-campus psychiatrists using Skype, a free videoconferencing software. The study replicated a real-world setting in which students used their own portable laptops with built-in webcams over wireless networks on campus. The quality of consultations was measured using a self-rated satisfaction questionnaire. We hypothesized that this Web-based model to enhance recognition and treatment of depressed college students is both feasible and acceptable.

2. Materials and Methods

2.1. Screening and Recruitment. Undergraduate and graduate students currently enrolled in universities in Massachusetts were recruited to participate in the Web-based screening survey for depression between December 2010 and December 2011 through Facebook (http://www.facebook.com/), Craigslist (http://craigslist.org/), and paper and electronic school flyers. Approximately 1,500 flyers were placed in student resident mailboxes at one local university in Boston. Students who participated in the study were entered in a raffle and had a 1 in 15 chance of winning a $20 gift card. All subjects provided informed, voluntary, written consent. The study and the use of Skype for a clinical consultation were approved by the Institutional Review Board.

The screening survey collected information on student demographics, including sex, year in college, and past and current history of depression and treatment, as well as the 9-item Patient Health Questionnaire (PHQ-9) for depression screening. A student was considered screen-positive for MDD if he or she scored 10 or above on the PHQ-9 or scored 1 or above on the PHQ-9 suicide item (question 9). If a student indicated any suicidality, the survey prompted the student to visit the nearest emergency room or call 911 before proceeding in the survey. If a student scored less than 10 on the PHQ-9 and did not endorse suicidality on the PHQ-9, he or she was identified as screening negative for MDD.

All students who completed the depression screening questionnaire received a direct link to an online depression toolkit at the conclusion of the survey regardless of their PHQ-9 score. The toolkit included links to two websites providing psychoeducational materials on depression, as well as information on a local suicide prevention helpline.

Participants who screened positive for MDD or suicidality were given an additional opportunity to schedule a Skype consultation with one of three research psychiatrists using "Doodle Meet Me" (http://www.doodle.com/about/meetMe.html), which showed clinicians' schedule availability in the following two weeks. To increase transparency, the final survey page included an explanation of the Skype consultation, as well as a direct hyperlink to the principal investigator's biography that provided detailed information of the clinician the students would speak with.

2.2. Web-Based Consultation. Measures were taken in this study to meet the Practice Guidelines for Video-Based Online Mental Health Services [29] of the American Telemedicine Association. Students provided a second informed, voluntary, written consent when scheduling the Web-based consultation. Prior to the videoconferencing session, a clinical research staff member verified the contact information of the student including a nonidentifying username, e-mail address, and phone number. The research staff member subsequently completed an online trial conversation with the student to test the connectivity and the functionality of the clinic's videoconferencing system. The online consultants are licensed psychiatrists who are experts in depression. The senior author (Albert Yeung) was responsible for most of the consultations. He has extensive experience in Skype-based clinical interviews and has performed more than 100 online consultations.

At the beginning of the one-hour Web-based consultation using Skype, the clinicians introduced themselves and identified the names of the students by asking them to present their school student identification card with a photo and the location of the student. Clinicians completed the sessions from their outpatient clinic offices and students were on their respective university campuses. The clinicians ensured that the participant was in a private room where the clinical discussion would not be easily overheard by others. The student used his or her own personal computer and webcam.

The consultation used a standardized clinical review of the history of present illness (including psychiatric, medical, psychosocial, and family history) and the mental status exam to generate the psychiatric diagnoses according to the Diagnostic and Statistical Manual of Mental Disorders (DSM-IV-TR), followed by a discussion of available options for treatment. In addition, the clinician solicited the student's feedback on the use of online screening and the consultation service. The details of the clinical interview were recorded and securely stored. At the conclusion of the consultation, clinicians sent a consultation report to the students' care providers if students signed a statement to release their medical information and made referrals as necessary.

All students who completed the one-hour Web-based consultation received a Skype satisfaction questionnaire within a week to inquire about the sound and visual of the Web-based interview, its helpfulness in understanding depression and starting treatment, and their opinions about the use of Web-based videoconferencing for mental health services.

Eight weeks after the completion of the initial survey, students who consented to be recontacted were e-mailed follow-up surveys, which included a second PHQ-9 questionnaire, questions about the use of online resources provided, any treatment sought by the student after the completion of initial survey, reasons for not seeking treatment, and obstacles to seeking treatment for depression. Again, students who responded were entered into a raffle with a 1 in 15 chance of winning a $20 gift card.

2.3. Instruments for Online Depression Screening. The 9-item Patient Health Questionnaire is a self-administered instrument that can be used to screen for patients with MDD in primary care settings. Each item in the questionnaire corresponds to one of the nine criteria upon which the DSM-IV-TR major depressive diagnosis is based. In a validation study of the PHQ-9, Kroenke and colleagues [30] showed that the instrument had a sensitivity of 88% and specificity of 88% for identifying MDD when using a total score of 10 or above as the threshold.

2.4. Software for Online Videoconferencing. Skype is a voice-over-Internet protocol service and software application that allows users to communicate by voice, video, and instant messaging over the Internet. Skype counts more than 300 million registered users [31] and is currently the most used desktop videoconferencing application [32]. The application can be downloaded free of charge on multiple platforms, including personal computers, tablets, and smart phones. Skype employs peer-to-peer communications, which means that computers exchange messages directly, without going through a third party server [33]. The students were asked to create a new Skype username that did not include identifying information such as birthday or name. The clinician also used the general clinic Skype account. Skype meets Advanced Encryption Standards, which meets the Federal Information Processing Standards for electronic transmission under HIPAA [34, 35].

3. Results

A total of 972 students consented to participate in this study. The majority of the respondents were female (71%) and Caucasian (67%). Freshmen (25%) and sophomores (24%) each made up a quarter of the total respondents, followed by juniors (17%) and seniors (17%) (Table 1). The screening survey was largely successful; approximately 10% of the students did not fully complete the assessment. Of the 861 students who completed the survey, 262 students (30.4%) screened positive for MDD based on a PHQ-9 score of 10 or above, and 151 students (17.5%) endorsed suicidal ideation on item number 9 of the PHQ-9.

Among those ($n = 285$) who screened positive for depression or had a positive response to the suicidality item of PHQ-9, 69 (24%) consented to participate in the Web-based psychiatric consultation and 17 (6% of eligible participants) successfully scheduled and completed the Skype consultation (Figure 1). The majority of students reported that the sound (87.5%) and video (81.3%) quality of the consultation were clear. Most students (81.3%) found the interview useful in understanding their depressive symptoms. Fewer students (18.8%) found the interview useful in starting treatment for depression. Overall, completers provided overwhelmingly positive feedback (93.8%) on the likelihood that psychologists and psychiatrists could successfully see patients via Web-based consultation service (Table 2).

Qualitative comments from the students also support the idea that Web-based consultation is an "effective" and "successful" alternative to an in-person clinic visit. One student commented, "It is relatively easy for me to go to a nearby hospital. But I know some of my friends who would have a much harder time doing that, so I would definitely recommend Skype as an appropriate substitute." Another student recommended the service especially for

Table 1: Demographics of college students who participated in online depression screening survey and Skype interview.

	Initial screening survey N (%)	Skype interview N (%)
Consented	972 (100)	17 (100)
Gender		
Male	220 (23)	3 (18)
Female	690 (71)	14 (82)
No response	62 (6)	0 (0)
Ethnicity		
Not Hispanic or Latino	775 (80)	14 (82)
Hispanic or Latino	77 (8)	3 (18)
Do not wish to provide an answer	9 (1)	0 (0)
Not known	111 (11)	0 (0)
Race		
Caucasian	652 (67)	13 (76)
Asian	84 (9)	3 (18)
Black	28 (3)	0 (0)
American Indian or Alaska native	4 (0)	0 (0)
Other	78 (8)	1 (6)
Do not wish to provide an answer	126 (13)	0 (0)
Year in college		
Freshman	242 (25)	7 (41)
Sophomore	230 (24)	4 (24)
Junior	161 (17)	4 (24)
Senior	163 (17)	0 (0)
5th year	43 (4)	1 (6)
Graduate student	41 (4)	0 (0)
Do not wish to provide an answer	92 (9)	1 (6)
Aware or previously diagnosed with depression		
No	456 (47)	1 (6)
Yes	306 (31)	12 (71)
Do not know	110 (11)	4 (24)
Do not wish to provide an answer	100 (10)	0 (0)
Previously received treatment for depression		
No	593 (61)	4 (24)
Yes	271 (28)	13 (76)
Do not know	9 (1)	0 (0)
Do not wish to provide an answer	99 (10)	0 (0)
If yes:		
Medication	56 (21)	2 (15)
Therapy	93 (34)	7 (54)
Both	115 (42)	4 (31)
Do not wish to provide an answer	7 (3)	0 (0)
Currently consider themselves suffering from depression		
No	472 (49)	1 (6)
Yes	171 (18)	8 (47)
Do not know	139 (14)	8 (47)
Do not wish to provide an answer	190 (20)	0 (0)
Currently receiving treatment for depression		
No	629 (65)	9 (53)
Yes	151 (16)	8 (47)
Do not know	4 (0)	0 (0)
Do not wish to provide an answer	188 (19)	0 (0)
If yes:		
Medication	55 (36)	3 (38)
Therapy	28 (19)	3 (38)
Both	61 (40)	2 (25)
Do not wish to provide an answer	7 (5)	0 (0)

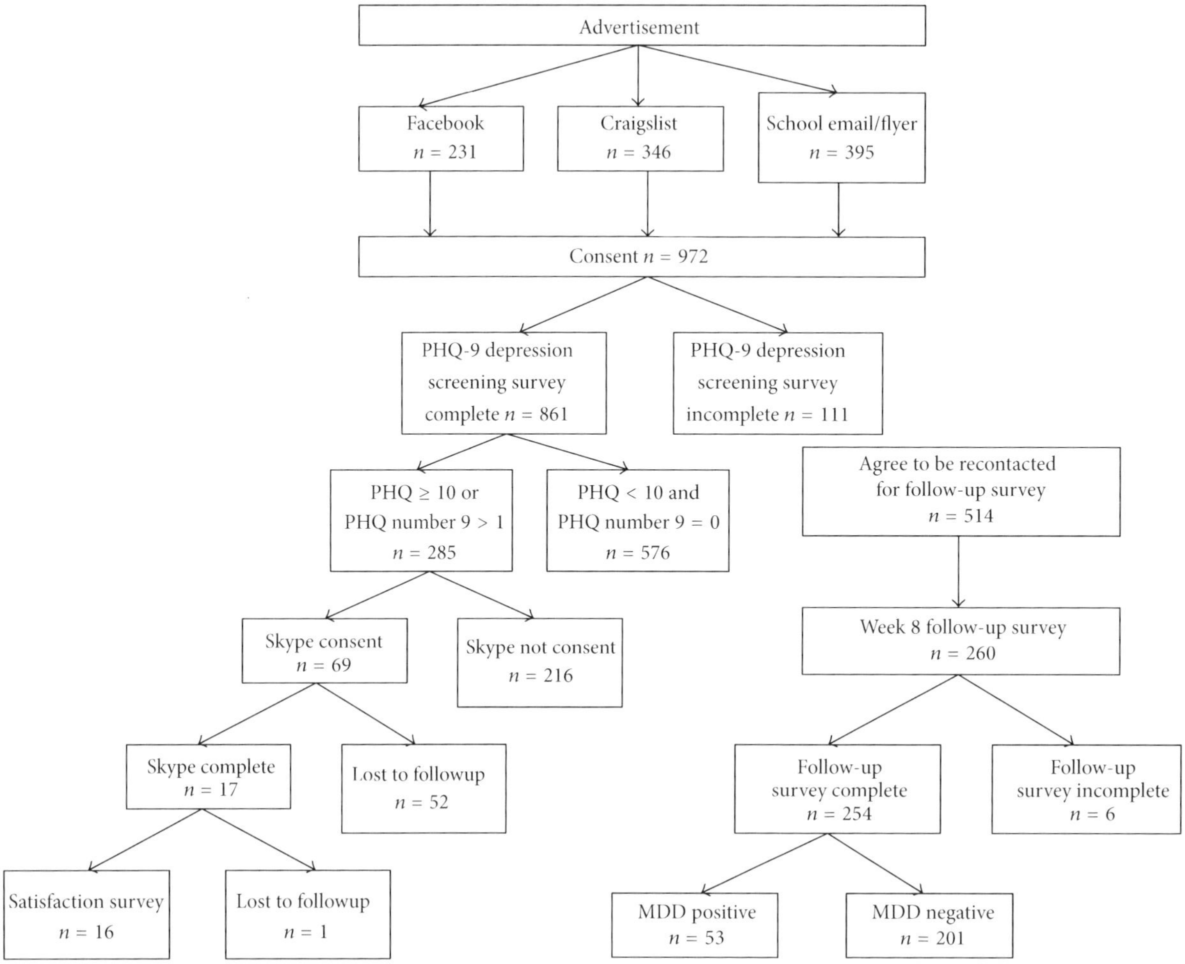

FIGURE 1: Subject participation and study flow.

those who "may not have the capability of leaving their houses." Students identified the benefit of being "able to connect with a doctor from my apartment where I was comfortable." One student commented that with the use of Web consultation, "I may have been able to start my treatment earlier." Students moreover noted the preference for visual cues, stating "body language and seeing someone interact in one-on-one situation is very important." With the use of the webcam from the students' computers, the consulting clinicians were not able to adjust webcams remotely during the interview. Yet, the consulting clinicians felt that this did not affect their ability to make psychiatric diagnosis and consult the students (personal communications with N.T., T.C., and A.Y.).

A total of 254 students completed the eight-week follow-up survey. According to the second PHQ-9, 53 students (20.9%) scored positive for depression. Forty-three students (16.9%) sought treatment for depression since completing the initial screening survey. Fifteen students (6%) used online resources including the depression toolkit. A total of 123 students (51.5%) indicated "too busy/I forgot" as the reason for not using online resources in the eight weeks following the screen. Thirty-three students (56.9%) indicated that they "did not experience any obstacles" when seeking depression treatment.

4. Discussion

This study shows that a comprehensive model of active outreach to college students via online screening, followed by student-initiated online scheduling and a psychiatric consultation using Skype, may be a feasible and acceptable model to improve the recognition and treatment of college students with depression.

This study demonstrates the safety and technical capability for students to use their personal computers and webcams to complete an online depression screening and psychiatric consultation. The use of the Web-based technology eliminated geographical barriers and saved transportation time as well as cost for such screening and consultations. This is of particular importance to college students who have limited time due to numerous academic and social commitments. Moreover, the symptoms of depression can inhibit patients from making the effort to visit a clinic in person. This service offered the option of consulting a professional from the comforts of their own dormitory rooms. A major advantage of the

Table 2: Descriptive statistics of Skype satisfaction survey.

	N (%)
Completed	16 (100)
Number 1: audio quality: was the sound clear?	
Clear	14 (87.5)
No opinion	2 (12.5)
Unclear	0 (0)
Number 2: visual quality: was the image clear?	
Clear	13 (81.3)
No opinion	2 (12.5)
Unclear	1 (6.3)
Number 3: was the interview useful in helping you understand your depression?	
Useful	13 (81.3)
No opinion	1 (6.3)
Not useful	2 (12.5)
Number 4: was the interview useful in helping you start treatment for your depression?	
Useful	3 (18.8)
No opinion	9 (56.3)
Not useful	4 (25.0)
Number 5: have you received treatment for depression within two months after the interview?	
Yes	7 (43.8)
No	9 (56.3)
If yes: (n = 7)	
Medication	
Therapy	3 (42.9)
Both	4 (57.1)
Number 6: do you think psychologists and/or psychiatrists can successfully see patients via Skype video-conferencing?	
Likely	15 (93.8)
No opinion	0 (0)
Unlikely	1 (6.3)
Number 7: if you were to see a psychiatrist or psychologist, would you prefer to be interviewed face to face or through videoconferencing?	
Face to face	12 (75.0)
Videoconferencing	1 (6.3)
No preference	3 (18.8)

videoconferencing therapy is that it allows for the exchange of visual and nonverbal communications between patients and therapists, unlike telephone or Web-based treatments [26]. These students' qualitative responses supported the use of videoconferencing over audioconferencing, which allowed visual cues such as eye contact, facial expressions, and body language.

Out of the 285 students who screened positive for depression or suicidality symptoms, 69 (24%) showed initial interest in a Skype interview. This finding is consistent with previous studies that found that many college students with significant depressive symptoms do not pursue professional help [36]. It is possible that some of the students who screened positive for depression were "false positives." They could be experiencing stress-related symptoms during an intense academic semester but not actually have a depressive disorder. However, it is also possible that students may feel comfortable filling out an anonymous survey but still hesitate to discuss their symptoms with a live clinician over a virtual medium. This is a public health challenge that may be related to the stigma regarding psychiatric illnesses [37], the lack of insight into the need for help [38], or concerns about potential administrative sanctions, such as mandatory leave or dismissal from school [17].

These concerns may be alleviated by adding a brief personalized psychoeducation component at the end of the screening material, as well as by providing more information on the content of the psychiatric consultation. An explanation of student's PHQ-9 depression score addressing which specific depressive symptoms the student might be experiencing and their short and long-term negative effects on their life may emphasize the need for professional intervention. A psychiatric consultation with a clinician will offer a more thorough evaluation of this score. The specific details of this consultation, such as what topics are discussed and what treatment options might be available following the session, also might reduce fears about seeing a psychiatrist for the first time. It should be made clear that confidentiality is protected. Informing potential participants of the high acceptability ratings among peers who have received such a consultation may make the service more approachable.

The low rate (25%) of completion of the consultation among interested subjects (17 out of 69 subjects) may be due to the limitation of time and the lack of mental health priority in that limited time. In the eight-week follow-up survey, 123 students (51.4%) indicated "Too busy/I forgot" as the reason for not using online mental health resources. Moreover, 33 students (56.9%) indicated that they "did not experience any obstacles" when seeking treatment for depression. Internal barriers may be playing as important of a role as external barriers to treatment. Yorgason et al. [39] also list the top reason for not using mental health services among college students as their lack of time. Although students were able to immediately schedule their consultation appointments, some students requested appointments one to two weeks after the screening visit, and many were unable to keep them. One session that encompasses both screen and consultation may be advisable [13]. This Web-based model could allow universities to employ outside providers for Web-based consultations or use current providers to practice from off-campus. By increasing clinician time, the service may be made more available during the times when students do not have classes or extracurricular commitments, such as in the early evening.

A more active outreach in the mediating step between the screen and online consultation may increase priority and flexibility of appointment times. In this study, while students were able to schedule an online consultation appointment immediately following the screen, this was a one-time opportunity.

Sending automated follow-up e-mails with a link to the online schedule service might increase participation by providing second and third opportunities. This also allows flexibility for college students with changing schedules to move their initial appointment as necessary. It is also possible to allow students to respond to this e-mail or Skype chat with clinical staff to address questions and concerns about the consultation. However, the focus of such a conversation would be to facilitate and encourage the online consultation rather than to address any psychiatric concerns.

Another concern could be raised by the modest number of participants (18.8%) who found the consultation useful for starting depression treatment. About half of the students were already mental health consumers and thus did not need a consultation with a specialist to help them start the treatment for depression. On the other hand, a week may not have been enough time to seek treatment after the consultation. Nonetheless, future studies should be restricted to students who are not receiving any active treatment to focus on depressed college students who are undertreated. A more direct communication between the psychiatrists and the university mental health clinic may be helpful. In this study, the psychiatrist offered consultation report for outside providers. With more concerted efforts between the on-campus clinic and outside providers, the Web-based psychiatric consultation could serve as a gateway to distinguish those students who need further treatment and motivate students' help seeking behavior by sending the report directly to an on-campus clinician.

The 47% of students currently receiving psychiatric treatment who sought this online consultation might suggest a self-selection bias. The experience of previously or currently seeing a clinician in person might have lowered barriers to seek help via online psychiatric consultation. As mentioned earlier, there may be stigma or fear of seeing a mental health clinician for the first time even through a virtual medium. There is a need to make transparent what occurs during the consultation and what options might be available following the session. While currently receiving psychiatric treatment, students screened positive for depression and sought an online consultation. This might indicate the usefulness of this model not only to recognize depression but also to augment an ongoing in-person treatment for students. Overall, the high acceptability rating (93.8%) among those who are currently receiving other psychiatric treatment as well as those who are not indicates the acceptability of this online consultation model.

Finally, there are advantages and disadvantages to using Skype as the platform for an online psychiatric consultation. The advantages of using the software include familiarity and ease of access from computers and multiple types of mobile applications for free [35]. Within the U.S., there are 47 million individuals who already use Skype [31] and do not need to sign up for a new service to speak with mental health professionals. More than half of the users are between the ages of 18–35 [31], which makes this software appropriate for a younger population, such as college students. The disadvantages of Skype involve its security concerns and HIPAA compliance. Skype utilizes 256-bit encryption, which meets the Advanced Encryption Standard specified by the U.S. National Institute of Standard of Technology [34]. Skype operates behind a firewall that can help protect it from unauthorized access [40]. Several experts have noted that it is harder to hack into Skype than into most telephone lines or brick and mortar offices with file cabinets; hacking into Skype requires high expertise and skills [35]. However, there is an ongoing debate as to whether Skype satisfies the HIPPAA Conduit Exception or not [35]. Critics of Skype indicate that Skype does not state on its website that it is HIPAA-compliant and does not offer Business Associate contracts to therapists or clinics that use it for telemental health purposes [35]. Future telepsychiatric consultations should monitor if Skype will address these concerns or should consider using a platform that has demonstrated HIPAA compliance.

5. Conclusions

In summary, we achieved some success using a comprehensive Internet-based screening and consultation model to increase recognition and treatment of depressed college students. High acceptability among completers demonstrates that the use of students' personal laptops, built-in webcams, and Skype is a potentially viable model to bring mental health services to college students. The students' qualitative comments suggest the importance of a real-time interaction with a clinician. The low participation rate among eligible students in this study suggests the need for more psychoeducation increase awareness of depression and the benefits of obtaining treatment for depression, as well as a flexible schedule that can adapt to the needs of busy college students. In addition, we recommend that all measures meet the American Telemedicine Association guidelines and that a videoconferencing platform that protects personal confidentiality be used.

This model is valuable for colleges with limited mental health resources on-campus and in their localities, as clinicians who are based at distant sites can now provide their services via Web-based videoconferencing. While we provided a one-time Web-based consultation in this current study, the model could be further developed to provide long-term symptom monitoring and to deliver continued treatment for students with MDD. Future studies on a larger scale and randomized controls are needed to demonstrate this model's efficacy, effectiveness, cost, and potential for expansion to other populations. With rapid increase in the use of webcam-equipped laptops, tablets, and smart phones among both patients and clinicians, this Web-based service may eventually benefit underserved individuals in university settings and beyond.

Acknowledgment

The authors thank university student mental health groups in local Boston area for helping with recruitment of subjects for the study.

References

[1] R. C. Kessler, P. Berglund, O. Demler et al., "The epidemiology of major depressive disorder: results from the national comorbidity survey replication (NCS-R)," *Journal of the American Medical Association*, vol. 289, no. 23, pp. 3095–3105, 2003.

[2] A. A. Ceyhan, E. Ceyhan, and Y. Kurtyilmaz, "Investigation of university students' depression," *Egitim Arastirmalari-Eurasian Journal of Educational Research*, vol. 36, pp. 75–90, 2009.

[3] J. M. Twenge, B. Gentile, C. N. DeWall, D. Ma, K. Lacefield, and D. R. Schurtz, "Birth cohort increases in psychopathology among young Americans, 1938–2007: a cross-temporal meta-analysis of the MMPI," *Clinical Psychology Review*, vol. 30, no. 2, pp. 145–154, 2010.

[4] E. J. Miller and H. Chung, "A literature review of studies of depression and treatment outcomes among U.S. College students since 1990," *Psychiatric Services*, vol. 60, no. 9, pp. 1257–1260, 2009.

[5] E. Heiligenstein, G. Guenther, K. Hsu, and K. Herman, "Depression and academic impairment in college students," *Journal of American College Health*, vol. 45, no. 2, pp. 59–64, 1996.

[6] A. Hysenbegasi, S. L. Hass, and C. R. Rowland, "The impact of depression on the academic productivity of university students," *Journal of Mental Health Policy and Economics*, vol. 8, no. 3, pp. 145–151, 2005.

[7] V. V. Grant, S. H. Stewart, and C. D. Mohr, "Coping-anxiety and coping-depression motives predict different daily mood-drinking relationships," *Psychology of Addictive Behaviors*, vol. 23, no. 2, pp. 226–237, 2009.

[8] W. E. Hawkins, R. J. McDermott, J. Seeley, and M. J. Hawkins, "Depression and maladaptive eating practices in college students," *Women and Health*, vol. 18, no. 2, pp. 55–67, 1992.

[9] H. E. Rawson, K. Bloomer, and A. Kendall, "Stress, anxiety, depression, and physical illness in college students," *The Journal of Genetic Psychology; Child Behavior, Animal Behavior, and Comparative Psychology*, vol. 155, no. 3, pp. 321–330, 1994.

[10] S. J. Garlow, J. Rosenberg, J. D. Moore et al., "Depression, desperation, and suicidal ideation in college students: results from the American Foundation of Suicide Prevention College Screening at Emory University," *Depression and Anxiety*, vol. 25, no. 6, pp. 482–488, 2008.

[11] A. C. Arria, K. M. Caldeira, K. B. Vincent, B. A. Winick, R. A. Baron, and K. E. O. 'Grady, "Discontinuous college enrollment: associations with substance use and mental health," *Psychiatric Services*, vol. 2, no. 64, pp. 165–172, 2013.

[12] A. K. Ibrahim, S. J. Kelly, C. E. Adams, and C. Glazebrook, "A systematic review of studies of depression prevalence in university students," *Journal of Psychiatric Research*, vol. 47, no. 3, pp. 391–400, 2013.

[13] E.-H. Kim, A. Coumar, W. B. Lober, and Y. Kim, "Addressing mental health epidemic among university students via web-based, self-screening, and referral system: a preliminary study," *IEEE Transactions on Information Technology in Biomedicine*, vol. 15, no. 2, pp. 301–307, 2011.

[14] D. Eisenberg, E. Golberstein, and S. E. Gollust, "Help-seeking and access to mental health care in a university student population," *Medical Care*, vol. 45, no. 7, pp. 594–601, 2007.

[15] S. J. Youn, N. Trinh, I. Shyu et al., "Using online social media, Facebook, in screening for major depressive disorder among college students," *Journal of Clinical and Health Psychology*, vol. 14, pp. 74–80, 2013.

[16] S. J. Garlow, J. Rosenberg, J. D. Moore et al., "Depression, desperation, and suicidal ideation in college students: results from the American Foundation for Suicide Prevention College Screening Project at Emory University," *Depression and Anxiety*, vol. 25, no. 6, pp. 482–488, 2008.

[17] A. Haas, B. Koestner, J. Rosenberg et al., "An interactive web-based method of outreach to college students at risk for suicide," *Journal of American College Health*, vol. 57, no. 1, pp. 15–22, 2008.

[18] E. L. Mailey, T. R. Wójcicki, R. W. Motl et al., "Internet-delivered physical activity intervention for college students with mental health disorders: a randomized pilot trial," *Psychology, Health and Medicine*, vol. 15, no. 6, pp. 646–659, 2010.

[19] M. G. Newman, L. E. Szkodny, S. J. Llera, and A. Przeworski, "A review of technology-assisted self-help and minimal contact therapies for anxiety and depression: is human contact necessary for therapeutic efficacy?" *Clinical Psychology Review*, vol. 31, no. 1, pp. 89–103, 2011.

[20] P. Cukor, L. Baer, B. S. Willis et al., "Use of videophones and low-cost standard telephone lines to provide a social presence in telepsychiatry," *Telemedicine Journal*, vol. 4, no. 4, pp. 313–321, 1998.

[21] H. Christensen, K. M. Griffiths, and A. Korten, "Web-based cognitive behavior therapy: analysis of site usage and changes in depression and anxiety scores," *Journal of Medical Internet Research*, vol. 4, no. 1, pp. 29–40, 2002.

[22] K. C. Cukrowicz and T. E. Joiner Jr., "Computer-based intervention for anxious and depressive symptoms in a non-clinical population," *Cognitive Therapy and Research*, vol. 31, no. 5, pp. 677–693, 2007.

[23] N. G. Choi, M. T. Hegel, M. L. Marinucci, L. Sirrianni, and M. L. Bruce, "Association between participant-identified problems and depression severity in problem-solving therapy for low-income homebound older adults," *International Journal of Geriatric Psychiatry*, vol. 27, no. 5, pp. 491–499, 2012.

[24] L. Farrer, A. Gulliver, J. K. Chan et al., "Technology-based interventions for mental health in tertiary students: systematic review," *Journal of Medical Internet Research*, vol. 15, no. 5, article e101, 2013.

[25] E. V. Khasanshina, W. L. Wolfe, E. N. Emerson, and M. E. Stachura, "Counseling center-based tele-mental health for students at a rural university," *Telemedicine and e-Health*, vol. 14, no. 1, pp. 35–41, 2008.

[26] E. K. Yuen, J. D. Herbert, E. M. Forman et al., "Acceptance based behavior therapy for social anxiety disorder through videoconferencing," *Journal of Anxiety Disorders*, vol. 27, pp. 389–397, 2013.

[27] K. L. Lichstein, F. Scoggins, S. J. Thomas et al., "Telehealth CBT for co-occurring insomnia and depressive symptoms in older adults," *Journal of Clinical Psychology*, vol. 69, pp. 1056–1065, 2013.

[28] N. G. Choi, M. T. Hegel, C. N. Marti et al., "Telehealth problem solving therapy for low-income homebound older adults," *American Journal of Geriatric Psychiatry*, 2013.

[29] American Telemedicine Association, "Practice Guidelines for Video-Based Online Mental Health Services," Washington,

DC, USA, 2013, http://www.americantelemed.org/docs/default-source/standards/practice-guidelines-for-video-based-online-mental-health-services.pdf?sfvrsn=6.

[30] K. S. Kroenke, R. L. Spitzer, and J. B. W. Williams, "The PHQ-9: validity of a brief depression severity measure," *Journal of General Internal Medicine*, vol. 16, no. 9, pp. 606–613, 2001.

[31] Skype, "Skype Audiencae Stats-Microsoft Advertising," 2013, http://advertising.microsoft.com/uk/WWDocs/User/display/cl/brand_subproperty/1589/global/Skype-Audience-Stats.pdf.

[32] L. De Cicco and S. Mascolo, "A mathematical model of the skype VoIP congestion control algorithm," *IEEE Transactions on Automatic Control*, vol. 55, no. 3, pp. 790–795, 2010.

[33] SANS Institute, "Skype: A Practical Security Analysis," 2008, http://www.sans.org/reading-room/whitepapers/voip/skype-pratical-security-analysis_32918.

[34] Skype, "Skype Security," 2013, http://www.skype.com/en/security/#encryption.

[35] Zur Institute, "Utilizing Skype to Provide TeleMental Health, E-Counseling, or E-Therapy: Reviewing the debate on Skype & HIPAA Compliance," http://www.zurinstitute.com/skype_telehealth.html.

[36] D. Eisenberg, J. Hunt, N. Speer, and K. Zivin, "Mental health service utilization among college students in the United States," *Journal of Nervous and Mental Disease*, vol. 199, no. 5, pp. 301–308, 2011.

[37] E. E. Golberstein, D. Eisenberg, and S. E. Gollust, "Perceived stigma and help-seeking behavior: longitudinal evidence from the healthy minds study," *Psychiatric Services*, vol. 60, no. 9, pp. 1254–1256, 2009.

[38] K. E. Zivin, D. Eisenberg, S. E. Gollust, and E. Golberstein, "Persistence of mental health problems and needs in a college student population," *Journal of Affective Disorders*, vol. 117, no. 3, pp. 180–185, 2009.

[39] J. B. Yorgason, D. Linville, and B. Zitzman, "Mental health among college students: do those who need services know about and use them?" *Journal of American College Health*, vol. 57, no. 2, pp. 173–181, 2008.

[40] University of Texas at Austin, "ISO Consensus Paper: Skype," 2009, http://security.utexas.edu/consensus/skype.html.

5

An Android-Based Heart Monitoring System for the Elderly and for Patients with Heart Disease

Paola Pierleoni, Luca Pernini, Alberto Belli, and Lorenzo Palma

Dipartimento di Ingegneria dell'Informazione, Universitá Politecnica delle Marche, Via Brecce Bianche, 60131 Ancona, Italy

Correspondence should be addressed to Luca Pernini; l.pernini@univpm.it

Academic Editor: Jocelyne Fayn

The current trend in health monitoring systems is to move from the hospital to portable personal devices. This work shows how consumer devices like heart rate monitors can be used not only for applications in sports, but also for medical research and diagnostic purposes. The goal pursued by our group was to develop a simple, accurate, and inexpensive system that would use a few pieces of data acquired by the heart rate monitor and process them on a smartphone to (i) provide detailed test reports about the user's health state; (ii) store report records; (iii) generate emergency calls or SMSs; and (iv) connect to a remote telemedicine portal to relay the data to an online database. The system developed by our team uses sophisticated algorithms to detect stress states, detect and classify arrhythmia events, and calculate energy consumption. It is suitable for use by elderly subjects and by patients with heart disease (e.g., those recovering from myocardial infarction) or neurological conditions such as Parkinson's disease. Easy, immediate, and economical remote health control can therefore be achieved without the need for expensive hospital equipment, using only portable consumer devices.

1. Introduction

Recent technological advances in electronic and biomedical engineering are making it possible to move health monitoring away from the hospital and the clinic to portable personal devices [1]. Smartphones and biometric sensors are now available to all. These devices, which are often used in sport-related applications, are gaining an important role in health research and monitoring, enabling fast measurement of health parameters, accurate diagnosis of a number of conditions, and a reduction in hospital admissions.

Monitoring of heart function, accurate diagnosis of cardiac conditions, and prevention of heart disease are important goals. The electrocardiogram (ECG) is the gold standard method to detect cardiovascular abnormalities. It is a noninvasive diagnostic technique that records the electrical activity of the heart and enables diagnosis of a number of abnormalities and conditions based on a few simple features. The system described herein does not use a multichannel electrocardiograph but a much less expensive heart rate (HR) monitor and provides three types of tests:

(i) stress test, based on HR variability (HRV) and instantaneous HR;

(ii) arrhythmia classification, based on R peak to R peak (RR) intervals;

(iii) energy consumption evaluation, based on resting HR and instantaneous HR.

HRV can be related to chronic and acute stress [2]. Reduced HRV has consistently been documented in patients with anxiety disorders and chronic or posttraumatic stress, irrespective of individual features [3], due to autonomic nervous system alterations. Several studies have demonstrated connections between a chronic stress state and the risk of cardiovascular disease (CVD) [4]. Fast and easy testing of the main parameters of heart activity is therefore quite useful in daily life. A real-time personal stress monitor can provide continuous information on the user's stress level at all times and in any place.

RR intervals are important measures in sinus rhythm classification and identification of arrhythmia episodes and allow detection of sinus arrhythmia, premature ventricular contraction, ventricular tachycardia, ventricular flutter or fibrillation, and second-degree atrioventricular block [5]. A portable system providing hourly testing of heart activity and detecting episodes of arrhythmia would be valuable for patients with CVD. Several techniques are capable of providing these results; some detect a single type of arrhythmia, whereas others detect multiple types. The former techniques include time-domain analysis, sequential hypothesis testing algorithm, threshold-crossing intervals, artificial neural networks, time-frequency analysis, fuzzy adaptive resonance theory mapping, and sequential detection algorithm; the latter approaches include multiway sequential hypothesis testing, wavelet analysis, artificial neural networks, complexity measure, multifractal analysis, wavelet analysis combined with radial basis function neural networks, and nonlinear dynamic modeling [5]. These methods rely on ECG signal analysis; however, the analysis is not always technically feasible due to signal noise and the high computational cost of real-time analysis. Moreover such systems detect only a small number of arrhythmia types. We describe a validated method that allows real-time classification of sinus rhythm type and detection and classification of different arrhythmia events by an approach based on RR intervals and instantaneous HR [5].

Instantaneous HR is an important index of recovery after myocardial infarction and of the effect of medication for a number of neurological diseases [6, 7]. It can also be used to estimate the calories burned by any type of activity. Currently, the most accurate methods for measuring energy expenditure are based on calorimeters and respirometers, but they are quite expensive and are not suitable for portable devices. The portability requirement is met by approaches based on the HR monitor and the accelerometer, which provide effective means to estimate individual's energy expenditure during a given activity. We describe a novel HR-based algorithm that despite being less accurate than the methods mentioned above is sufficient for the application, which provides only an index of an individual's level of activity.

A number of similar systems and applications have already been devised, but none integrates powerful algorithms that process HR and the tachogram into an easy-to-use application that provides clear and immediate test reports to the user and to medical personnel. Moreover most existing systems merely display the raw data acquired by one or more wearable sensors [8], whereas others use sensors in the smartphone to show the raw data [9].

Another remarkable and innovative feature of the device described herein is that, unlike existing systems, which contain a single type of signal processing algorithm, it provides three different tests [10], that is, stress test, real-time classification of sinus rhythm type, and detection and classification of different arrhythmia events. This feature allows documenting correlations between stressful situations and arrhythmia episodes and enables CVD patients, who are prescribed exercise, to measure real-time calorie consumption. The test reports can then be sent to and stored in an online database that can be searched by a physician.

This paper shows how data about an individual's health state can be collected by real-time sampling and analysis of a few parameters using noninvasive, inexpensive, and portable devices.

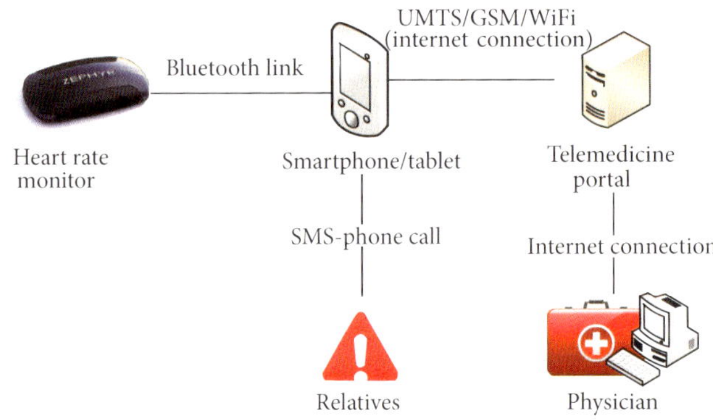

Figure 1: System architecture.

2. Materials and Methods

The HR monitor used in this work is a Zephyr HxM-BT device (Zephyr Technology Corporation) that was chosen for its modest cost, high usability, and good performances. An application for Android OS, which is widely applied in portable devices all over the world, was developed by our team. Its main tasks include data processing; reporting of test results to the user; test scheduling during the day; dialing of automatic emergency calls or sending an SMS in case of critical user conditions; and data storage in a telemedicine portal database (Figure 1). The application also provides the controls, settings, views, and Bluetooth connection management required for easy system use and clear test reporting.

2.1. Data Acquisition and Storage. A Bluetooth connection between a smartphone or a tablet and the HR monitor provides secure data acquisition. The HR monitor used in this work transmits data packets containing information acquired by biosensors at a frequency of 1 Hz [11]; a routine implemented in the Android application extracts from each packet the following information: instantaneous HR, last 15 heartbeat time stamps, and last heartbeat progressive number. Unless a test is in progress the smartphone display shows only the HR. The test results are then saved to an internal SQLite database and may be sent to an online MySql database via Wi-Fi or a 3G connection of the Android device using Json format and Php web pages.

2.2. Stress Test. HRV analysis in the time domain is based on the calculation of a number of statistical indices over an appropriate data acquisition window [12]. A first key feature that needs to be calculated is the standard deviation of the RR interval (SDNN): this is the square root of variance and is related to all the cyclical components connected to the variability detected during the observation period. It is important to note that HRV variance depends on the length of the observation period; measurement repeatability and comparability require this period to be established in advance

Table 1: Thresholds for detection of stress state.

Variable	Threshold	Unit
HR_{AVG}	>85	Beats/min
pNN50	<7	%
SDNN	<55	ms
rMSSD	<45	ms

Table 2: Thresholds for supraventricular sinus rhythm classification.

Sinus rhythm type	HR (bpm)
Bradycardia	HR < 60
Normal	60 ≤ HR ≥ 100
Tachycardia	HR > 100

[13]. A standard duration (e.g., 5 minutes) therefore needs to be set. The next feature to be extracted is the square root of the mean squared differences of successive RR intervals (rMSSD). The last collected feature is the proportion that is obtained by dividing the number of interval differences of successive RR intervals greater than 50 milliseconds (ms) by the total number of RR intervals, in the observation window (pNN50). These data and the average HR (HR_{AVG}) are the key stress test parameters and are based on a decision threshold for each feature.

Since in the case of stress testing the analysis requires the heartbeat time stamps, the algorithm stores these values: a number of R peak time stamps are extracted from each packet depending on the heartbeats that have been detected after the latest packet has been received. This control is enabled by checking the heartbeat number extracted from each packet. Then the RR intervals are calculated in real time from the time stamps and stored.

At the beginning of the algorithm (Figure 2), there are $i = 0$ packet received and $n = 0$ heartbeats detected. After the arrival of the ith packet, the first control is whether the index is <2. If this is true the system must wait for the next packet before processing the data; if it is false the control is on the heartbeat number (HBN). If the difference from last HBN to previous HBN is 0, no new heartbeats have been detected and the algorithm waits for the next packet. If the difference is 1, 2, 3, or 4, new heartbeats have been detected and the relevant RR intervals are calculated and stored. The limit is 4 heartbeats because the maximum HR measurable by the HR monitor is 240 beats/minute or 4/second. The next control involves index i which is compared with the predetermined duration of the analysis. In fact, this index is also used as the timer of the algorithm in relation to the frequency of 1 packet received/second. If the index is less than the duration of the observation window the system waits for the next data packet before repeating the steps; otherwise, it calculates all the statistical features and compares them with the threshold, to determine whether a stress state is present. The decision is reached by majority vote: if three of the four values exceed (HR_{AVG}) or are lower than (other features) the thresholds (Table 1) [14], the stress state is considered to be present [15].

It is important to note that SDNN is calculated at 5-minute intervals regardless of the duration of the analysis and then averaged over that duration, because this parameter changes with the length of the interval and because the relevant threshold is referred to as a 5-minute window [13]. The evolution of the tachogram is plotted on the phone display and the test results are finally shown and stored in a local database. The application also allows alerting a distant person (e.g., a relative) by dialing an emergency call with a prerecorded message or sending an SMS to a favorite number if a stress state is detected. The test results can also be stored in the patient's account in a telemedicine database. The real-time stress analysis algorithm, which includes the formulas and the HRV thresholds mentioned above, has been wholly developed by our research team.

2.3. Detection of Episodes of Arrhythmia. Arrhythmia may occur in a healthy heart with minimal consequences. It may present as respiratory sinus arrhythmia, a natural periodic variation in HR, or it may be an index of a severe heart condition [16]. An automatic device providing real-time arrhythmia detection and rhythm classification therefore has the potential to be highly useful in the daily monitoring of patients with heart conditions.

The method described herein provides sinus rhythm type classification and detection and classification of different arrhythmia events using an approach based on RR intervals and instantaneous HR [5]. It is based on three algorithms running in parallel.

2.3.1. Sinus Rhythm Classification. The most immediate analysis provided by the system is classification of the supraventricular rhythm as normal, bradycardia, or tachycardia.

The algorithm calculates the HR_{AVG} during the observation window (Figure 3), with the user at rest. It extracts the instantaneous HR of each packet and adds up to a total value HR_{TOT}. The HR_{AVG} is then obtained by dividing the HR_{TOT} by the duration of the observation window, that is, the total number of packets received, and is compared with two thresholds: the rhythm is classified as bradycardia if HR_{AVG} is <60 beats per minute (bpm), normal if is comprised between 60 and 100 bpm, and tachycardia if is >100 bpm (Table 2) [17].

2.3.2. Sinus Arrhythmia Detection. Sinus arrhythmia is also detected by our system. It is a common supraventricular rhythm and is related to breathing: HR increases during inspiration (Bainbridge reflex) and decreases during expiration (vagal effect). It affects especially young people, where it is not considered pathological.

Our algorithm uses RR intervals (Figure 4): since each packet contains $k < 4$ new beats, the relative RR intervals are calculated and compared with the actual RR_{MAX} and RR_{MIN} values and if necessary replaced with them. When the total number of packets received matches the predetermined observation window, the difference between the longest and the shortest RR intervals is calculated to check if it is >0.16 seconds (s) [18]. If this is true, sinus arrhythmia is considered to be present and a report is generated on the phone display.

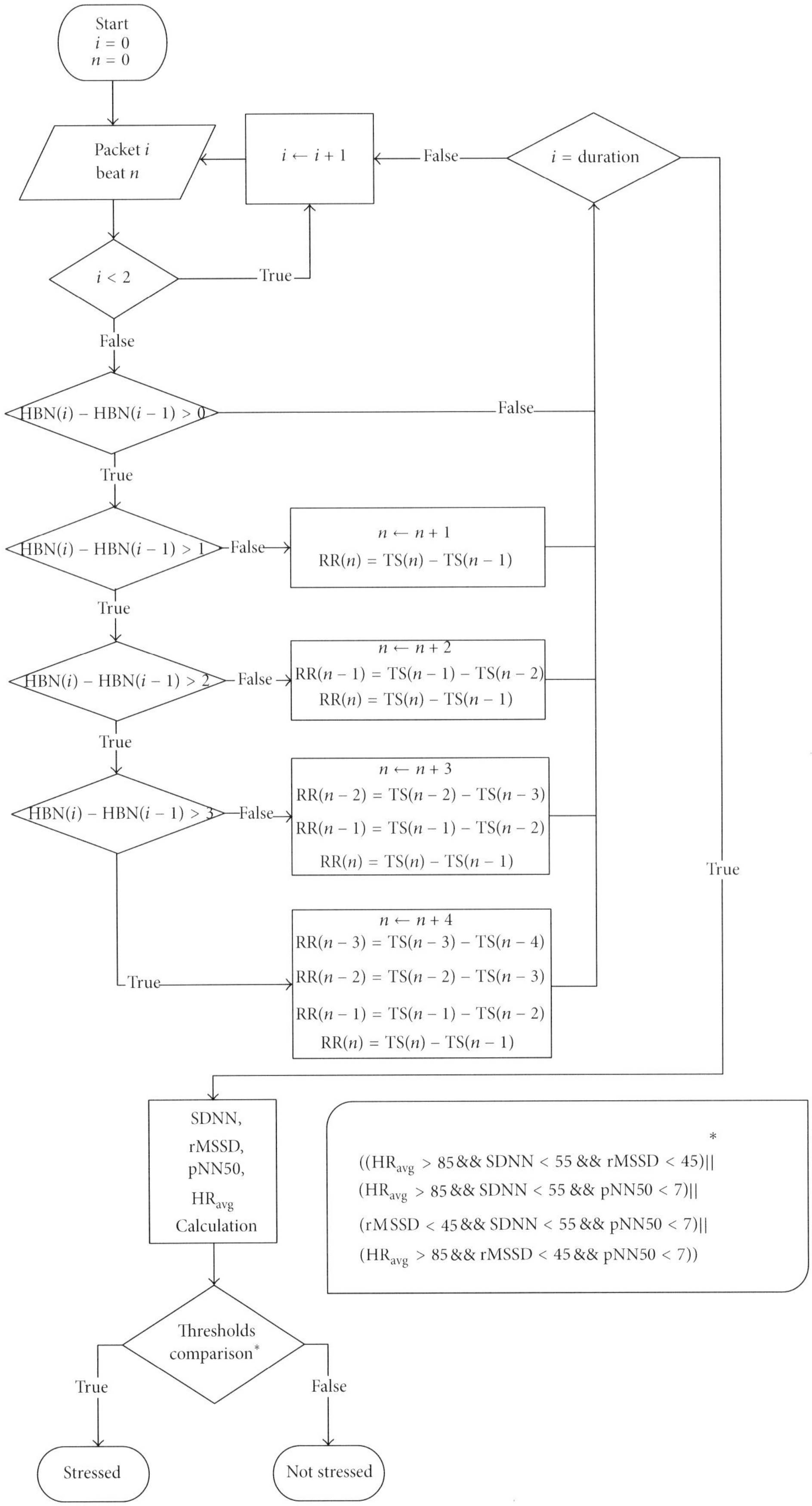

FIGURE 2: Stress test algorithm block diagram.

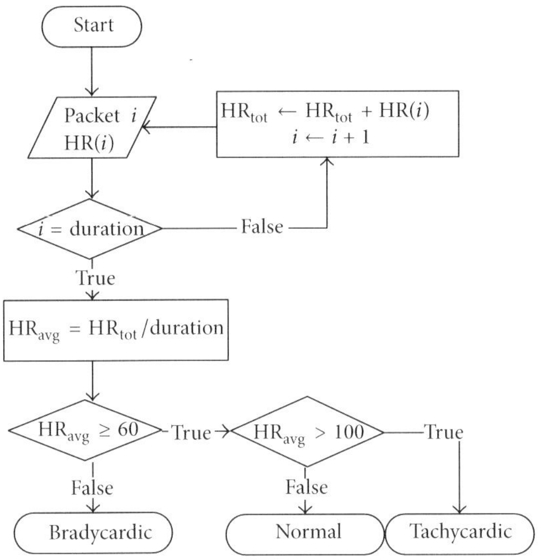

FIGURE 3: Sinus rhythm classification block diagram.

The sinus rhythm classification and sinus arrhythmia detection algorithms have been wholly developed by our team for real-time use.

2.3.3. Detection of Other Arrhythmia Types. Other types of arrhythmia can be detected and classified using a more complex algorithm. The method implemented in our device involves two steps: arrhythmia beat classification and arrhythmia episode classification. The episodes that can be classified include ventricular premature systole, ventricular bigeminy, ventricular trigeminy, ventricular couplet, ventricular tachycardia, ventricular flutter/fibrillation, and 2nd degree heart block.

This algorithm also uses RR intervals. It is based on the algorithm described by Tsipouras et al. [5]; we improved it adding real-time implementation. The first step is beat classification (Figure 5). This preliminary task is based on a 3-RR interval window (RR_1, RR_2, and RR_3) that slides one beat at a time, where the RR interval to be classified is the middle one. This beat is initially considered as normal and may subsequently be assigned to another category based on three rules related to medical-clinical data. There are four categories: (1) normal sinus beat (N); (2) premature ventricular contraction (PVC); (3) ventricular flutter/fibrillation (VF); and (4) 2nd degree heart block (BII). These acronyms are used in the MIT-BIH database. The three rules are as follows.

Rule 1. VF: it is activated if $RR_1 > 1.8RR_2$ and if the duration of RR_2 is less than 0.6 s. In this case RR_2 is considered as the beginning of a VF episode and subsequent windows are tested for the following two conditions:

(i) Condition 1.1: the duration of each RR-interval in the window is <0.7 s;

(ii) Condition 1.2: the overall duration of the $RR_1 + RR_2 + RR_3$ window is <1.7 s;

If one of the two conditions is met the middle RR interval is classified as category (3). The rule is based on classification of the whole VF episode, not a single beat, and is applied to m consecutive windows. A VF episode will be detected only if the m index of windows containing beats classified as category (3) is ≥4. The algorithm continues with the next rule, coming back to the $i - m$ window if neither condition is true for at least 4 consecutive windows or if Rule 1 is not verified.

Rule 2. PVC, category (2): this state is present if one of the following conditions is true:

(i) Condition 2.1: if $RR_1 > 1.15RR_2$ and $RR_3 > 1.15RR_2$, the RR_2 interval is classified as an isolated PVC;

(ii) Condition 2.2: if $|RR_1 - RR_2| < 0.3$ s and both RR_1 and RR_2 are <0.8 s and $1.2(RR_1 + RR_2)/2 < RR_3$, then we have a PVC couplet;

(iii) Condition 2.3: if $|RR_2 - RR_3| < 0.3$ s and both RR_1 and RR_2 are less than 0.8 s and $1.2(RR_2 + RR_3)/2 < RR_1$, then we have a PVC couplet.

Rule 3. BII, category (4): if conditions 3.1 and 3.2 are both true, the RR_2 interval is assigned to this category:

(i) Condition 3.1: 2.2 s $< RR_2 <$ 3.0 s;

(ii) Condition 3.2: $|RR_1 - RR_2| < 0.2$ s or $|RR_2 - RR_3| <$ 0.2 s.

The algorithm is repeated for all subsequent windows. The rules are mutually exclusive and must be applied in the reported sequence. After a beat has been classified by one rule its classification cannot be changed by another.

The results of beat classification are used as input of the automaton (Figure 6) for detection and classification of the arrhythmia episode. The rhythm classification categories and relevant MIT-BIH symbols are normal sinus rhythm N, ventricular premature systole VPS, ventricular bigeminy B, ventricular trigeminy T, ventricular couplet C, ventricular tachycardia VT, ventricular flutter/fibrillation VFL, and 2nd degree heart block BII. The default rhythm is normal, unless an episode of one of the above rhythms is detected. Episodes start with a distinctive beat—for instance, a PVC beat is the first beat for B, T, and VT episodes; VF for VFL episodes; and BII for BII episodes—and are characterized by a specific sequence pattern; they then end with a nonspecific beat. B has a PVC-N-PVC-N-· · · -N-PVC pattern, T has a PVC-N-N-PVC-N-N-· · · -PVC-N-N-PVC pattern, the pattern of VC is PVC-PVC-not PVC, and the pattern of VT is PVC-PVC-PVC-· · · -VC structure (≥3 consecutive PVCs). A major challenge to be met by the automaton is discrimination among these arrhythmia types, due to the similarity of the initial phase of each episode. VF episodes start with a VF beat and the number of consecutive VF beats determines its duration. The same applies to BII episodes. The states of the automaton are as follows.

(i) State 1: start of the automaton: the automaton remains in this state as long as the input is an N beat. It moves to states 2, 7, or 8 if a PVC, a VF, or a BII beat occurs, respectively.

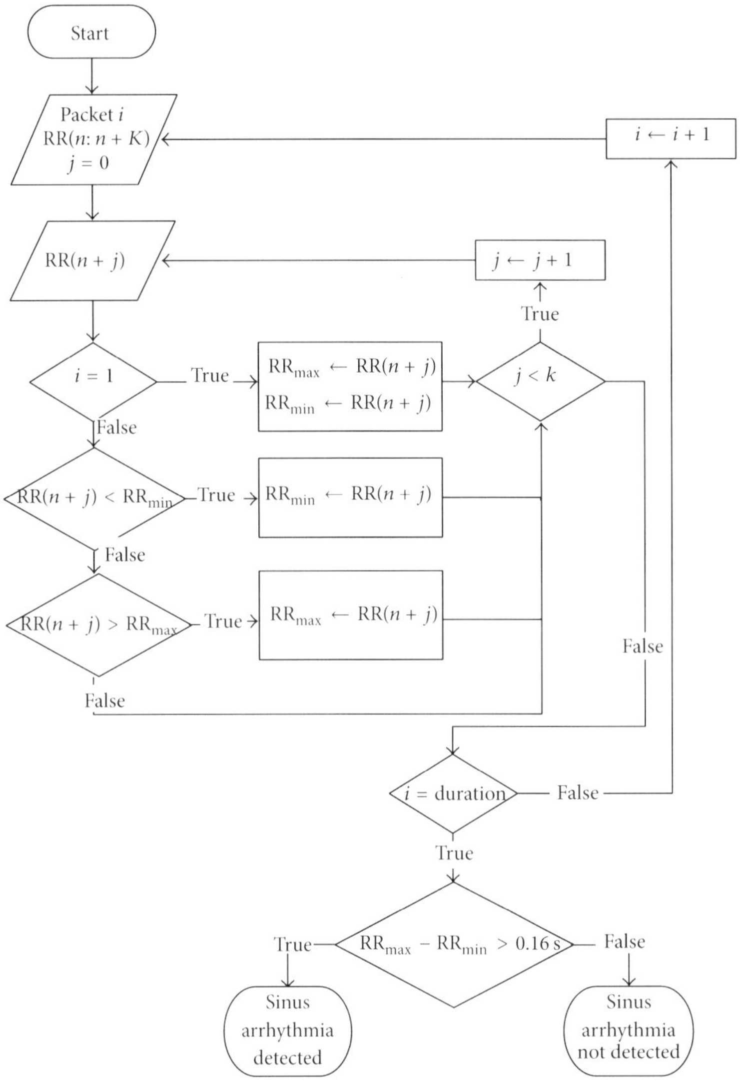

FIGURE 4: Sinus arrhythmia detection block diagram.

(ii) State 2: possible B, T, and C and single VPS or VT: the automaton goes to state 3 if the next beat is N; to state 5 if the next beat is a PVC; or to state 1 if the next beat is neither an N nor a PVC.

(iii) State 3: possible B and T and single VPS: if the next beat is a PVC and B is detected the automaton returns to state 1. If the next beat is N, it moves to state 4; if the beat is none of the above types, it moves to 1 and no episode is detected.

(iv) State 4: possible T and single VPS: if the next beat is a PVC, a T is detected, whereas if the beat is N, a single VPS is detected; otherwise, nothing is detected and the automaton returns to state 1.

(v) State 5: possible C and VT: if the next beat is not a PVC, C is detected and the automaton returns to state 1; if it is a PVC, the automaton moves to state 6.

(vi) State 6: VT is detected: if the beat is a PVC, the automaton remains in state 6 until the VT episode has ended. If the next beat is a VF or a BII, the automaton moves, respectively, to state 7 or 8; if it is different, it moves to state 1.

(vii) State 7: VFL is detected: if the next beat is a VF, the automaton remains in state 7 and the episode is considered to continue. In any other case the automaton returns to state 1.

(viii) State 8: BII is detected: if the next beat is a BII, the automaton remains in state 8 and the episode is considered to continue. In any other case the automaton returns to state 1.

The automaton returns to state 1, and the previous episode is considered as completed (and is reported by the system if it has reached the minimum required HBN); if an unexpected beat occurs, the new episode is ignored.

2.4. Evaluation of Energy Consumption. The approach described herein requires knowledge of the user's weight, height,

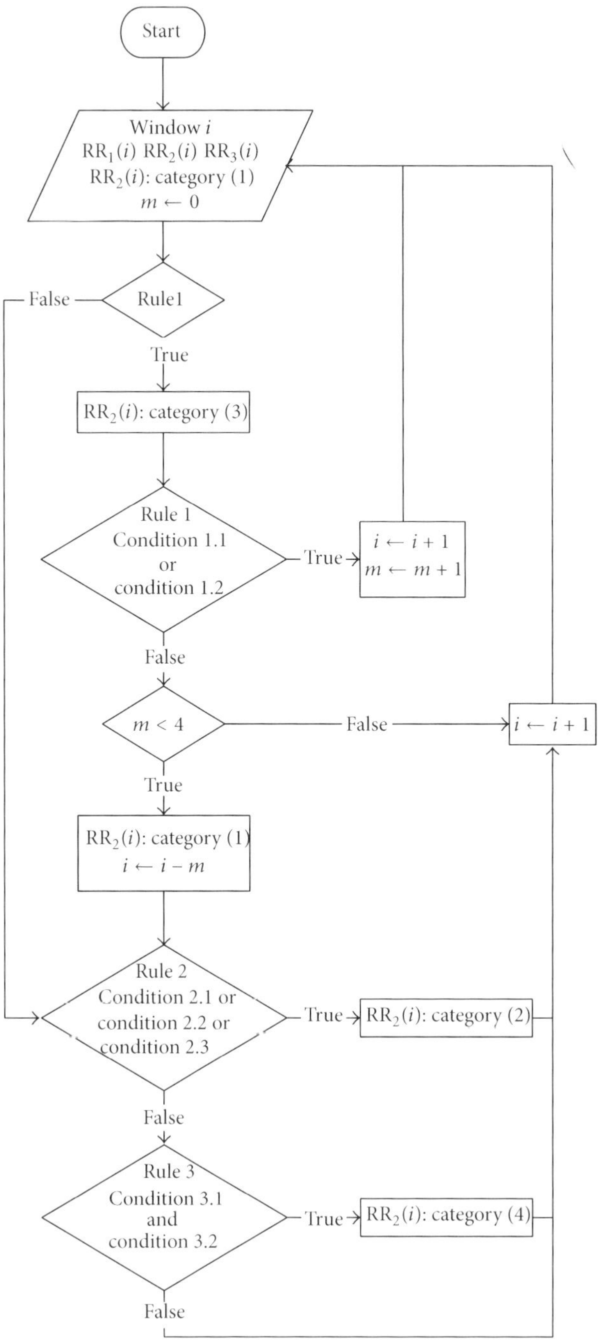

FIGURE 5: Arrhythmia beat classification block diagram.

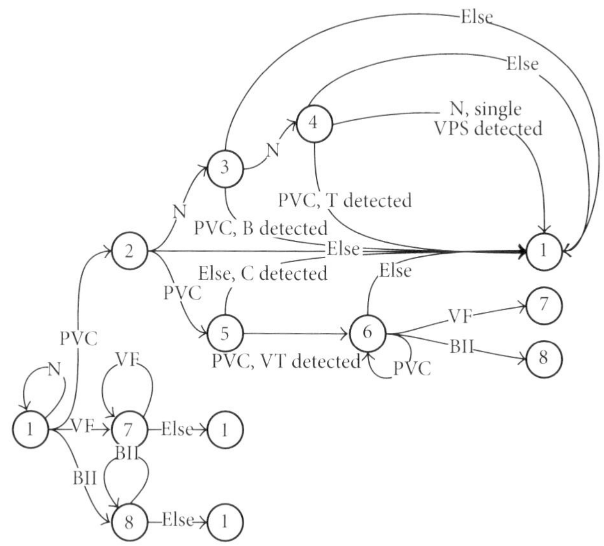

FIGURE 6: Arrhythmic episode classification by the automaton.

gender, age, and resting HR. Calorie consumption is then calculated by integrating the HR value over the observation period. The algorithm used in our application is evolution of the algorithm developed by Lee and coworkers [19] and exploits the computational abilities of current smartphones: HR is continuously monitored instead of being sampled at predetermined time points. Real-time analysis is the main improvement over the previous method. Notably, the new approach can be extended to any type of physical activity.

The method developed by Lee and coworkers requires entering resting HR, initial HR, final HR, and total duration of the analysis. This entails a number of limitations.

(i) The requirement of knowing total analysis duration and final HR precludes calculation in real time.

(ii) It assumes that the final HR is the peak value in the entire exercise; any pauses or final cooling down may thus affect the calculation.

The previous method [19] makes integration to calculate energy consumption: three types of instantaneous energy consumptions are computed by functions that are linearly dependent on HR and are subsequently integrated over the total duration of the analysis. The method involves three calculation steps:

(i) calorie consumption at rest over the entire activity;

(ii) calorie consumption after starting the exercise and up to the peak HR (10% of total duration);

(iii) calorie consumption during maximum sustained HR (90% of total duration).

Therefore, pauses or interruptions of any type are not accommodated.

The method developed by our team analyzes 10-second windows and involves two steps:

(i) calculation of calorie consumption at rest;

(ii) calculation of calorie consumption during exercise based on the mean HR sampled in the interval.

The two steps provide the final calorie consumption value, which is updated every 10 s by adding the two new values. The equation for estimating energy expenditure at rest (step (i)) is

$$K_{1_i}\,[\text{kcal}] = t\left[\left(\text{hr}_1 - \text{hr}_0 + 20.25\right) + C\right] \times \left(0.01808s + 0.00895\left(1 - s\right)\right), \tag{1}$$

where K_{1i} is the energy consumption of the ith interval in kilocalories, hr_0 is the HR at rest, hr_1 is the HR at the beginning of analysis, C is a coefficient of basal metabolic rate (per second in this case), s is a value depending of gender (1 for male, 0 for female), and t is the interval duration (in s).

The basal metabolic rate allows calculating energy expenditure based on user physical features [20]:

$$\begin{aligned} \text{bmr} &= (655 + 9.6w + 180h - 4.7a)(1 - s) \\ &\quad + (66 + 13.7w + 500h - 6.8a)s, \end{aligned} \tag{2}$$

where w is the user's weight (in kg), h is the height (in m), and a is the age (in years).

The equation calculating calorie consumption per second of exercise in steps (ii) and (iii) is

$$\begin{aligned} Y\left[\frac{\text{kcal}}{\text{s}}\right] &= \left[B_m(\text{hr}_x - \text{hr}_0) + C + 0.3645\right]s \\ &\quad + \left[B_f(\text{hr}_x - \text{hr}_0) + C + 0.1812\right](1 - s), \end{aligned} \tag{3}$$

where hr_x is the HR at the start or at the end of exercise, whereas B_m and B_f are

$$\begin{aligned} B_m &= \frac{0.0109\text{LBM}}{h^2} - 0.0023\%\text{FAT} - 0.0007a - 0.0211, \\ B_f &= \frac{0.014\text{LBM}}{h^2} - 0.0012\%\text{FAT} - 0.01254. \end{aligned} \tag{4}$$

LBM is lean body mass, equal to

$$\text{LBM} = w(1 - \%\text{FAT}). \tag{5}$$

%FAT is the percentage body fat [21]:

$$\%\text{FAT} = \frac{(1.2\text{BMI} + 0.23a - 10.8s - 5.4)}{100}. \tag{6}$$

BMI is the body mass index [22]:

$$\text{BMI} = \frac{w}{h^2}. \tag{7}$$

The calculation involved in step (iii) is as follows (step (ii) is not used in our method):

$$K_{3i} = (Y(\text{hr}_i) - Y(\text{hr}_s))t, \tag{8}$$

where hr_i is the mean HR value in the ith interval and t is interval duration. K_{3i} is also calculated for each interval.

Total K_1 and K_3 values are then added to obtain K_{tot}:

$$K_{\text{tot}} = \sum_{i=0}^{N}(K_{1i} + K_{3i}) \tag{9}$$

assuming N as the windows number.

Figure 7 shows the calculations described above. K_{tot} is the grey area and K_1 is the sum of K_{1i}.

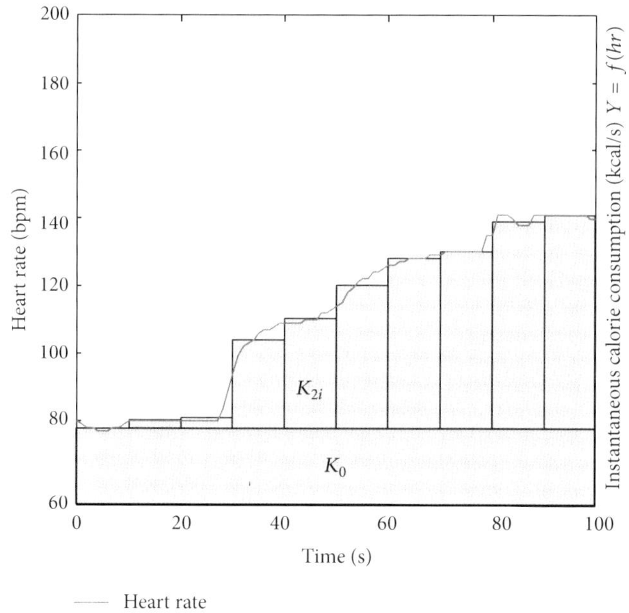

FIGURE 7: Calorie consumption calculation method.

2.5. Application Details. The other functionalities developed by our team include a Bluetooth connection, graphical interfaces, user settings, and alarm management.

The Bluetooth connection between smartphone and HR monitor is established using Android Bluetooth APIs and the Java library of the pulse sensor [23]. The only requirement for the connection is pairing the two devices via the Android settings menu. After selection of a user command that prompts the appearance of a connection button on the screen, the application searches for the device, which is listed in the bonded device list, and a Bluetooth socket is established. A connection thread listens for incoming packets and saves them in a buffer. Finally, the required information is extracted from the packets and sent to the class assigned to the processing using the *obtainMessage* method (Handler class).

The user can interact with the application through a main interface, a menu interface, and the settings interface (Figure 8). The main interface contains buttons for device connection and disconnection via Bluetooth and shows several items of information: the connection status, the battery status of the connected pulse sensor, the instantaneous HR, and the progress and results of current tests. It may also show the HR trend or the tachogram (RR interval trend); these charts are created using the *aChartEngine* library and implement zooming and scrolling functionalities.

The menu interface allows activating/disabling the different analysis algorithms, clearing the chart, accessing the settings menu, viewing data history, and quitting.

Using the Service class, a background part of the application reminds the user to perform any scheduled tests during the day.

The settings interface makes it possible to enter user features (age, weight, height, resting HR, and gender), set test duration, manage alert messages and calls (activation, phone

TABLE 3: Results of the stress test algorithm.

Condition	Number of subjects	PSS mean score	PSS variance
Not stressed	13	22.3	5.6
Stressed	7	27.6	4.7

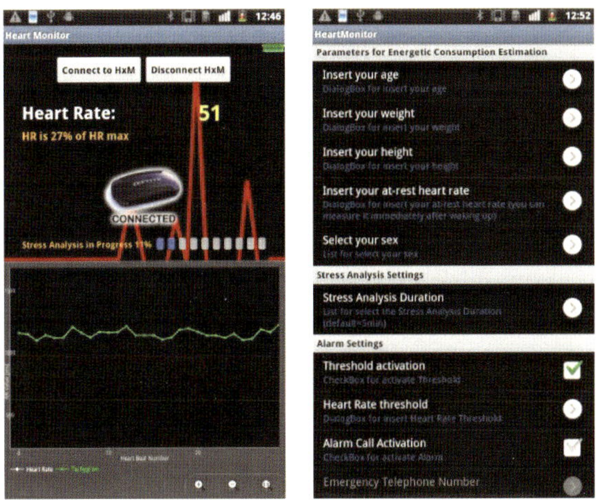

FIGURE 8: Application interfaces: main interface and settings interface.

number, and preconfigured text messages), and schedule tests.

Alerts are sent to a remote phone using *SmsManager* and *TelephonyManager*.

Finally HR, RR interval signals, and test reports can be saved to *.txt files and to a local SQLite database, ready to be sent in Json format to a telemedicine portal consisting of a MySql database and Php web pages.

3. Results and Discussion

3.1. Stress Test Results. The stress test was assessed in a trial involving 20 healthy individuals (6 female and 14 male university students aged 23–27 years without neurological disorders) who had abstained from coffee and alcoholic beverages for 12 hours. Participants underwent analysis by our application for 10 minutes and the test results were not shown. They subsequently completed the validated 10-item Perceived Stress Scale (PSS) questionnaire [24]. The test data and the results of the questionnaire are reported in Table 3, where subjects are divided into stressed and nonstressed based on test results and the mean PSS score is reported for the two groups. The same data are shown in Figure 9 in a traditional box-plot, where the dots are the median values and the squares the mean values.

The two datasets were assumed to have normal distribution. The resulting t value is 4.49, $P = 0.0003$ (Student's t-test). The mean PSS scores of the two groups were significantly different ($P < 0.01$).

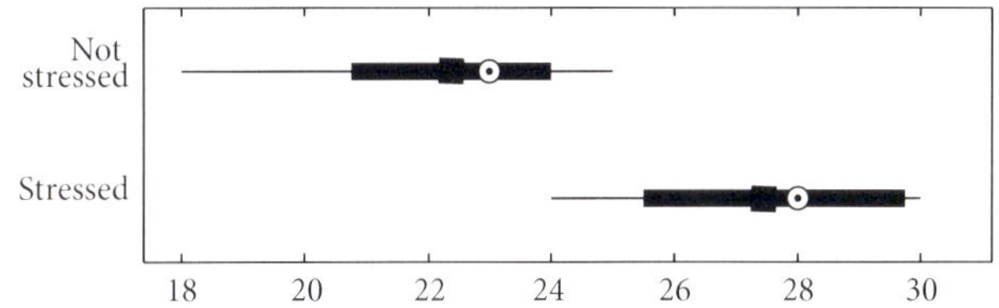

FIGURE 9: Statistical box-plot. x-axis: results of the PSS questionnaire; y-axis: participants divided by the algorithm into "stressed" and "nonstressed."

TABLE 4: Results of the sinus rhythm classification and the sinus arrhythmia detection algorithm.

Sinus rhythm	Number of subjects	Confirmed by ECG
Normal	18	100%
Bradycardic	5	100%
Tachycardic	2	100%
Arrhythmia	16	100%

3.2. Results of Arrhythmia Episode Detection. Sinus rhythm classification and sinus arrhythmia detection were tested in 25 healthy students aged 23–29 years. The experiment involved 10-minute parallel testing with our device and an ECG. The algorithm output simply described the subject's cardiac rhythm and whether he/she presented sinus arrhythmia. The ECG tracings were assessed by a cardiologist and compared to the test results reported by our application. The two sets of test reports matched, demonstrating that the algorithm is 100% accurate in sinus rhythm classification and sinus arrhythmia detection. As regards the sinus rhythm, 18 participants had a normal rhythm, 5 had a bradycardic rhythm, and 2 had a tachycardic rhythm. Moreover, 16/25 subjects presented sinus arrhythmia, which is common among the young. These data are reported in Table 4.

The detection and classification of arrhythmia events have previously been tested by Tsipouras and coworkers [5], who found very high sensitivity and specificity. We tested our real-time Java implementation by an offline simulation using as input the values available on the MIT-BIH database rather than the signal acquired from the heart monitor. We found 94% accuracy in detection and classification of arrhythmia episodes, the same result obtained by Tsipouras et al. [5].

3.3. Results of Energy Consumption Evaluation. The energy estimation algorithm described herein was compared with the method used by Garmin Ltd. This method was chosen as the reference because Garmin is widely considered a leader in its sector. In addition a large amount of data that can be used for comparisons is available on the Garmin Connect platform.

For this test we used offline implementation of our algorithm that simulates real-time device operation. The algorithm was applied to 10 different HR acquisitions relating to 10 subjects and three different types of activity (available on the Garmin Connect web platform). The results are shown in Table 5. The results obtained by our device are very close to

TABLE 5: Results of the energy expenditure algorithm.

Activity	Garmin method (kcal)	Our method (kcal)
Walking	745	610
Walking	430	382
Running	669	747
Running	545	515
Running	1222	1102
Running	930	766
Cycling	755	820
Cycling	2533	1968
Cycling	564	515
Cycling	532	537

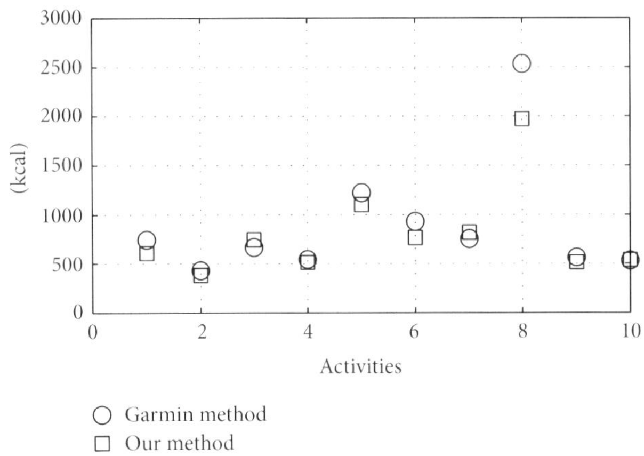

FIGURE 10: Comparison of calorie calculation data from the Garmin method and our algorithm.

those obtained by Garmin's method (Figure 10). The Pearson linear correlation coefficient between the two datasets is $r = 0.9865$. Since the test used merely indicative information about user activity levels, the results are quite acceptable.

3.4. Application Usability and Usefulness. The final feature that needed to be tested was user perception. To do this we administered to the 20 participants involved in stress test validation an additional questionnaire, the 10-item System Usability Scale (SUS) [25], which is a platform-independent model widely used in subjective software evaluation. The mean values, converted values, and standard deviation (Std) for each question as well as total SUS scores are reported in Table 6. The total per cent score is 75.625, which corresponds to a B grade and is therefore a good result [26]. The Std values are quite small, entailing narrow spread around the mean. In more general and objective terms, users and patients who have used the application during the test expressed their satisfaction in the use. Importantly, prolonged use of the application did not evidence bugs or unexpected system crashes.

TABLE 6: Results of the System Usability Scale (SUS) questionnaire.

Question	Mean value	SUS converted value	Std
Q1	3.75	2.75	0.79
Q2	2.2	2.8	0.95
Q3	4.2	3.2	0.7
Q4	1.75	3.25	0.79
Q5	3.35	2.35	0.81
Q6	1.95	3.05	0.89
Q7	4.6	3.6	0.6
Q8	2.3	2.7	0.66
Q9	4.05	3.05	0.83
Q10	1.5	3.5	0.6
Total score		% score	
30.25		75.625	

4. Conclusions

This paper describes a real-time heart monitoring system suitable for a variety of users including elderly individuals and patients with CVD. The system is based on a simple, inexpensive, and wearable device whose functionalities are comparable to those of more expensive and sophisticated clinical devices. The system's high-level performances are related to a set of complex algorithms that have been implemented in the Android device. The stress test, heart rhythm classification, and sinus rhythm detection algorithms have been developed entirely by our group, whereas the arrhythmia classification and detection algorithm and the algorithm evaluating energy expenditure employ known methods that were improved to suit the real-time and mobile conditions of the present application.

The stress test and the arrhythmia algorithms proved to be able to identify a stress state and episodes of arrhythmia. Clearly, the computer software cannot replace a physician, but it does provide information and alerts. The energy expenditure algorithm calculates calorie consumption in real time; it is based on an existing method that was improved by our team and extended to cover a number of general conditions (exercise with breaks, exercise with cooling down, and normal daily activities). These features make the device suitable for users who need to monitor calorie consumption during the day due to health reasons.

An additional novel feature of the device is that it integrates three different algorithms for HR and tachogram processing in a single mobile application that (i) provides remote monitoring of patients outside the hospital, (ii) is easy to use, and (iii) provides clear test reports to users and medical staff. All the data about the patient's health status can be stored in an online database.

The HRV and arrhythmia algorithms provide useful information about patients with a range of diseases. For example it has been reported that there may be a close association between reduced HRV and the severity of Parkinson's disease (PD) [27]. Indeed, PD affects the diurnal autonomic cardiovascular regulation, whose alteration seems to be more profound in patients with more severe disease. The result of these changes is a reduced HRV, but current knowledge of the long-term consequences of certain HR features and HRV, for example, circadian regulation, is limited. We are currently collecting heart activity data from PD patients at the Regional Hospital Department of Rehabilitation (Ancona, Italy) with a view both to validate our system and to test the hypothesis of a correlation between PD and abnormal HRV.

We are also testing the algorithms developed for our device and the scope for its application to a number of conditions and uses in view of its marketing in the near future.

Acknowledgment

The authors are grateful to Dr. S. Modena for the language revision (http://www.silviamodena.com/).

References

[1] M. Milošević, M. T. Shrove, and E. Jovanov, "Applications of smartphones for ubiquitous health monitoring and wellbeing management," *Journal of Information Technology and Applications*, vol. 1, no. 1, 2011.

[2] J. Kulmala and E. Hynynen, *Heart Rate Variability in Chronic and Acute Stress*, 2011.

[3] C. M. M. Licht, E. J. C. de Geus, F. G. Zitman, W. J. G. Hoogendijk, R. van Dyck, and B. W. J. H. Penninx, "Association between major depressive disorder and heart rate variability in the Netherlands study of depression and anxiety (NESDA)," *Archives of General Psychiatry*, vol. 65, no. 12, pp. 1358–1367, 2008.

[4] J. Macleod, G. D. Smith, P. Heslop, C. Metcalfe, D. Carroll, and C. Hart, "Psychological stress and cardiovascular disease empirical: demonstration of bias in a prospective observational study of Scottish men," *British Medical Journal*, vol. 324, no. 7348, pp. 1247–1251, 2002.

[5] M. G. Tsipouras, D. I. Fotiadis, and D. Sideris, "An arrhythmia classification system based on the RR-interval signal," *Artificial Intelligence in Medicine*, vol. 33, no. 3, pp. 237–250, 2005.

[6] R. Piotrowicz and J. Wolszakiewicz, "Cardiac rehabilitation following myocardial infarction," *Cardiology Journal*, vol. 15, no. 5, pp. 481–487, 2008.

[7] C. L. Comella, G. T. Stebbins, N. Brown-Toms, and C. G. Goetz, "Physical therapy and Parkinson's disease: a controlled clinical trial," *Neurology*, vol. 44, no. 3 I, pp. 376–378, 1994.

[8] A. Bourouis, M. Feham, and A. Bouchachia, "A new architecture of a ubiquitous health monitoring system," 2012.

[9] O. Postolache, P. S. Girão, M. Ribeiro et al., "Enabling telecare assessment with pervasive sensing and Android OS smartphone," in *Proceedings of the IEEE International Symposium on Medical Measurements and Applications (MeMeA '11)*, 293, p. 288, May 2011.

[10] S. Gradl, P. Kugler, C. Lohmuller, and B. Eskofier, "Real-time ecg monitoring and arrhythmia detection using android-based mobile devices," in *Proceedings of the IEEE Annual International Conference of the Engineering in Medicine and Biology Society (EMBC '12)*, pp. 2452–2455, 2012.

[11] ZephyrTechnologyCorporation, "Bluetooth hxm api guide," 2011.

[12] A. Camm, M. Malik, J. Bigger et al., "Heart rate variability: standards of measurement, physiological interpretation and clinical use. task force of the european society of cardiology and the north american society of pacing and electrophysiology," *Circulation*, vol. 93, no. 5, pp. 1043–1065, 1996.

[13] M. Malik, "Heart rate variability," *Annals of Noninvasive Electrocardiology*, vol. 1, no. 2, pp. 151–181, 1996.

[14] H. Yang, J. Lee, K. Lee et al., "Application for the wearable heart activity monitoring system: analysis of the autonomic function of HRV," in *Proceedings of the 30th Annual International Conference of the IEEE Engineering in Medicine and Biology Society (EMBS '08)*, pp. 1258–1261, August 2008.

[15] A. Andreoli, R. Gravina, R. Giannantonio, P. Pierleoni, and G. Fortino, "SPINE-HRV: a BSN-based toolkit for heart rate variability analysis in the time-domain," in *Wearable and Autonomous Biomedical Devices and Systems for Smart Environment*, vol. 75 of *Lecture Notes in Electrical Engineering*, pp. 369–389, Springer, Berlin, Germany, 2010.

[16] A. L. Goldberger, *Clinical Electrocardiography: A Simplified Approach*, Elsevier Health Sciences, 2012.

[17] R. A. O'Rourke, V. Fuster, and R. Alexander, *Hurst. Il Cuore, Il Manuale*, McGraw Hill, 2003.

[18] K. Najarian and R. Splinter, *Biomedical Signal and Image Processing*, Taylor & Francis, 2nd edition, 2012.

[19] M.-H. Lee, H.-K. Lee, K. Choi, S. Bang, J. Kim, and S. Kim, "Method of measuring calorie consumption for portable apparatus," in *Proceedings of the 27th Annual International Conference of the Engineering in Medicine and Biology Society (IEEE EMBS '05)*, pp. 5203–5206, Shanghai, China, January 2006.

[20] J. A. Harris and F. G. Benedict, "A biometric study of human basal metabolism," *Proceedings of the National Academy of Sciences of the United States of America*, vol. 4, no. 12, p. 370, 1918.

[21] S. H. Cohn, A. N. Vaswani, S. Yasumura, K. Yuen, and K. J. Ellis, "Improved models for determination of body fat by in vivo neutron activation," *The American Journal of Clinical Nutrition*, vol. 40, no. 2, pp. 255–259, 1984.

[22] World Health Organization, *BMI Classification 2010*, vol. 27, 2013, http://www.who.int/features/factfiles/obesity/facts/en/.

[23] Zephyr Technology Corporation, "Hxm bt android api user guide," 2011.

[24] S. Cohen, T. Kamarck, and R. Mermelstein, "A global measure of perceived stress," *Journal of Health and Social Behavior*, vol. 24, no. 4, pp. 385–396, 1983.

[25] J. Brooke, "Sus—a quick and dirty usability scale," *Usability Evaluation in Industry*, vol. 189, p. 194, 1996.

[26] A. Bangor, P. Kortum, and J. Miller, "Determining what individual sus scores mean: adding an adjective rating scale," *Journal of Usability Studies*, vol. 4, no. 3, pp. 114–123, 2009.

[27] N. Covassin, A. B. Neikrug, L. Liu et al., "Relationships between clinical characteristics and nocturnal cardiac autonomic activity in Parkinson's disease," *Autonomic Neuroscience*, 2012.

6

Attracting Child Psychiatrists to a Televideo Consultation Service: The TeleLink Experience

Tiziana Volpe,[1] Katherine M. Boydell,[1,2,3,4] and Antonio Pignatiello[4,5]

[1] *Community Health Systems Resource Group, The Hospital for Sick Children, 555 University Avenue, Toronto, ON, Canada M5G 1X8*
[2] *Child Health Evaluative Sciences, Research Institute, The Hospital for Sick Children, 555 University Avenue, Toronto, ON, Canada M5G 1X8*
[3] *Dalla Lana School of Public Health, University of Toronto, 155 College Street, 6th Floor, Toronto, ON, Canada M5T 3M7*
[4] *Department of Psychiatry, Faculty of Medicine, University of Toronto, 250 College Street, 8th Floor, Toronto, ON, Canada M5T 1R8*
[5] *Department of Telepsychiatry, TeleLink Mental Health Program, The Hospital for Sick Children, 555 University Avenue, Toronto, ON, Canada M5G 1X8*

Correspondence should be addressed to Tiziana Volpe; tiziana.volpe@sickkids.ca

Academic Editor: George Demiris

Objective. Identify aspects of psychiatry work that are rewarding, as well as those that are challenging, from the perspective of psychiatrists and residents participating in televideo consultation services. *Method.* A web-based survey was distributed to psychiatrists within the Division of Child Psychiatry at the University of Toronto. Also, semistructured interviews were conducted with six child psychiatrists providing services to a telepsychiatry program. Finally, a focus group interview was held with four psychiatry residents. *Results.* Child psychiatrists are very comfortable conducting assessments via televideo. Factors identified as being important in the decision to participate in telepsychiatry include assisting underserved communities, supportive administrative staff, enhanced rural provider capacity, financial incentives, and convenience. The study's qualitative phase identified four themes in the decision to participate in telepsychiatry: (1) organizational, (2) shared values, (3) innovation, and (4) the consultation model. *Conclusion.* The success of televideo consultation programs in attracting child psychiatrists to provide consultation services to underresourced communities makes an important contribution to psychiatric workforce shortages. Understanding what aspects of telepsychiatry are most appreciated by consulting psychiatrists and residents offers useful strategies to telepsychiatry administrators and medical school educators seeking to attract, train, and retain psychiatry practitioners.

1. Background

There is an emerging concern about the shortage of child psychiatrists in Canada and elsewhere [1, 2], a problem that is expected to worsen in the coming years. As availability of psychiatric expertise diminishes, access to timely and appropriate specialty mental health care for children and youth is endangered. In Ontario, Canada, the problem of access is particularly problematic in rural communities and complicates provision of mental health services [3]. The ratio of child psychiatrists to children with mental health needs is approximately 1:6,148 [4]. However, only 2% of child psychiatrists practice primarily in areas with populations of less than 20,000, though approximately 18% of the population lives in rural areas [4]. The shortage of resources and support services in rural communities means that children requiring urgent care often are frequently placed in residential care outside of their community [5].

Live interactive videoconferencing technology offers an innovative opportunity to address the shortage of child psychiatrists in Canada [6]. The use of interactive video technology is endorsed by The Canadian Academy of Child Psychiatry [2]. Also, the Canadian Standing Senate Committee on Social Affairs, Science, and Technology [7] recommends that telepsychiatry be used in rural and remote communities for consultations, education, and training of mental health practitioners.

2. The TeleLink Mental Health Program

In 1997, The Hospital for Sick Children (SickKids), in Toronto, Ontario, undertook a pilot project to provide mental health support to primary care settings through videoconferencing. Fully operational in 2000, the program evolved to become the TeleLink Mental Health Program. The program aims to enhance the knowledge, skill set, and confidence of children's mental health practitioners using videoconferencing and other technologies by providing timely, equitable access to bilingual (English and French) specialist services.

Videoconferencing between recipient "far" sites and TeleLink "hub" site occurs by way of Internet Protocol (IP), (maximum bandwidth 384 Kbits/second). Two or more sites can be connected simultaneously, and videos, powerpoint, and scanned documents may be transmitted. The hub site is equipped with five stationary studios, each utilizing a 50 inch plasma or LCD monitor, and one mobile unit containing a 17 inch LCD monitor. Both hub and far sites can be viewed simultaneously, and all cameras have local and remote pan-tilt-zoom control. Polycom or Tandberg videoconferencing units enable the data transmission. Infrastructure support is provided by core staff at the hub and a designated telepsychiatry coordinator at far sites.

Referral routes are multiple: 15 primary children's mental health agencies in rural Ontario (including satellite locations); three community hospitals; one youth detention centre; one community youth justice diversion program; and community physicians. Models of service delivery include clinical consultation and/or short-term follow-up, professional to professional consultation, shared care, program consultation, and education and training. As a consultative program, responsibility for the case remains primarily with the referring agency or physician, with the consulting psychiatrist neither accepting ongoing responsibility for primary care, nor prescribing medication. Referring clinicians complete a mental health assessment before the consultation. Supporting documentation such as past psychological/psychoeducational evaluations, school reports, and screening tools, is also requested. It is highly encouraged that the client's primary clinician/case manager be present during the session; other participants may include parents/caregivers and others involved in the child's care.

Since its inception, the TeleLink Mental Health Program has successfully recruited a stable core of consulting child psychiatrists. Twenty-three child psychiatrists within the Division of Child and Adolescent Psychiatry at the University of Toronto provide the bulk of services through a regular weekly or monthly roster, as determined by the consultant's interest, availability, and commitment. An additional 16 faculty members are called on regularly for specific consultations and educational sessions, depending on their expertise and availability. Every faculty member must have active privileges at The Hospital for Sick Children.

The recruitment of child psychiatrists into the TeleLink Mental Health Program has grown since its inception. However, little is known about the factors that may influence the decision of residents and child psychiatrists to work with rural and remote communities via televideo. In a child and youth mental health system that is fragmented, underfunded, and with a critical shortage of specialists in rural areas, it is important to identify the factors that could enhance recruitment into telepsychiatry and contribute to the expansion of telepsychiatry services to rural and remote communities. This study identifies aspects of psychiatry work that are most rewarding, as well as those that are challenging, from the perspective of psychiatrists and residents participating in televideo consultation services.

3. Methods

To enhance our understanding of psychiatrists' decisions to participate in the provision of services via televideo, this study used a mixed method design, combining quantitative and qualitative methods. For the quantitative component, a web-based survey was developed using SurveyGizmo online software. For the qualitative phase, in-depth interviews and a focus group were conducted following Denzin's [8] interpretive interactionist framework.

3.1. Data Collection. The survey was distributed via e-mail to all child psychiatrists ($n = 80$) within the Division of Child and Adolescent Psychiatry at the University of Toronto. The distribution sample was based on the fact that the TeleLink Program is well promoted within the division and all faculty members are eligible to participate in the Program. The survey included questions related to their experiences with the TeleLink Program (see Tables 1–5). Twenty-six responses (32.5%) were received, a response rate exceeding expectations for web-based surveys (27.4%) [9, 10].

The survey used was developed specifically for this study. It was created by the authors based on their collective experience in the field [6], literature review, and consultation with key stakeholders. Its design was informed by a social ecological framework that highlights the need to address phenomena from the interaction among many factors at the individual, relationship, community, and societal level [11].

Focus groups and semistructured individual interviews were conducted to provide a more detailed examination of the survey questions. Invitations to participate in a focus group were sent to all division child and adolescent psychiatrists ($n = 80$) and all psychiatry residents ($n = 26$) located at The Hospital for Sick Children at the time of data collection. Despite multiple attempts to engage focus group participants, our efforts to recruit psychiatrists were unsuccessful. As such, one focus group was held with four psychiatry residents. For the individual interviews, eight individuals involved or familiar with pediatric telepsychiatry services were approached, both in Ontario and internationally. Six individuals agreed to participate; four providing services to the TeleLink Program in Ontario and two providing services to programs outside the country, one in the United States and one in Australia.

Table 1: Frequency of assessments ($n = 26$).

How often do you provide assessments to the TeleLink Program?	Percentage
Never	23.1%
Rarely (less than 6 times per year)	19.2%
Occasionally (6–12 times per year)	23.1%
Frequently (more than 12 times per year)	34.6%

Table 2: Comfort with conducting assessments via televideo ($n = 25$).

How comfortable are you conducting assessments via televideo?	Percentage
Not comfortable (1–4)	20%
Moderately comfortable (5–7)	20%
Very comfortable (8–10)	60%

Table 3: Comfort with video equipment and technology ($n = 25$).

How comfortable are you with the video equipment and technology?	Percentage
Not comfortable (1–4)	4%
Moderately comfortable (5–7)	40%
Very comfortable (8–10)	56%

This sampling strategy, focused on "information-rich cases" [12], was selected as most productive in helping us understand the factors that influence the decision to participate in a telepsychiatry program and those that may be unique to the TeleLink Program. Interviews lasted approximately 40–60 minutes and were conducted either face-to-face or by telephone. A semistructured interview guide directed the interviews and focus group discussion (see Table 6). As with the survey, the interview guide was informed by the authors' previous work, the literature, and consultation with key informants.

3.2. Data Analysis. Survey response data were analyzed using simple frequency statistics and graphic representations. An open-ended text report assisted in the analysis of multiple choice questions as well as verbatim responses. Qualitative interviews were audiotaped and transcribed. The interview and field note transcripts were analyzed using an interpretive interactionist framework [8]. The first step of the analytic process is bracketing, followed by construction and contextualization of findings. Bracketing involves isolating the essential elements under investigation, a process commonly known as coding. The process of construction classifies, orders, and reassembles the phenomenon back into a coherent whole. Finally, with contextualization, greater meaning is sought across individual experiences.

4. Results

4.1. Part 1: Online Survey. The 26 survey respondents consisted of 14 (53.8%) males and 12 females (46.2%), ranging in age from under 34 to over 65 and averaging 47.1 years. There was a range of experience in working as a child psychiatrist, from 1 to 47 years, with a median of 21 years. Over 80% of respondents ($n = 21$) indicated that more than 50% of their practice was dedicated to working with children and adolescents. The type of services provided included outpatient (88%), consultation (80%), private practice (40%), in-patient (36%), and others (32%).

Survey respondents were all familiar with the TeleLink Program but diverse in terms of their experience with the Program. While more than one third indicated that they provide frequent consultation services of more than 12 per year (34.6%), there were respondents who had never provided services (23.1%) (Table 1). The majority (68%) indicated that telepsychiatry is an important innovation that allows access to much needed resources in underserviced communities and that it is important for psychiatric trainees to develop expertise in providing consultation. To this end, 68% of respondents recommend that the University's curriculum committee make telepsychiatry mandatory for subspecialty training. Those who resist mandatory telepsychiatry training believe that people are more likely to choose it if it is not forced upon them.

Working with TeleLink technology was not identified as a significant barrier. As reported in Tables 2 and 3, respondents indicate that they are moderately (20%) to very comfortable (60%) conducting assessments via televideo (with 72% selecting 7 or above on a 10-point Likert scale), as well as with operating the video equipment and associated technology (40% and 56%, resp.).

At least 50% of respondents identify a number of factors as being very important or important in their decision to provide psychiatric services via televideo, including the ability to provide services to underserviced communities, the support they receive from TeleLink administrative staff, contributing to the enhancement of rural provider capacity, and maintaining ongoing relationships with rural providers, financial incentives, and convenience (Table 4). The novelty of the technology, privileges associated with a hospital appointment, and the opportunity to be a part of a larger group of professionals were of relatively lower importance. The management of the Program, supporting TeleLink's mission, working within a consultation model, trying out telepsychiatry on a trial basis and diversification of income sources were not identified at all as influencing the decision to become involved.

Survey respondents were asked to indicate the extent to which they agreed with a series of statements about the delivery of psychiatric services via televideo (Table 5). The majority (76%) agreed/strongly agreed that the technology was secure and confidential although about one-third (33.3%) expressed concerns about safety and liability issues. More than half (56%) desired more feedback about the helpfulness of the consultation. There was some need expressed for more knowledge about the particular culture of the community (20%) and for more awareness of the specific resources available in rural communities (52%).

Respondents were asked to identify the circumstances that would allow them to provide more hours to the TeleLink

TABLE 4: Decisions to provide telepsychiatry services-importance rankings ($n = 25$).

How important are the following in your decision regarding whether or not to provide services to the TeleLink Program?	Very important	Important	Neutral	Somewhat important	Not at all important	Not applicable
Flexibility regarding number of hours I provide to the program	40% 10	32% 8	8% 2	8% 2	8% 2	4% 1
Given only cases that match my area of expertise	24% 6	36% 9	20% 5	16% 4	0% 0	4% 1
Support provided by telepsychiatry staff	36% 9	60% 15	0% 0	0% 0	0% 0	4% 1
Comfortable environment	24% 6	52% 13	20% 5	0% 0	0% 0	4% 1
Convenience	32% 8	44% 11	16% 4	4% 1	0% 0	4% 1
Financial incentives	20% 5	60% 15	12% 3	0% 0	0% 0	8% 2
Opportunity to be part of larger group of professionals	8% 2	36% 9	36% 9	12% 3	0% 0	8% 2
Enhance capacity of local providers	32% 8	52% 13	8% 2	4% 1	0% 0	4% 1
Privileges associated with a hospital appointment	4% 1	8% 2	32% 8	4% 1	32% 8	20% 5
Novelty of the medium/technology	4% 1	8% 2	36% 9	8% 2	36% 9	8% 2
Maintaining ongoing relationship with rural agency	24% 6	36% 9	24% 6	0% 0	8% 2	8% 2
Providing service to underserved areas	52% 13	44% 11	0% 0	4% 1	0% 0	0% 0

Program. Responses included flexibility to see the child on more than one occasion, increased time for teaching and training, and review of documents, opportunity to work more closely with community physicians and to have their follow-up and support.

4.2. Part 2: Qualitative Interviews and Focus Group. For the qualitative phase of the study, participants were asked to discuss their involvement in a telepsychiatry program and the factors that may encourage or deter their participation. Four main factors were identified: (1) organizational; (2) shared values; (3) innovation; and (4) the consultation model.

(1) Organizational Factors. An important component in recruiting and retaining consulting psychiatrists is the support provided by the program's executive and administrative staff. This result is supported in the survey data, with 96% of respondents identifying staff support as very important or important in their decision to participate in a telepsychiatry Program. Interview participants identified "*friendly staff, welcoming environment and comfortable set-up*" as influencing factors. Consultants with the TeleLink Program cited "*effective leadership*" by the TeleLink medical director, and his visibility within the department of psychiatry as important aspects of participation. Psychiatrists noted that strong administrative and technical support ensures worry-free consultation sessions.

As revealed in the survey data, the TeleLink Program's ability to provide a flexible work environment and willingness to adapt to consultant needs emerged as a deciding factor. In the qualitative interviews, further exploration revealed that prospective consultants, uncertain about participating, appreciated the offer of a trial period without obligation. Further tailoring included flexibility regarding the number of hours worked per week or month and the type of cases offered. Participants acknowledged that it "*takes time*" to become comfortable with televideo, and the option to try it out on a trial basis is a facilitator. For one international participant, the increasing demands on pediatric teaching hospitals and the psychiatry department make participation in telepsychiatry difficult to negotiate.

While most consultants find participating in the TeleLink Program convenient, those located at a distance from the Program's head office find it inconvenient and costly given commuting times and parking costs. One international participant notes that her institution schedules several televideo consultations in one day, similar to a half-day clinic, to make participation more attractive to consulting psychiatrists.

(2) Shared Values. In keeping with survey respondents, interviewees indicate that a shared sense of purpose and belief in the mission of telepsychiatry is an important aspect of participation. Involvement in telepsychiatry allows consultants the opportunity to improve access to mental health services in rural and remote communities and support local health

TABLE 5: Psychiatric services via televideo (n = 25).

To what extent do you agree or disagree with the following statements regarding the provision of psychiatric services via televideo?	Strongly disagree	Disagree	Neutral	Agree	Strongly agree	Not applicable
Technology is sufficiently secure and confidential	0% 0	12% 3	12% 3	36% 9	40% 10	0% 0
I am concerned about safety & liability issues	8.3% 2	37.5% 9	20.8% 5	20.8% 5	12.5% 3	0% 0
Having others in room with patient is helpful in conducting an assessment	0% 0	0% 0	16% 4	48% 12	36% 9	0% 0
It is difficult to build rapport with others via televideo	8% 2	32% 8	24% 6	32% 8	4% 1	0% 0
I lack knowledge of the culture of rural communities to provide effective assistance	16% 4	48% 12	16% 4	20% 5	0% 0	0% 0
Information received prior to consultation is sufficient to conduct a proper assessment	0% 0	4% 1	32% 8	52% 13	8% 2	4% 1
I have insufficient knowledge regarding the resources available in rural communities	4% 1	24% 6	20% 5	44% 11	8% 2	0% 0
Need more feedback from rural agencies about helpfulness of my recommendations	0% 0	8% 2	28% 7	40% 10	16% 4	8% 2

TABLE 6: Qualitative semistructured interview questions.

How often do you provide assessments to the TeleLink Program?
How did you become involved in the TeleLink Program?
What aspects of the program's organization/service delivery model facilitate and/or deter participation by psychiatrists and/or psychiatric residents?
What are your thoughts regarding the provision of psychiatric services to rural and remote communities via televideo? How does that influence your decision to participate in the Program?
How comfortable are you conducting assessments via televideo? How comfortable are you with the video equipment and technology?
What circumstances or changes to the TeleLink Program would encourage you to provide some or more hours?
If consulting to the TeleLink Program, what circumstances or changes would lead you to offer fewer hours?

practitioners. Also in keeping with survey data, interview participants value the opportunity to enhance the knowledge and skills of rural clinicians, recognizing it as "*an innovative way to extend your skills beyond your local practice, and serve great benefits to rural communities.*" Psychiatrists providing regular service to particular sites develop a strong connection and beneficial relationship with the rural clinicians and wider community.

The sense of contributing to a shared mission and a collective pride in program accomplishments is attributed to the staff retention rates. The fact that a program is well supported within the psychiatry department and showcased nationally and internationally enhances its profile. One consultant with TeleLink stated that the "*synchronicity of purpose*" between the Program and its consultants is the vital ingredient in recruiting dedicated child and adolescent psychiatrists. He goes on to say that "*retention is not just about money*", but rather creating "*an environment where an individual feels comfortable, recognized, contributory to the mission.*"

(3) Innovation. The role of innovation and technological advances in bringing scarce psychiatric resources to underserved communities emerged as a key factor to both the quantitative and qualitative participants. While survey data suggests that only 12% of respondents identify "novelty" of the technology as important or very important in their decision to provide services via televideo, 96% reported the opportunity to provide services to rural communities as important/very important. In our individual interviews, participants explore this theme further, acknowledging the increasing use of "*electronic connections*" such as Skype and Facebook in modern culture, the appeal this has for younger generations, and its potential role in attracting medical students to the field of psychiatry. Psychiatry residents in the focus group session concur, describing the delivery of mental health services via televideo as a creative way to deliver a scarce resource to communities in need.

In both interview and focus group data, the TeleLink Program is credited with offering psychiatric residents unique training opportunities (each of the core child residents at the University of Toronto must participate in two telepsychiatry consultations, during their six-month rotation). In particular, it is seen as addressing important learning gaps, including how to do a consultation, work collaboratively, and use televideo technology effectively. According to the psychiatric residents, participating in telepsychiatry sessions is rewarding, particularly if the consulting psychiatrist provides opportunities to participate on camera and ask questions. Being outside of the camera's view was difficult, awkward, and not as rewarding. According to one participant, this positive experience may be "*one of the little things that tip them towards child psychiatry.*"

Both interview and survey data reveal a high level of comfort with technology among consultants, with many stating little or no differences between video and face-to-face consultations. Others identify the immediacy of the service as important, as well as the ability to follow-up with patients via video. While participants noted that the technology does not interfere with performing a mental health assessment, some difficulties were identified such as poor picture quality, audio lag, uncertainty in operating the equipment, and unstable internet connections in remote communities. Also, one participant noted that room setup and camera placement at the far sites are not always ideal. Despite these difficulties, one participant states that the advantages of telepsychiatry "*far outweigh these small disadvantages*", while another dismisses them as "*minor quibbles*."

(4) The Consultation Model. A consultation model of service delivery was the fourth theme to emerge from the qualitative phase of research. Though this theme was not selected by survey respondents as an important factor in their decision to work with TeleLink, 92% strongly agreed or agreed with the statement "*I am comfortable with the consultation model of service delivery*" and 56% identified "*I am only given cases that match my area of expertise*" as important or very important to their participation. Also, 80% identified telepsychiatry as a valuable resource to communities with limited access to specialized mental health care. In the interviews, psychiatrists indicate that the consultation model of service delivery encourages participation since the consulting psychiatrist does not accept ongoing responsibility for primary care, nor does he or she prescribe medication or do treatment. With a full-time job and regular patient load elsewhere, interview participants appreciate the opportunity to expand their practice without having to take on new patients. The financial incentives are attractive, as is the possibility to diversify their income sources.

The majority of interview participants indicate that conducting psychiatric assessments via televideo does not significantly differ from those conducted face-to-face. Forty percent of survey respondents agreed or strongly agreed with this. One experienced psychiatrist, new to telepsychiatry, however, expresses a preference for face-to-face encounters and the need for more than one consultation session to do a thorough assessment. An added concern was the lack of feedback from rural clinicians regarding the effectiveness of his recommendations, stating "*I have no idea whether any of this is making any difference in kids' lives because I have not seen any follow-up data .... I have never seen a kid more than once.*"

Other concerns emerging from the qualitative data include the lack of information regarding resources in rural communities, rural clinicians who may be inexperienced due to high turnover rates, and having to "*tread carefully*" so as not be seen as a "*big shot coming in telling us* [*rural clinicians*] *what to do.*" There was also a lack of knowledge regarding liability and safety issues, clinical follow-up procedures, and funding mechanisms, with one consultant stating "*What is the renumeration? I do not know how I get paid; I do not know what it is. It is not all that transparent for some people.*" Many of these themes echo concerns expressed by survey respondents, as reported earlier. Despite these concerns, study participants acknowledge that, by providing timely, equitable access to specialist services, the TeleLink Program fills an important gap in the children's mental health system, "*distributing (psychiatric expertise) to a wide area.*"

5. Discussion

The delivery of psychiatric services using videoconferencing technology is an efficient, cost-effective [13–16], and user-friendly [17] approach that has been recommended for expansion in jurisdictions across Canada [7]. However, it has been noted that the growth and advancement of telepsychiatry programs may be constrained by human resource factors [7], including psychiatry workforce shortages [2, 18] and resistance from specialists to participate in such programs [19, 20]. As such, it is important to understand what factors may encourage or deter specialists from engaging with telepsychiatry programs. The TeleLink Mental Health Program offers a compelling case as it has regular access to approximately 40 child psychiatrists and, since its inception in 2000, retained much of its original workforce. The main factors contributing to this success as identified by study participants provide important strategies for the field in attracting and retaining child psychiatrists to a telepsychiatry program.

For both survey and interview participants, organizational factors were identified as crucial to their participation in the TeleLink Program. Features such as efficient administrative staff, convenient setup, flexible work hours, and financial compensation allowed consulting psychiatrists to deliver services with minimal workload. In the literature, time, money [19], and technical skills [21] are identified as barriers to the uptake of telemedicine. This study and others [22, 23] indicate that such barriers can be significantly reduced by providing dedicated administrative and technological support. Also, adequate funding is critical, with 80% of survey participants identifying financial compensation as important or very important to their participation. For consultants working primarily in locations at a distance from the host site, costs associated with commuting could be mitigated by offering multiple consultations per visit, or offsite service provision, where feasible.

A second set of factors linked to telepsychiatry participation is related to the technology itself. The majority of survey and interview participants reported being comfortable with the equipment and technology, as well as conducting assessments via televideo. However, results suggest that more could be done to improve technical aspects and provider comfort. As reported in a recent literature review [24], problems related to nonverbal communication and audiovisual quality are seen as drawbacks to telepsychiatry and that more needs to be done to improve infrastructure issues [19]. Also, training, ongoing technical support [25], and more user-friendly technology [26] have been shown to facilitate acceptance. Comfort levels could also be improved through better communication and information exchange, for example, providing consultants with information regarding available resources in local communities as well as postconsultation feedback regarding the appropriateness and usefulness of their recommendations. Finally, providing potential recruits and new consultants with an orientation package would help promote the program and provide answers to common questions, such as remuneration schemes and security issues.

A third factor in attracting consulting psychiatrists is active participation in postgraduate training; since 2005, all psychiatry residents at the University of Toronto are required to participate in at least two telepsychiatry consultations with the TeleLink Program. Additionally, three- and six-month electives are offered to interested residents [6]. This strategy is supported by survey respondents who believe that an organized effort is needed to introduce medical students and residents to specialized pediatric training early in their training, with 68% recommending that the University's curriculum committee make telepsychiatry mandatory for subspecialty training. In focus group data, psychiatry residents indicated that the opportunity to actively participate in televideo consultations was exciting and strengthened their interest in this model of psychiatric work. These data align with research that suggests exposure to positive training opportunities, and participation in psychiatry electives may enhance recruitment into psychiatry [27]. Given the downward trend in psychiatric recruitment [28–30], it behooves telepsychiatry programs to work with medical schools and psychiatric recruitment officers. To this end, the Canadian Mental Health Commission has encouraged the inclusion of telemental health instruction in medical schools [7].

6. Implications

This study aimed to gather objective data regarding how a telepsychiatry program in Toronto, Canada, is able to attract and keep child psychiatric consultants to the program, in the context of declining psychiatric recruitment and the difficulty in attracting psychiatrists to do this work, as indicated informally by similar programs in Canada and elsewhere. These results help us understand what aspects of telepsychiatry are most likely to attract and retain psychiatry practitioners, as well as aspects most appreciated by consulting psychiatrists and residents. Also, this study helps inform the effective recruitment of new graduates to the field, a current challenge for the TeleLink Program. In response to this challenge, the University of Toronto's Department of Psychiatry has made adult telepsychiatry a key goal and has asked the TeleLink Program to assist in setting up the program and attracting consulting psychiatrists. The results of this study will assist with this endeavour.

More research is needed to better understand residents' experiences of participating in the TeleLink Program, and more specifically what might attract them to continue to work in telepsychiatry after graduation. Future research would include a multicentered study involving other telepsychiatry programs in Ontario and across Canada.

7. Conclusion

This study offers important insights into addressing possible barriers in attracting psychiatrists and residents to a telepsychiatry program. It also provides an opportunity to think about wider recruitment and retention issues in the field of psychiatry. Understanding what aspects of the TeleLink Mental Health Program are most appreciated by consulting psychiatrists and what attracts residents to the Program offers useful strategies to telepsychiatry administrators and medical school educators seeking to attract, train, and retain psychiatry practitioners.

Acknowledgments

The authors have no real or perceived conflict of interests or affiliations with industry. Funding for this project was provided via the TeleLink Program at The Hospital for Sick Children in Toronto, a Program funded by the Ontario Ministry of Children and Youth Services. Antonio Pignatiello is the Medical Director of the TeleLink Program and as such receives a stipend for this role.

References

[1] C. M. Wilks, M. Oakley-Brown, and B. L. Jenner, "Attracting psychiatrists to a rural area—10 years on," *Rural and Remote Health*, vol. 8, no. 1, p. 824, 2008.

[2] Z. Parker, M. Steele, W. Junek et al., "Child psychiatry in Canada: physician resources," Position Statement, Canadian Academy of Child Psychiatry Physician Resources, Ottawa, Canada, 2002.

[3] A. F. Cook and H. Hoas, "Hide and seek: the elusive rural psychiatrist," *Academic Psychiatry*, vol. 31, no. 6, pp. 419–422, 2007.

[4] M. M. Steele and V. V. Wolfe, "Child psychiatry practice patterns in Ontario," *Canadian Journal of Psychiatry*, vol. 44, no. 8, pp. 788–792, 1999.

[5] A. E. R. Sheldon-Keller, J. R. Koch, A. C. Watts, and P. J. Leaf, "The provision of services for rural youth with serious emotional and behavioral problems: Virginia's Comprehensive Services Act," *Community Mental Health Journal*, vol. 32, no. 5, pp. 481–495, 1996.

[6] A. Pignatiello, K. M. Boydell, J. Teshima, T. Volpe, P. Braunberger, and D. Minden, "Transforming child and youth mental health via innovative technical solutions," *Healthcare Quarterly*, vol. 14, no. 2, pp. 92–102, 2011.

[7] M. J. L. Kirby and W. J. Keon, *Out of the Shadows at Last: Transforming Mental Health, Mental Illness and Addiction Services in Canada*, Standing Committee on Social Affairs, Science and Technology, Ottawa, Canada, 2006.

[8] N. Denzin, *Interpretive Interactionism*, Sage, Newbury Park, Calif, USA, 1989.

[9] D. Dillman, *Mail and Internet Surveys: The Tailored Design Method*, Wiley, New York, NY, USA, 2000.

[10] N. Kwak and B. Radler, "A comparison between mail and web surveys: response pattern, respondent profile, and data quality," *Journal of Official Statistics*, vol. 18, no. 2, pp. 257–273, 2002.

[11] U. Bronfenbrenner and G. W. Evans, "Developmental science in the 21st century: emerging questions, theoretical models,

research designs and empirical findings," *Social Development*, vol. 9, no. 1, pp. 115–125, 2000.

[12] M. B. Miles and A. M. Huberman, *Qualitative Data Analysis*, Sage, Thousand Oaks, Calif, USA, 2nd edition, 1994.

[13] D. R. Elford, H. White, K. St John, B. Maddigan, M. Ghandi, and R. Bowering, "A prospective satisfaction study and cost analysis of a pilot child telepsychiatry service in Newfoundland," *Journal of Telemedicine and Telecare*, vol. 7, no. 2, pp. 73–81, 2001.

[14] K. Myers and S. Cain, "Practice parameter for telepsychiatry with children and adolescents," *Journal of the American Academy of Child and Adolescent Psychiatry*, vol. 47, no. 12, pp. 1468–1483, 2008.

[15] R. O'Reilly, J. Bishop, K. Maddox, L. Hutchinson, M. Fisman, and J. Takhar, "Is telepsychiatry equivalent to face-to-face psychiatry? Results from a randomized controlled equivalence trial," *Psychiatric Services*, vol. 25, no. 6, pp. 836–843, 2007.

[16] D. D. Persaud, S. Jreige, C. Skedgel, J. Finley, J. Sargeant, and N. Hanlon, "An incremental cost analysis of telehealth in Nova Scotia from a societal perspective," *Journal of Telemedicine and Telecare*, vol. 11, no. 2, pp. 77–84, 2005.

[17] D. J. Ermer, "Experience with a rural telepsychiatry clinic for children and adolescents," *Psychiatric Services*, vol. 50, no. 2, pp. 260–261, 1999.

[18] J. K. Sargeant, T. Adey, F. McGregor et al., "Psychiatric human resources planning in Canada," *Canadian Journal of Psychiatry*, vol. 55, no. 9, pp. 1–20, 2010.

[19] J. J. Moffatt and D. S. Eley, "Barriers to the up-take of telemedicine in Australia—a view from providers," *Rural and Remote Health*, vol. 11, no. 1, article 1581, 2011.

[20] N. Menachemi, D. E. Burke, and D. J. Ayers, "Factors affecting the adoption of telemedicine—a multiple adopter perspective," *Journal of Medical Systems*, vol. 28, no. 6, pp. 617–632, 2004.

[21] A. Fitzgerald, M. Bailey, A. C. Smith et al., "Child development services: a multidisciplinary approach to professional education via videoconference," *Journal of Telemedicine and Telecare*, vol. 8, supplement 3, pp. 19–21, 2002.

[22] A. C. Smith and L. C. Gray, "Telemedicine across the ages," *Medical Journal of Australia*, vol. 190, no. 1, pp. 15–19, 2009.

[23] A. C. Smith, A. Isles, R. McCrossin et al., "The point-of-referral barrier—a factor in the success of telehealth," *Journal of Telemedicine and Telecare*, vol. 7, supplement 2, pp. 75–82, 2001.

[24] L. Pesämaa, H. Ebeling, M. Kuusimäki, I. Winblad, M. Isohanni, and I. Moilanen, "Videoconferencing in child and adolescent telepsychiatry: a systematic review of the literature," *Journal of Telemedicine and Telecare*, vol. 10, no. 4, pp. 187–192, 2004.

[25] J. Watson, L. Gasser, I. Blignault, and R. Collins, "Taking telehealth to the bush: lessons from north Queensland," *Journal of Telemedicine and Telecare*, vol. 7, supplement 2, pp. 20–23, 2001.

[26] P. M. Yellowlees and C. Kennedy, "Telemedicine: here to stay," *Medical Journal of Australia*, vol. 166, no. 5, pp. 262–265, 1997.

[27] K. Manassis, M. Katz, J. Lofchy, and S. Wiesenthal, "Choosing a career in psychiatry: influential factors within a medical school program," *Academic Psychiatry*, vol. 30, no. 4, pp. 325–329, 2006.

[28] Canadian Resident Matching Service, 2011, Ottawa, Canada, http://www.carms.ca/eng/r1_about_intro_e.shtml.

[29] H. Katschnig, "Are psychiatrists an endangered species? Observations on internal and external challenges to the profession," *World Psychiatry*, vol. 9, no. 1, pp. 21–28, 2010.

[30] F. S. Sierles and M. A. Taylor, "Decline of U.S. medical student career choice of psychiatry and what to do about it," *American Journal of Psychiatry*, vol. 152, no. 10, pp. 1416–1426, 1995.

7

Increasing Physical Activity Efficiently: An Experimental Pilot Study of a Website and Mobile Phone Intervention

Kjærsti Thorsteinsen,[1] Joar Vittersø,[2] and Gunnvald Bendix Svendsen[3]

[1] *Tromsø Telemedicine Laboratory, Department of Psychology, University of Tromsø, 9037 Tromsø, Norway*
[2] *Department of Psychology, University of Tromsø, 9037 Tromsø, Norway*
[3] *Brand Management, Telenor ASA, Snarøyveien 30, 1331 Fornebu, Norway*

Correspondence should be addressed to Kjærsti Thorsteinsen; kjarsti.thorsteinsen@uit.no

Academic Editor: Manolis Tsiknakis

The main objective of this pilot study was to test the effectiveness of an online, interactive physical activity intervention that also incorporated gaming components. The intervention design included an activity planner, progress monitoring, and gamification components and used SMS text as a secondary delivery channel and feedback to improve engagement in the intervention content. Healthy adults ($n = 21$) recruited through ads in local newspapers (age 35–73) were randomized to the intervention or the control condition. Both groups reported physical activity using daily report forms in four registration weeks during the three-month study: only the experiment condition received access to the intervention. Analyses showed that the intervention group had significantly more minutes of physical activity in weeks five and nine. We also found a difference in the intensity of exercise in week five. Although the intervention group reported more minutes of physical activity at higher intensity levels, we were not able to find a significant effect at the end of the study period. In conclusion, this study adds to the research on the effectiveness of using the Internet and SMS text messages for delivering physical activity interventions and supports gamification as a viable intervention tool.

1. Introduction

Being physically active is one of the most important predictors of mental and physical health [1]. In order to benefit from the positive effects of physical activity and avoid the negative effects of physical inactivity, it is important that we adhere to the World Health Organization's (WHO) recommendations for physical activity [2]. One problem is that some of us lack knowledge of the recommendations to be physically active for 30 minutes at a moderate intensity on most, preferably all, days of the week [3]. A more complex and tangible problem is that most of us fail to do so, even though we are fully aware of the consequences [3–5]. Researchers and clinicians working with behavior change have acknowledged that there is a gap between knowing what we should do and actually doing it. Thus, interventions to help people change their undesirable behavior and embrace more healthy habits have been developed.

Up-to-date intervention researchers utilize new opportunities for delivery of health promotion interventions brought on by advances in technology. Computer-tailoring an intervention and disseminating it through the Internet using a website, by e-mail and short mobile service (SMS) text messages, is a promising health education strategy [6–12]. This way people can get access to individually tailored advice, regardless of geographical and temporal barriers, and without the cost of a one-by-one consultation [13–15]. Still, one recent review found that the most effective interventions were delivered face to face [16]. One of the main challenges at this time is to maintain use of the interventions over time, as many studies of online computer-tailored interventions report an initial effect that wears off [6, 13, 17–21]. The decreased effect over time could be a result of decreased exposure to the intervention because of static content and boredom when the novelty of the system wears off [17, 21]. Thus, planning interventions that can maintain engagement over time is important. In a prestudy, potential consumers' intention to use a physical activity intervention (delivered online through the Internet and mobile phone) was influenced by perceived usefulness and expecting to have fun while using the system [22]. Ease of use, social support, and interactive features have also been reported to be important for usage of such systems [23, 24]. Naturally, previous studies have found that only active users of physical activity interventions improve their physical activity levels [25, 26]. Further developing and incorporating easy, social, and fun to use components in physical activity interventions is therefore an important way to increase usage and intervention exposure, consequently potentially produce more effective interventions.

One way to make interventions more fun is to add a game dimension. Gaming elements in nongame contexts of behavior change are an increasingly popular strategy to solve the adherence problem in health-related behavior [27, 28]. In what is known as gamification [29], interactivity is obligatory and making it easy and fun to use is part of the design process. Social components can also be integrated. Gaming components that require the participant to log in and register activity in order to make advancement in the game provide an extra incentive to use the intervention. However, so far there are not many interventions that utilize this opportunity.

Using SMS as a secondary delivery method has been shown to increase the effectiveness of website interventions [10, 30, 31]. Interventions using SMS as the primary delivery channel have also shown promising results for health care interventions [11]. In 2013 there were almost as many mobile-cellular subscriptions as people in the world [32]. Because people bring their mobile phones anywhere, they are perfect for instantaneous delivery of short intervention messages directly to individuals at any time, place, or setting. Also, they provide a means to give real-time feedback and just-in-time support for behavior change that could help the effectiveness of the intervention through improved adherence [33]. Although SMS messaging has been shown to be a viable intervention tool, there is a need for more research [34–36].

The present study reports a pilot test of an interactive, computer-tailored website physical activity intervention, with additional SMS text messages. The intervention was named Lifestyle Tool and is described further in the Method section. The goal of Lifestyle Tool was to motivate users of the program to incorporate physical activity in their daily routine, as doing so increases the chances of maintaining exercise over time [37]. The system was designed to be easy and fun to use and it incorporated social and individual gaming components to increase motivation and engagement. In order to closely monitor when the effect of the intervention occurred and how its influence projected over time, we wanted to assess participants' physical activity regularly. A three-month randomized controlled pilot trial with regular registration periods was conducted to compare the efficacy of the intervention on improving levels of physical activity in overall healthy adults with a control group. We hypothesized that participants randomized to the intervention condition would improve in physical activity more than the control group but that the effect would be greatest on the first measurement after implementation.

2. Materials and Method

2.1. Participants and Procedure. Participants were recruited through an advertisement in local newspapers in the town of Tromsø, Norway, in December 2008, which inspired 55 individuals to make initial contact and request more information about the study. The potential participants received additional information over e-mail and were asked to respond to a small set of initial questions such as age and gender. Additionally, using a short stages-of-change questionnaire [38], they reported on their level of physical activity. Inclusion criteria were access to the Internet and owning a mobile phone in addition to general good health (e.g., not having any known medical diseases). Of the 55 individuals that first made contact, 31 agreed to participate in the study and were invited to an information meeting in January 2009. The 31 participants were randomly assigned to either an experimental condition (the Lifestyle group) or a control condition. To ensure equal representation of age, gender, and physical activity level in the two groups the answers to the initial questions over e-mail were used to stratify the participants in sets. Based on the stages-of-change questionnaire [38] participants were given a contemplation score; precontemplation, contemplation, preparation, action, or maintenance. Participants belonging to precontemplation, contemplation, and preparation stages were put in one set (passive, $N = 14$); participants belonging to the action and maintenance stages were put in the other set (active, $N = 17$). Two sets were also created based on age (below/above average) and gender (male/female). Members from each set were then randomly assigned to the two experimental groups, 19 to the Lifestyle group, 12 to the control group. A flow chart of the grouping process following the Consort guidelines [39] is provided in Figure 1.

Participants were blinded to group allocation and not aware of the existence of another group. Both groups received identical envelopes by mail consisting of a consent form and daily report forms of physical activity which they were asked to complete one week before the initial information meeting. A total of 23 participants met at the information meeting and handed in consent and baseline (week 1) daily report forms.

Two participants from the Lifestyle group dropped out after the meeting. Thus, the final sample consisted of 21 participants—11 men and 10 women—who ranged in age from 35 to 73 years ($M = 55.3$, $SD = 11.2$). The Lifestyle group consisted of 12 participants; the control group consisted of 9 participants. However, one of the participants in the control group was far more active than the others (with physical activity scores more than three standard deviations above the rest) in weeks 5, 9, and 13. He was identified as an outlier and removed from subsequent analyses. This left 8 participants in the control group and 12 participants in the Lifestyle group.

The small sample size puts serious limitations to the statistical power of our study. For example, using 2-sided test and 5% significance level showed that we had 54% power to reject the null hypothesis of equal means if the population mean difference is 1.0 with a standard deviation for both groups of 1.0 (based on a calculation using the PASS 12 software) [40].

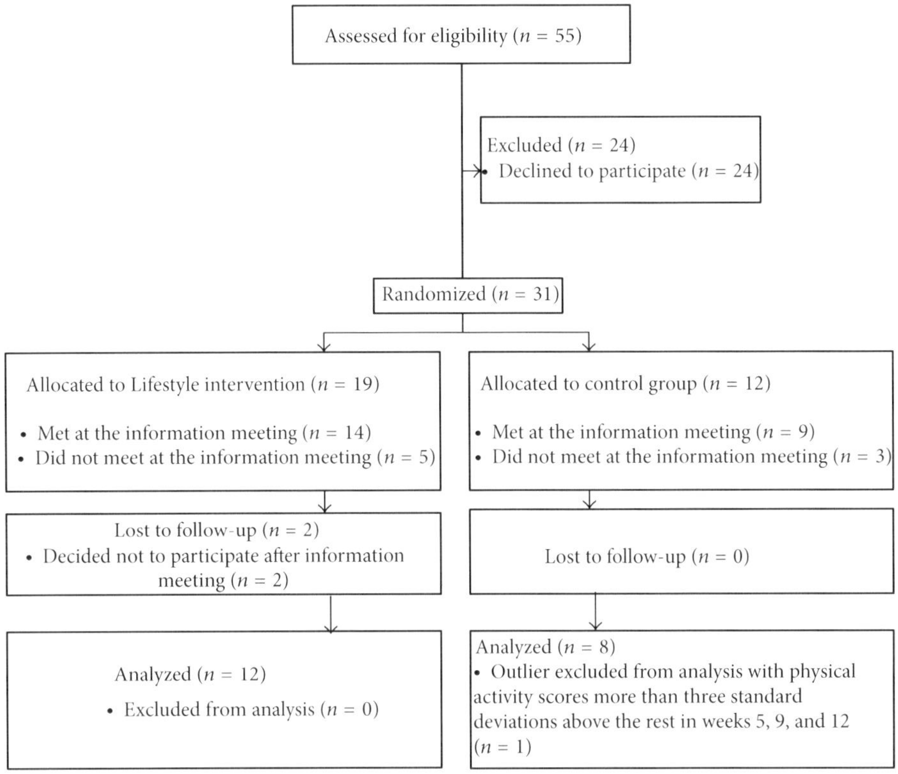

FIGURE 1: Participant flow diagram.

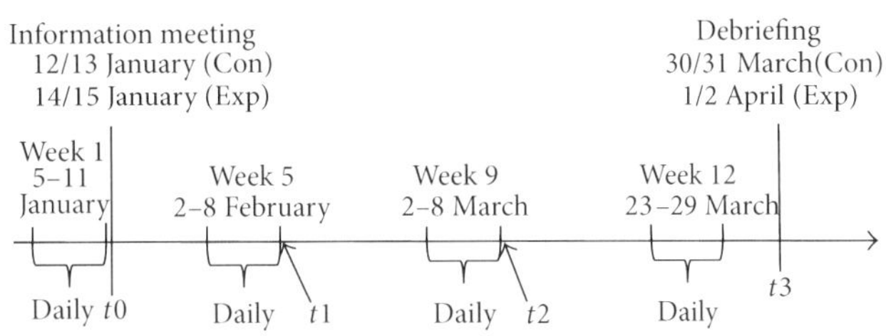

FIGURE 2: Study timeline. Registration of physical activity every night of weeks 1, 5, 9, and 12.

At the initial meetings (that were held separately for the two groups) both groups received general information about the study. In addition, the Lifestyle group was given information about—and basic training in using—Lifestyle Tool, and they were asked to create a personal account on the Lifestyle Tool website the next day. All of the participants in the Lifestyle group made an account on the Lifestyle portal within three days from the initial meeting.

Participants in both groups completed daily report forms of physical activity (described in Section 2.3) every night of the week, roughly every four weeks over three months. They also filled out a set of questionnaires with 61–79 items at the information meeting (*t*0), at the end of registration weeks five and nine (*t*1 and *t*2) and at the debriefing (*t*3; see study timeline in Figure 2). The answers to these questionnaires are not included in any of the analyses, thus they are not further described in this paper. Participants in the Lifestyle group were encouraged to use the Lifestyle Tool intervention during the three-month period the study lasted. As reward for their participation, all participants took part in a lottery for three gift certificates of 5000 Norwegian Kroner (approximately 900$) at the end of the study.

2.2. Intervention. The intervention Lifestyle Tool consisted of a rule-based website designed to help people plan and monitor their physical activity in order to become more physically active. Participants in the Lifestyle group created a user-account on the Lifestyle Tool portal which gave them access to their personal page. On the first log-in they were asked to fill out the behavioral regulation in exercise questionnaire (BREQ-2: [41, 42]) which assessed motivational level for physical activity. When logged on the personal page of Lifestyle Tool, participants had access to a physical activity calendar where they could fill in and plan their physical activities. The program made a graphical representation of the accomplished physical activity each week, with the recommended guidelines [2] plotted in the same chart. This gave participants an opportunity to monitor their own level of physical activity in relation to the guidelines (self-monitoring) and set specific goals [43, 44]. Participants also received text messages by SMS from a message library with educational information of the benefits of being physically active and the potential harmful risks of being inactive, in addition to concrete tips on what to do. The messages were tailored using personalization and adaption [45]. Messages were personalized by referring to the participants by their first name, which is thought to activate the process of self-referent encoding (superior memory of information with reference to the self). The information content was individually adapted to match participants age and gender, and the number of messages each participant received each week was based on their motivational level for physical activity (measured with the BREQ-2 questionnaire).

To make Lifestyle Tool more interactive and fun to use, we included a game-component in which participants received points for completed activities. When participants had registered an activity, the system generated a reminder-text by SMS 30 minutes before the activity should start according to the plan. Then, 30 minutes after the activity ended the system generated a new SMS text asking the following. (1) To which degree did you complete the activity according to the plan? (2) How exhausting was it? And (3) how pleased are you with what you have accomplished? The responses to the first two questions in addition to the length of the activity gave the basis for how many points the participant received for a given activity. The answers to these questions also determined the feedback-message that was sent automatically, designed to positively reinforce complying behavior or help improve compliance in the future. Accumulated points were visible on the participants' personal site in addition to a hierarchical category status level. The status level was based on how many points a participant had, ranging from novice to enthusiast. By earning points the participants went up the ladder.

Lifestyle Tool also included two gaming components designed to increase the motivation for being physically active and helping participants to set goals: social contract and competition. The social contract component consisted of an agreement between two or more participants. When participants accepted a contract proposal they committed to complete all of their planned physical activities within a period of time (the time-window was determined by the initiator of the agreement). If they were successful in adhering to the agreement participants received bonus-points (50% of the points they earned in this period were added to the regular points). No bonus points were handed out to participants who violated the contract. The competition component had two alternatives. Participants could initiate a competition where the winner was (a) the first one to be *xx* minutes physically active, or (b) the most physically active (most minutes of physical activity) in a period of time (set by the initiator). Also here, successful participants received bonus points (75% extra for first place, 50% extra for second place, and 25% extra for third place). In addition, they received medals for first (gold), second (silver), and third (bronze) places. Medals won were visible on the participants' personal page. The Lifestyle group participants received messages when they were invited to join a competition or engage in a social contract by SMS text and under "Messages" on their personal page in Lifestyle.

2.3. Measures. The outcome of primary interest in the study was change in physical activity behavior after the intervention was implemented. Daily report forms were used to assess physical activity. Participants reported what kind of physical activity they had completed that day (example given "walked fast to work"), the duration in minutes they engaged in this activity, and how strenuous each activity was using Borg's ratings of perceived exertion scale (RPE-scale; [46]) for a maximum of five activities each day. Borg's RPE scale ranges from 6 (no exertion at all) to 20 (maximal exertion). The scale is designed in such a way that approximate pulse can be found by multiplying the reported number with ten (e.g., if you score an activity as 8, your pulse during this activity would be around 80). It measures perceived exertion, which is the heaviness and strain experienced subjectively in physical activity, and is widely used as a measure of perceived physical exertion [47]. Using daily report forms constitutes a sort of day reconstruction method which relies on short recall periods. This method has the benefit of reducing errors and biases of recall [48]. One participant recorded car driving and shopping as exercise, while another recorded working. These activities were removed before further analyses were conducted. The daily report forms were completed every night of study weeks 1, 5, 9, and 12. Physical activity in minutes was added together to make a sum score for the weekly exercise minutes. The reported Borg scores for each activity were averaged to compute the average Borg score of each week. In addition, physical activity in minutes was combined with their respective Borg score (that is Borg x minutes) to compute an effectual physical activity score that was averaged.

2.4. Statistical Analyses. Data analyses were performed with SPSS for Windows (version 21, IBM corp.). The difference in physical activity minutes, Borg, and effectual physical activity between the control and the Lifestyle group in weeks 5, 9, and 12 was evaluated using an analysis of variance with a covariate (ANCOVA). Week 1 measures were included as a covariate in the model to control for the effect of initial physical activity. In all tests, differences were considered statistically significant if the P value was less than 0.05.

3. Results

The Lifestyle group participants registered 1046 activities in the physical activity (PA) planner. All of the participants used the PA planner, with a range from 31 to 178 activities for each of the participants, $M = 87.17$, $\mathrm{SD} = 44.24$. All of the Lifestyle group participants also tried out the contest component and eight of the twelve participants participated in at least one social contract.

The two groups started out with the same physical activity minute in the first measurement week (baseline): $M = 473.83$, $\mathrm{SD} = 237.95$ for the Lifestyle group and $M = 485.50$, $\mathrm{SD} = 221.40$ for the Control group, $F(1,18) = 0.030$, $P = 0.913$. The Borg intensity level was also equivalent for the two groups at this time point: $M = 12.53$, $\mathrm{SD} = 1.85$ for the Lifestyle group and $M = 12.41$, $\mathrm{SD} = 0.85$ for the control group, $F(1,18) = 0.030$, $P = 0.865$. After the onset of the intervention the Lifestyle group performed consistently more physical activity, at a higher intensity, than the control group. However, the differences between the two groups were not always significant (see Table 1).

TABLE 1: Analyses of covariance for means in minutes exercising, Borg, and minutes * Borg between the Lifestyle and the control group for the four measurement weeks. Significant ($P < 0.05$) F's in Bold.

	Minutes					Borg					Borg * Minutes				
	Lifestyle		Control			Lifestyle		Control			Lifestyle		Control		
	M (SD)	CI	M (SD)	CI	F	M (SD)	CI	M (SD)	CI	F	M (SD)	CI	M (SD)	CI	F
Week 1	473.83 (237.95)	322.65–625.02	485.50 (221.40)	300.40–670.60	0.012	12.53 (1.85)	11.35–13.71	12.41 (0.85)	11.79–13.12	0.030	159.36 (73.29)	112.79–205.93	176.64 (85.60)	105.08–248.20	0.234
Week 5	576.67 (235.29)	427.17–726.16	413.13 (224.42)	225.51–600.74	**4.739**	13.52 (1.98)	12.19–14.85	12.01 (2.00)	10.34–13.69	**5.208**	196.84 (109.01)	127.57–266.10	150.44 (196.84)	69.11–231.77	1.231
Week 9	660.25 (359.60)	431.77–888.73	377.25 (167.39)	237.31–517.19	**4.510**	13.25 (1.85)	12.07–14.43	11.95 (1.55)	10.51–13.39	3.213	247.53 (137.65)	160.07–334.99	114.95 (72.12)	54.65–175.24	**6.115**
Week 12	574.42 (434.74)	298.20–850.64	501.88 (232.90)	307.16–696.59	0.264	13.34 (2.22)	11.85–14.83	12.75 (1.08)	11.85–13.65	1.731	210.69 (156.13)	111.49–309.90	178.69 (89.56)	103.82–253.56	0.616

Note: week 1 measures of minutes, Borg, and Borg * minutes are included as a covariate in the analyses for week 5, 9, and 12.

As can be seen from Table 1, the Lifestyle group reported significantly more minutes of physical activity than the control group in week 5 (Lifestyle M = 576.67, SD = 235.29 versus control group M = 413.13, SD = 224.42, $F(1, 17)$ = 4.739, P = 0.044) and week 9 (Lifestyle group M = 660.25, SD = 359.60 versus control group M = 377.25, SD = 167.39, $F(1, 17)$ = 4.510, P = 0.049). In week 12 the difference between the two groups was no longer significant. In week 5 (the first measurement week after the intervention started), the Lifestyle group (M = 13.52, SD = 1.98) performed physical activity at a significantly higher Borg intensity level than the control group (M = 12.01, SD = 2.00), $F(1, 16)$ = 5.208, P = 0.037. In the other weeks there were no significant differences for the intensity of the exercise. For effectual physical activity (Borg $*$ minutes) there was a significant difference between the Lifestyle group (M = 247.53, SD = 137.65) and the control group (M = 114.95, SD = 72.12) only in week 9, $F(1, 17)$ = 6.115, P = .024.

4. Discussion

The present pilot study suggests that including gaming elements and SMS-text in an interactive, computer-tailored physical activity intervention is useful. All of the participants in the Lifestyle group registered physical activity in the online planner and received points when reporting back afterwards using SMS text. All of them also joined one or more competitions and the majority joined at least one social contract.

An initial boost in minutes of physical activity was observed. In week 5 the participants who received the intervention performed significantly more physical activity minutes than the control group and the effect was sustained in week 9. However, the effect was gone in the last registration week of the study period as observed elsewhere [21]. Corroborating this, newer studies and reviews continue to report declining effects over time [19, 49, 50]. The initial effect is promising. Despite few participants and high activity level at baseline (both groups exercised more than the recommended minimum amount in registration week 1), there was a significant increase in physical activity for the intervention group compared with the control group in weeks 5 and 9. By three months, although the Lifestyle group still performed more minutes of physical activity than the control group, the effect was not significant. The Lifestyle group also consistently reported performing more strenuous physical activity than the control group, and this difference was significant in week 5. In week 9 the combination of Borg and minutes was higher for participants in the Lifestyle group compared to the control group: participants receiving the intervention completed more physical activity at a higher intensity level than participants in the control group at this time. The intervention seems to have encouraged participant to do more moderate and vigorous exercise which is positive considering the dose-response relation between physical activity and health benefits [1].

Our results are supplement to the growing evidence supporting the effectiveness of online tailored physical activities for increasing physical activity [18–20, 51] and suggest using gamification and SMS texts as viable tools that need further investigation [52, 53].

This pilot study has some limitations. First, as this was an initial study with a small number of participants there are constraints regarding generalizing the results. However, finding a significant effect of the intervention even with only a small sample size attests to the robustness of the reported effects, at least for the population from which our sample was recruited. Because of the small sample size we were not able to analyze which components of the interventions were most effective in increasing physical activity. Feedback from participants suggested that the gaming components, especially the individual competition (advancing to the next status level for physical activity) and social competition (winning a competition), were highly motivating. Future studies with larger populations should identify which components are more effective.

Second, recruiting was done by self-selection; interested participants responded to an ad in the paper. This leaves us with highly motivated participants, and perhaps not those that need it the most [54]. Both the control and the Lifestyle group exercised more than the recommended guidelines at baseline (week 1) even though about half reported being passive three weeks before the baseline measure was completed. One possible explanation could be that the study started in January, which for some could mean a New Year resolution to exercise more. Also it could be a measurement effect; the daily report forms of physical activity (which both groups completed) would trigger awareness of own physical activity level which is an important starting point for behavior change [55–57]. However, even though the baseline measure was high, participants using Lifestyle Tool increased their physical activity and maintained a higher physical activity level than the control group throughout the study period.

Third, in this study, we used self-reports to measure physical activity. Although using daily report forms would reduce memory bias and thus yield more accurate reports than retrospective questions, participants still could report more physical activity than they actually completed (e.g., social bias). Measuring physical activity objectively; for example, using novel sensing technology already available in cell phones should be a goal for future studies.

In conclusion, using gamification in physical activity interventions is a fun and engaging way to help people achieve behavior change. The effect seems to drop off after some weeks though. Further development of gaming components in combination with using the mobile phone to stay connected with participants could help solve the adherence problem in intervention research. However, more research is needed in order to identify which components are more effective. The new technology increases opportunities to reach people where they are and when they need it. The entrance of smart phones allows further sophistication of interventions for health promotion and disease prevention; the challenge is to utilize the available technology optimally [26, 58]. However, text-messaging will likely continue to be used [59], especially in less developed countries.

Acknowledgments

This work was supported by the Norwegian Research Council (Grant no. 174934) and Telenor. The authors thank Arne Munch-Ellingsen and Anders Schürmann for developing and running the Intervention website and SMS data bank; they also thank Yngvil Søholt for her assistance in developing the layout for the Website and her involvement in the early phases of the Lifestyle Tool project.

References

[1] D. E. Warburton, C. W. Nicol, and S. S. Bredin, "Health benefits of physical activity: the evidence," *Canadian Medical Association Journal*, vol. 174, no. 6, pp. 801–809, 2006.

[2] World Health Organization, *Global Recommendations on Physical Activity for Health*, World Health Organization, Geneva, Swizerland, 2010.

[3] J. R. Morrow Jr., J. A. Krzewinski-Malone, A. W. Jackson, T. J. Bungum, and S. J. FitzGerald, "American adults' knowledge of exercise recommendations," *Research Quarterly for Exercise and Sport*, vol. 75, no. 3, pp. 231–237, 2004.

[4] W. L. Haskell, I.-M. Lee, R. R. Pate et al., "Physical activity and public health: updated recommendation for adults from the American college of sports medicine and the american heart association," *Medicine and Science in Sports and Exercise*, vol. 39, no. 8, pp. 1423–1434, 2007.

[5] M. Sjöström, P. Oja, M. Hagströmer, B. J. Smith, and A. Bauman, "Health-enhancing physical activity across European Union countries: the Eurobarometer study," *Journal of Public Health*, vol. 14, no. 5, pp. 291–300, 2006.

[6] L. M. Neville, B. O'Hara, and A. Milat, "Computer-tailored physical activity behavior change interventions targeting adults: a systematic review," *International Journal of Behavioral Nutrition and Physical Activity*, vol. 6, article 30, 2009.

[7] W. Kroeze, A. Werkman, and J. Brug, "A systematic review of randomized trials on the effectiveness of computer-tailored education on physical activity and dietary behaviors," *Annals of Behavioral Medicine*, vol. 31, no. 3, pp. 205–223, 2006.

[8] B. H. Marcus, B. A. Lewis, D. M. Williams et al., "A comparison of internet and print-based physical activity interventions," *Archives of Internal Medicine*, vol. 167, no. 9, pp. 944–949, 2007.

[9] B. S. Fjeldsoe, A. L. Marshall, and Y. D. Miller, "Behavior change interventions delivered by mobile telephone short-message service," *The American Journal of Preventive Medicine*, vol. 36, no. 2, pp. 165–173, 2009.

[10] H. Cole-Lewis and T. Kershaw, "Text messaging as a tool for behavior change in disease prevention and management," *Epidemiologic Reviews*, vol. 32, no. 1, pp. 56–69, 2010.

[11] S. Faghanipour, E. Hajikazemi, S. Nikpour, S. A.-S. Shariatpanahi, and A. F. Hosseini, "Mobile phone short message service (SMS) for weight management in iranian overweight and obese women: a pilot study," *International Journal of Telemedicine and Applications*, vol. 2013, Article ID 785654, 5 pages, 2013.

[12] H. Spittaels, I. de Bourdeaudhuij, J. Brug, and C. Vandelanotte, "Effectiveness of an online computer-tailored physical activity intervention in a real-life setting," *Health Education Research*, vol. 22, no. 3, pp. 385–396, 2007.

[13] G. J. Norman, M. F. Zabinski, M. A. Adams, D. E. Rosenberg, A. L. Yaroch, and A. A. Atienza, "A review of eHealth interventions for physical activity and dietary behavior change," *The American Journal of Preventive Medicine*, vol. 33, no. 4, pp. 336.e16–345.e16, 2007.

[14] B. A. Lewis, D. M. Williams, C. J. Neighbors, J. M. Jakicic, and B. H. Marcus, "Cost analysis of Internet versus print interventions for physical activity promotion," *Psychology of Sport and Exercise*, vol. 11, no. 3, pp. 246–249, 2010.

[15] M. L. A. Lustria, J. Cortese, S. M. Noar, and R. L. Glueckauf, "Computer-tailored health interventions delivered over the web: review and analysis of key components," *Patient Education and Counseling*, vol. 74, no. 2, pp. 156–173, 2009.

[16] V. S. Conn, A. R. Hafdahl, and D. R. Mehr, "Interventions to increase physical activity among healthy adults: meta-analysis of outcomes," *The American Journal of Public Health*, vol. 101, no. 4, pp. 751–758, 2011.

[17] C. Vandelanotte, K. M. Spathonis, E. G. Eakin, and N. Owen, "Website-delivered physical activity interventions: a review of the literature," *The American Journal of Preventive Medicine*, vol. 33, no. 1, pp. 54–64, 2007.

[18] R. Hurling, M. Catt, M. de Boni et al., "Using internet and mobile phone technology to deliver an automated physical activity program: randomized controlled trial," *Journal of Medical Internet Research*, vol. 9, no. 2, article e7, 2007.

[19] M. Gotsis, H. Wang, D. Spruijt-Metz, M. Jordan-Marsh, and T. W. Valente, "Wellness partners: design and evaluation of a web-based physical activity diary with social gaming features for adults," *JMIR Research Protocols*, vol. 2, no. 1, article e10, 2013.

[20] L. J. Carr, S. I. Dunsiger, B. Lewis et al., "Randomized controlled trial testing an internet physical activity intervention for sedentary adults," *Health Psychology*, vol. 32, no. 3, pp. 328–336, 2013.

[21] M. A. Napolitano, M. Fotheringham, D. Tate et al., "Evaluation of an internet-based physical activity intervention: a preliminary investigation," *Annals of Behavioral Medicine*, vol. 25, no. 2, pp. 92–99, 2003.

[22] G. B. Svendsen, Y. Søholt, A. Munch-Ellingsen, D. Gammon, and A. Schürmann, "The importance of being useful and fun: factors influencing intention to use a mobile system motivating for physical activity," in *Proceedings of the 42nd Hawaii International Conference on System Sciences (HICSS '09)*, pp. 1–10, Big Island, Hawaii, USA, January 2009.

[23] S. L. Ferney and A. L. Marshall, "Website physical activity interventions: preferences of potential users," *Health Education Research*, vol. 21, no. 4, pp. 560–566, 2006.

[24] C. Davies, K. Corry, A. van Itallie, C. Vandelanotte, C. Caperchione, and W. K. Mummery, "Prospective associations between intervention components and website engagement in a publicly available physical activity website: the case of 10,000 steps Australia," *Journal of Medical Internet Research*, vol. 14, no. 1, article e4, 2012.

[25] A. W. Hansen, M. Grønbæk, J. W. Helge, M. Severin, T. Curtis, and J. S. Tolstrup, "Effect of a web-based intervention to promote physical activity and improve health among physically inactive adults: a population-based randomized controlled trial," *Journal of Medical Internet Research*, vol. 14, no. 5, article e145, 2012.

[26] M. Kirwan, M. J. Duncan, C. Vandelanotte, and W. K. Mummery, "Using smartphone technology to monitor physical

activity in the 10,000 steps program: a matched case-control trial," *Journal of Medical Internet Research*, vol. 14, no. 2, article e55, 2012.

[27] D. King, F. Greaves, C. Exeter, and A. Darzi, "'Gamification': influencing health behaviours with games," *Journal of the Royal Society of Medicine*, vol. 106, no. 3, pp. 76–78, 2013.

[28] B. A. Primack, M. V. Carroll, M. McNamara et al., "Role of video games in improving health-related outcomes: a systematic review," *The American Journal of Preventive Medicine*, vol. 42, no. 6, pp. 630–638, 2012.

[29] S. Deterding, D. Dixon, R. Khaled, and L. Nacke, "From game design elements to gamefulness: defining gamification," in *Proceedings of the 15th International Academic MindTrek Conference: Envisioning Future Media Environments*, pp. 9–15, ACM, New York, NY, USA, 2011.

[30] T. L. Webb, J. Joseph, L. Yardley, and S. Michie, "Using the internet to promote health behavior change: a systematic review and meta-analysis of the impact of theoretical basis, use of behavior change techniques, and mode of delivery on efficacy," *Journal of Medical Internet Research*, vol. 12, no. 1, article e4, 2010.

[31] A. Soureti, P. Murray, M. Cobain, M. Chinapaw, W. van Mechelen, and R. Hurling, "Exploratory study of web-based planning and mobile text reminders in an overweight population," *Journal of Medical Internet Research*, vol. 13, no. 4, article e118, 2011.

[32] International Telecommunication Union, *World in 2013: ICT Facts and Figures*, International Telecommunication Union, Geneva, Switzerland, 2013.

[33] S. M. Kelders, R. N. Kok, H. C. Ossebaard, and J. E. van Gemert-Pijnen, "Persuasive system design does matter: a systematic review of adherence to web-based interventions," *Journal of Medical Internet Research*, vol. 14, no. 6, article e152, 2012.

[34] G. A. O. O'Reilly and D. Spruijt-Metz, "Current mHealth technologies for physical activity assessment and promotion," *The American Journal of Preventive Medicine*, vol. 45, no. 4, pp. 501–507, 2013.

[35] J. Wei, I. Hollin, and S. Kachnowski, "A review of the use of mobile phone text messaging in clinical and healthy behaviour interventions," *Journal of Telemedicine and Telecare*, vol. 17, no. 1, pp. 41–48, 2011.

[36] S. Krishna, S. A. Boren, and E. A. Balas, "Healthcare via cell phones: a systematic review," *Telemedicine and e-Health*, vol. 15, no. 3, pp. 231–240, 2009.

[37] A. L. Dunn, B. H. Marcus, J. B. Kampert, M. E. Garcia, H. W. Kohl III, and S. N. Blair, "Comparison of lifestyle and structured interventions to increase physical activity and cardiorespiratory fitness: randomized trial," *The Journal of the American Medical Association*, vol. 281, no. 4, pp. 327–334, 1999.

[38] B. H. Marcus, V. C. Selby, R. S. Niaura, and J. S. Rossi, "Self-efficacy and the stages of exercise behavior change," *Research Quarterly for Exercise and Sport*, vol. 63, no. 1, pp. 60–66, 1992.

[39] K. F. Schulz, D. G. Altman, and D. Moher, "CONSORT 2010 statement: updated guidelines for reporting parallel group randomised trials," *The British Medical Journal*, vol. 340, article c332, 2010.

[40] J. Hintze, "PASS 12," http://www.ncss.com/.

[41] D. Markland and V. Tobin, "A modification to the behavioural regulation in exercise questionnaire to include an assessment of amotivation," *Journal of Sport and Exercise Psychology*, vol. 26, no. 2, pp. 191–196, 2004.

[42] E. Mullan, D. Markland, and D. K. Ingledew, "A graded conceptualisation of self-determination in the regulation of exercise behaviour: development of a measure using confirmatory factor analytic procedures," *Personality and Individual Differences*, vol. 23, no. 5, pp. 745–752, 1997.

[43] S. Michie, C. Abraham, C. Whittington, J. McAteer, and S. Gupta, "Effective techniques in healthy eating and physical activity interventions: a meta-regression," *Health Psychology*, vol. 28, no. 6, pp. 690–701, 2009.

[44] C. J. Greaves, K. E. Sheppard, C. Abraham et al., "Systematic review of reviews of intervention components associated with increased effectiveness in dietary and physical activity interventions," *BMC Public Health*, vol. 11, article 119, 2011.

[45] A. Dijkstra, "Working mechanisms of computer-tailored health education: evidence from smoking cessation," *Health Education Research*, vol. 20, no. 5, pp. 527–539, 2005.

[46] G. Borg, *An Introduction to Borg's RPE-Scale*, Mouvement Publications, Ithaca, NY, USA, 1985.

[47] G. Borg, *Borg's Perceived Exertion and Pain Scales*, Human Kinetics, Champaign, Ill, USA, 1998.

[48] D. Kahneman, A. B. Krueger, D. A. Schkade, N. Schwarz, and A. A. Stone, "A survey method for characterizing daily life experience: the day reconstruction method," *Science*, vol. 306, no. 5702, pp. 1776–1780, 2004.

[49] L. M. Hamel, L. B. Robbins, and J. Wilbur, "Computer- and web-based interventions to increase preadolescent and adolescent physical activity: a systematic review," *Journal of Advanced Nursing*, vol. 67, no. 2, pp. 251–268, 2011.

[50] L. F. Kohl, R. Crutzen, and N. K. de Vries, "Online prevention aimed at lifestyle behaviors: a systematic review of reviews," *Journal of Medical Internet Research*, vol. 15, no. 7, article e146, 2013.

[51] H. Spittaels, I. de Bourdeaudhuij, and C. Vandelanotte, "Evaluation of a website-delivered computer-tailored intervention for increasing physical activity in the general population," *Preventive Medicine*, vol. 44, no. 3, pp. 209–217, 2007.

[52] J. Fanning, S. P. Mullen, and E. McAuley, "Increasing physical activity with mobile devices: a meta-analysis," *Journal of Medical Internet Research*, vol. 14, no. 6, article e161, 2011.

[53] B. S. Fjeldsoe, Y. D. Miller, and A. L. Marshall, "MobileMums: a randomized controlled trial of an SMS-based physical activity intervention," *Annals of Behavioral Medicine*, vol. 39, no. 2, pp. 101–111, 2010.

[54] M. W. Verheijden, M. P. Jans, V. H. Hildebrandt, and M. Hopman-Rock, "Rates and determinants of repeated participation in a web-based behavior change program for healthy body weight and healthy lifestyle," *Journal of Medical Internet Research*, vol. 9, no. 1, article e1, 2007.

[55] E. M. van Sluijs, M. N. van Poppel, J. W. Twisk, and W. van Mechelen, "Physical activity measurements affected participants' behavior in a randomized controlled trial," *Journal of Clinical Epidemiology*, vol. 59, no. 4, pp. 404–411, 2006.

[56] B. H. Marcus, L. H. Forsyth, E. J. Stone et al., "Physical activity behavior change: issues in adoption and maintenance," *Health Psychology*, vol. 19, no. 1, supplement, pp. 32–41, 2000.

[57] N. D. Weinstein, A. J. Rothman, and S. R. Sutton, "Stage theories of health behavior: conceptual and methodological issues," *Health Psychology*, vol. 17, no. 3, pp. 290–299, 1998.

[58] R. M. Kaplan and A. A. Stone, "Bringing the laboratory and clinic to the community: mobile technologies for health

8

Scheduling in Sensor Grid Middleware for Telemedicine Using ABC Algorithm

T. Vigneswari[1,2] and M. A. Maluk Mohamed[2]

[1] *Kings College of Engineering, Punalkulam, Tamilnadu 613303, India*

[2] *System Software Group, M.A.M College of Engineering, Tiruchirappalli, Tamilnadu 621105, India*

Correspondence should be addressed to T. Vigneswari; jayasuriyaus@yahoo.com

Academic Editor: Fei Hu

Advances in microelectromechanical systems (MEMS) and nanotechnology have enabled design of low power wireless sensor nodes capable of sensing different vital signs in our body. These nodes can communicate with each other to aggregate data and transmit vital parameters to a base station (BS). The data collected in the base station can be used to monitor health in real time. The patient wearing sensors may be mobile leading to aggregation of data from different BS for processing. Processing real time data is compute-intensive and telemedicine facilities may not have appropriate hardware to process the real time data effectively. To overcome this, sensor grid has been proposed in literature wherein sensor data is integrated to the grid for processing. This work proposes a scheduling algorithm to efficiently process telemedicine data in the grid. The proposed algorithm uses the popular swarm intelligence algorithm for scheduling to overcome the NP complete problem of grid scheduling. Results compared with other heuristic scheduling algorithms show the effectiveness of the proposed algorithm.

1. Introduction

Telemedicine plays a very important role in patient management and has been effectively used for intrahospital transport of patients. Live monitoring of patients across hospitals creates new challenges. Similar issues arise as where to process the data captured in real time. Sensor grid can overcome some of the challenges faced in telemedicine.

Human life can be made more comprehensive by equipping it with modern diagnosis which utilizes the advancement in the field of information and communication and this arena is termed as telemedicine. Sensor grid is one among the computing methods which can be used efficiently to provide such a service. Grid computing [1, 2] is a growing distributed computing paradigm which enables coordinated sharing of heterogeneous resources across the globe. Sensor networks have [3] group of sensor nodes that are deployed to receive real time values about the parameters which they sense. Sensor grid [4] is the integration of sensor network and grid computing by which both of the paradigms can complement each other with their own strengths.

The advantages of merging sensor network and grid computing to form sensor grids [5, 6] include the following.

(i) Large amount of real time data generated by sensors can be processed and stored in the grid.

(ii) Set of sensors can be shared by different user based on the application they are using.

(iii) Pervasive seamless access to sensor data is made possible.

A sensor grid architecture to monitor patients who have undergone transplantation surgery is proposed in our previous work which includes the architecture for the sensor middleware [7, 8]. Scheduling component is a significant constituent in the proposed middleware. In general, scheduling discovers resources and allocates suitable tasks on appropriate resource to meet the requirement of the job handled. The major criteria for a good scheduling algorithm are response time, optimized resource utilization, load balancing, and meeting QoS constraints.

The scheduler in grid assigns jobs to the resources in an optimum way. Jobs arrive at the grid environment specifying the requirement about the resources. The assignment of jobs to the resources should be optimal to minimize the makespan, minimize the cost of allocated resources, and maximize the throughput [9]. Grid monitoring [10] collects the status and performance details of a large-scale distribution system. The parameters such as load on the system, number of jobs in the running state, and the performance of each job in running state are gathered to notify the behavior of the grid environment to the consumers.

Various scheduling algorithms have been proposed in literature for the grid environment. All algorithms fall into the taxonomy proposed in [11]. The first level in taxonomy is local versus global scheduling algorithms. In local scheduling, scheduler schedules the processes available on a single CPU. Global scheduler allocates processes to multiple CPUs. Grid scheduling uses global scheduling. Global scheduling uses static and dynamic scheduling. In static scheduling, the information about the jobs and resources are available at the time of scheduling. In dynamic scheduling, it is impossible to predict the arrival time and resource request of jobs, earlier to the time of scheduling. First in first out (FIFO), balance constrained techniques, and cost constrained techniques are some of the techniques which have been used in grids [12].

Due to the NP completeness of grid scheduling, metaheuristics techniques like particle swarm optimization (PSO), ant colony optimization (ACO), genetic algorithm (GA), and artificial bee colony (ABC) have been used effectively for grid scheduling [13–16].

This paper proposes ABC algorithm that can be used in scheduling of resource for the middleware discussed in [8] to provide a scheduling solution which optimizes the makespan of the submitted task.

2. Related Works

Telemedicine architecture using a sensor with P2P overlay has been proposed and a middleware has been developed for the abovementioned architecture. Among the middleware components, scheduling plays an inevitable role such that a proper scheduling may save a life. The data sets from the sensor should be scheduled to a computational resource for execution in the SaaS. The SaaS may send alert if the vital signs are abnormal and doctor reviews the patient immediately. An analysis of execution times of scheduling algorithms in [17] shows that taboo search algorithm is a suitable choice for applications including telemedicine involving static scheduling. The creation time is relatively small and simultaneously average execution time of the schedule is minimal. The total processor cycle consumption model [18] has shown to be useful for independent and coarse-grain task scheduling, that is, scheduling in which the computation time in grid nodes is superior to data transmission time.

A resource-performance-fluctuation-aware workflow scheduling algorithm proposed in [19] considers dynamic resource performance fluctuation in the grid, and scheduling is performed according to its knowledge of the fluctuation. This new algorithm works in an offline way which allows it to be easily set up and run with lower cost. The variation in the computing capability of heterogeneous nodes is also reflected on our proposed algorithm. A scheduling algorithm based on PSO [20] is proposed for task scheduling problem on computational grids. The proposed system reduced minimum completion time (MCT). In [21], adaptive workload balancing algorithm (AWLB) was incorporated into the distributed analysis environment (DIANE) user-level scheduling (ULS) environment. This gives the capability to select resources by the AWLB which is most suitable for the application, and the ULS environment is equipped with an advanced strategy to optimize resource usage. Optimization of the workload performed by the AWLB is adaptable to the resource characteristics (CPU power, memory, network bandwidth, input/output (I/O) speed, etc.) and to the corresponding application requirements.

Two models to predict job completion time in a service grid were proposed by Gao et al. [22]. The single service model predicts job completion time in a grid providing only one service type. Multiple services model predicts job completion time in a grid offering multiple types of services. To confront new challenges in grid environment job scheduling, Fidanova and Durchova [23] presented a heuristic scheduling algorithm designed to achieve high throughput computing in a grid environment. The authors proposed ACO which guarantees load balancing.

Fidanova [24] introduced a grid computing tasks scheduling algorithm based on simulated annealing (SA). Tasks are first collected in a set and then scheduled. So task arrival time is unimportant. Tasks scheduled on the same machine form a local queue related to the machine. Tasks queue is sent on to the machine when running tasks from a previous queue. Thus, sending time does not influence makespan time.

Scheduling workflows problem regarding quality of service (QoS) requirements is challenging. Though there are algorithms for grid workflow scheduling, most tackle problems with a single QoS parameter or with smaller workflows. An ACO algorithm to schedule large-scale workflows with various QoS parameters was proposed by Chen and Zhang [25] which enabled users to specify their QoS preferences and also define minimum QoS thresholds for specific applications. The algorithm's objective is to find a solution meeting all QoS constraints and optimizing the user-preferred QoS parameter. Based on workflow scheduling characteristics, 7 new heuristics for ACO approach were designed and an adaptive scheme that allowed artificial ants to select pheromone value based heuristics was proposed. Experiments done on ten workflow applications with 120 tasks demonstrate the proposed algorithm's effectiveness.

Di Martino and Mililotti [26] designed a two-level scheduling system, with the first level being formed by a computing nodes set (the sites participating in the grid)—each with a local scheduling policy—and a second level formed by super scheduler. The local scheduler accepts one job at a time and allocates it on local hardware regarding current (local) information. Results of grid jobs allocation simulation were presented. Garg and Singh [27] proposed the design/implementation of hierarchical discrete particle swarm optimization (H-DPSO) for grid environment's dependent task scheduling. In HDPSO, particles are dynamic, hierarchically arranged with good particles lying above and having much influence on swarm. The biobjective version of the problem is to minimize makespan and total cost simultaneously when optimization criteria were considered. The H-DPSO based scheduler was evaluated through various application task graphs. Simulation analysis shows that H-DPSO based scheduling for grid computing is highly viable and effective.

A binary artificial bee colony (BABC) algorithm for grid computing scheduling was proposed by Kim et al. [28]. An efficient binary artificial bee colony extension of BABC that incorporates a flexible ranking strategy (FRS) to improve balance between exploration and exploitation was proposed. The FRS generates and uses new solutions for diversified search in early generations and speeds up convergence in latter generations. Two variants to minimize the makespan were introduced. A fixed number of best solutions are employed with FRS in the first, while in the second the number of best solutions is reduced with every new generation. Simulation results for benchmark job scheduling issues reveal that the proposed method's performance is better than alternatives like SA, GA, and PSO.

Khanli et al. [29] presented a reliable job scheduler using resource fault occurrence history (RFOH) in grid computing. To improve the reliability, RFOH stored the number of faults occurring and number of jobs in execution. Based on the RFOH information genetic algorithm (GA) was used to find an optimum schedule. Pooranian et al. presented GLOA (a new job scheduling algorithm for grid computing) [30]. Group leader optimization algorithm (GLOA) is an optimization algorithm inspired by the role of leaders in a social group. The problem space was separated into multiple small parts, and each part was processed separately to find an optimal solution in parallel. GLOA was used to find an optimum schedule for the arrival of jobs with available resources. GLOA reached optimal solution quickly. Result showed that makespan was lower when comparingto all other traditional scheduling algorithms.

Karimi and Motameni presented tasks scheduling in computational grid using a hybrid discrete particle swarm optimization (HDPSO) [31]. The initial solution was obtained by Min-Min algorithm. For each job, the set of minimum completion time on all the available processors were found. Then, for each task, processor was selected which gave minimum expected completion time. Simulations were conducted with a specific number of jobs, and the processing time for each processor was preassumed. Makespan and throughput were taken for evaluating the performance of the scheduling. Results were compared with algorithms such as Min-Min and Max-Min algorithms. Comparison showed that HDPSO algorithm gave minimum makespan and maximum throughput. Mandloi and Gupta presented adaptive job scheduling for computational grid based on ACO with genetic parameter selection [32].

Selvi and Umarani presented comparative study of GA and ABC for job scheduling [33]. For efficient job scheduling in a grid environment, functions similar to genetic operations and bees behaviour were combined. Numerical results showed that hybrid GA-ABC job scheduling gave high accuracy and efficiency with minimum job completion time when comparing to GA and ABC scheduling algorithms.

Apart from these generic scheduling algorithms, some algorithms in context with telemedicine are also investigated. A sensor schedule service [34] injects the sensors in the targets based on the request from user. The sensor schedule is designed in a way such that it provides availability, fidelity, and QoS along with economy. Service-oriented grid [35] has been developed by GEMSS project to support the provision of medical simulation services by service providers to clients such as hospitals. It uses queue scheduling with advanced reservation for allocating resources. Arogyasree [36] introduced a context-aware scheduling which schedules patients to appropriate doctor based on the ailment they can handle with lesser response time. A grid middleware [37] that practices event based communication in in vivo sensor nodes consists of a lightweight rendezvous algorithm. This algorithm schedules temperature for in vivo sensor nodes deployed for joint operation of hyperthermia, radiotherapy, and chemotherapy.

3. Structural Overview

Sensors attached to the patient's body send the vital sign values to the grid through a mobile device. The grid is designed as a two-layered P2P architecture to avoid centralized control. The peer to peer arrangement of grid nodes also improves scalability and fault tolerance. The first layer is the structured P2P layer used for analyzing the vital sign parameters. An application to analyze the values is made available in the grid nodes as SaaS. During the analysis if the SaaS finds that the parameter values exceed beyond normal values, an alert message is sent to the physician. The physician advises proper medication accordingly. The sensors are also abstracted as objects and stored in this layer. The second layer is a structured P2P layer for storing the vital parameter values. The patient or physician can retrieve the data from the database to know the history of a particular patient. This data can be shared with proper access rights. Distributed pipe communication is used for all the communications that take place between the sensors and grid nodes. The architectural overview is shown in Figure 1.

The proposed middleware is shown in Figure 2 and has been designed to achieve the scope of the above given architecture. The sensor data is sent to a data acquisition system (DAS) which acts as a mobile base station. Then a data conversion element in the middleware converts into xml format so that it can be used in grid. The scheduling component allocates computational resource for analyzing these data sets in the SaaS. The nodes participating in the grid are grouped into zones based on their locality. The grid archive system stores the patient history in a database with timestamp for continuous monitoring.

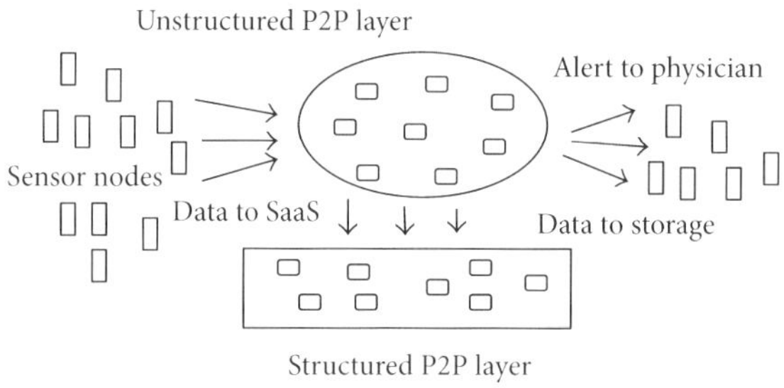

FIGURE 1: Structural overview.

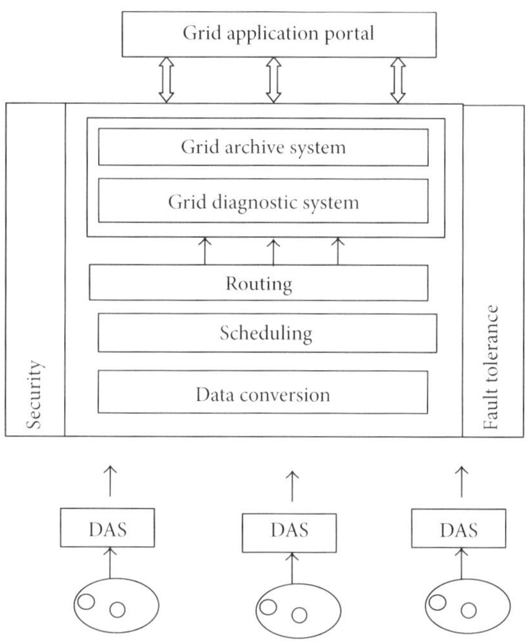

FIGURE 2: Middleware architecture.

4. Scheduling Algorithm

The middleware proposed by us aids in continuous monitoring of patients and sends alerts to the doctors if the patients vital sign values are abnormal. The data sets from DAS should be scheduled to a computational resource to analyze the data. The scheduling component should efficiently use the resources. In this regard, we have adapted ABC for resource scheduling.

4.1. Methodology. Artificial bee colony algorithm is based on the social behavior of honey bee colonies, and it can be applied to several optimization problems [14]. Honey bees share information about the location, quantity, and quality of foods. This information sharing activity can be used for resource management problems of grid scheduling. There are three types of honey bees in a bee colony. They are onlooker bees, employed bees, and scout bees. Employed bees search the locations of food in parallel and inform other bees by dancing. Onlooker bees evaluate and select the best solution among the solutions given by all the employed bees. Scout bees start a new search for solution [38].

4.2. Artificial Bee Colony Algorithm (ABC). A bee colony is considered a swarm with bees as individual agents. Each low-level component bee works through a global level swarm component to form a system. Thus, system's global behaviour is determined from individual's local behaviour where interactions/coordination among individuals lead to an organized system characterized by interacting collective behaviour through labour division, distributed simultaneous task performance, self-organization, and specialized individuals. Information exchange among bees results in formation of tuned collective knowledge [39].

ABC is designed to handle numerical optimization problems [40]. It is based in two natural processes: recruitment of bees to a food source and source abandonment. The difference between ABC and other swarm intelligence algorithms is that, in the former, problem's solutions are represented by food sources, not bees. In comparison, bees act as variation operators discovering new food sources based on existing ones. Three bee types are considered in ABC: employed, onlooker, and scout bees. The employed bees are equal in number to the number of food sources with an employed bee being assigned to each food source. On reaching the source, the bee calculates a new solution and retains the best solution (using greedy heuristics). When a source fails to improve after many iterations, it is dumped and replaced by food source located by a scout bee, which in turn involves a random calculation of a new solution.

4.3. The Procedure of ABC. Classical ABC includes 4 phases [41].

Initialization Phase. Food sources, with SN population size, are generated randomly by scout bees. The artificial bee number is NP. Each food source x_m is a vector to optimization problem, x_m has D variables, and D is searching space dimension of objective function needing optimization. Initiation food sources are produced randomly by

$$x_m = l_i + \text{rand}(0, 1) * (u_i - l_i), \quad (1)$$

where u_i and l_i are upper and lower bound of the objective function's solution space and rand(0, 1) is a random number within the range [0, 1].

Employed Bee Phase. Employed bees fly and locate a new food source in the food source's neighbourhood. A high quantity food source is selected. A neighbour food source v_{mi} is determined/calculated by

$$v_{mi} = x_{mi} + \phi_{mi}(x_{mi} - x_{ki}), \quad (2)$$

where x_k is randomly selected food source, i is randomly chosen parameter index, and ϕ_{mi} is a random number within range [−1, 1]. The food source fitness is essential to find a global optimal. In ABC, fitness is computed using (3), after which a greedy selection is applied between x_m and v_m:

$$\text{fit}_m(x_m) = \left\{ \begin{array}{l} \dfrac{1}{1 + f_m(x_m)}, f_m(x_m) > 0 \\ 1 + |f_m(x_m), f_m(x_m) < 0| \end{array} \right\}, \quad (3)$$

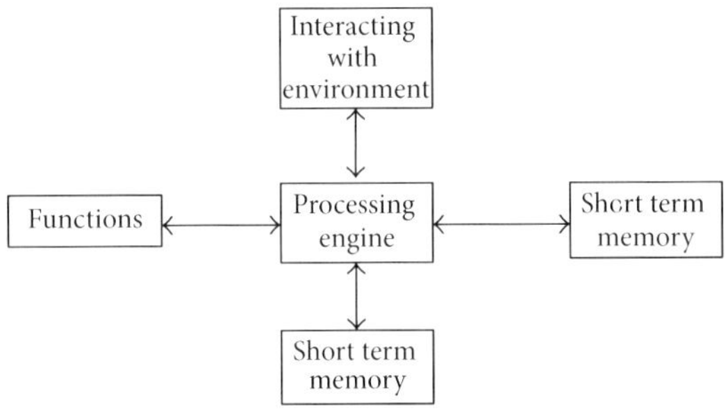

FIGURE 3: Architecture of artificial bee colony system.

where $f_m(x_m)$ is the objective function value of x_m. In this work, makespan and available bandwidth based objective function were used.

Onlooker Bee Phase. Onlooker bees see waggle dance in dance area and calculate food sources profitability and randomly choose a higher food source. Food source quantity is evaluated by profitability (P_m) of all food sources. P_m is determined by

$$P_m = \frac{\text{fit}_m(x_m)}{\sum_{m-1}^{\text{SN}} \text{fit}_m(x_m)}, \quad (4)$$

where $\text{fit}_m(x_m)$ is the fitness of x_m. The objective function and fitness function used in this work are the same.

Scout Phase. The scouts randomly search for new solutions. If solution x_i is abandoned, a new solution x_m is discovered. x_m is defined by

$$x_m = l_i + \text{rand}(0,1) * (u_i - l_i), \quad (5)$$

where x_m is new generated food source, rand(0, 1) is a random number within range [0, 1], and u_i and l_i are upper and lower bound of objective function's solution space.

The architecture of an ABC system is shown in Figure 3.

In the algorithm's first step, $\vec{x}_i$ $(i = 1, \ldots, \text{SN})$ solutions are randomly produced where SN is total number of food sources. In the algorithm's second step, for every employed bee, whose total number equals half the number of food sources, a new source is produced through (2). In the algorithm's third step, an onlooker bee chooses a food source with probability given by (4) and produces a new source in chosen food source site by (2). Onlookers are distributed to good food sources only, thus eliminating suboptimal solutions. If number of iterations by which a source cannot be improved is bigger than a predetermined limit, source is considered exhausted. Employed bee linked to exhausted source is now a scout searching randomly in the problem domain by

$$x_{ij} = x_j^{\min} + (x_j^{\max} - x_j^{\min}) * \text{rand}. \quad (6)$$

Simulations are conducted with 25 jobs, and the resources are grouped into 5 clusters. Using dynamic arrival time of jobs with different requirement of resources, the proposed ABC scheduling algorithm is run five times. During every run, makespan value is recorded. Figure 4 shows the obtained average makespan and Figure 5 shows the individual makespan obtained in each run.

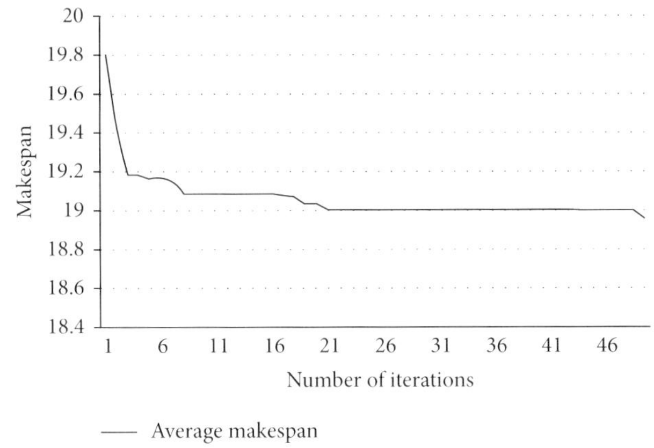

FIGURE 4: Average makespan.

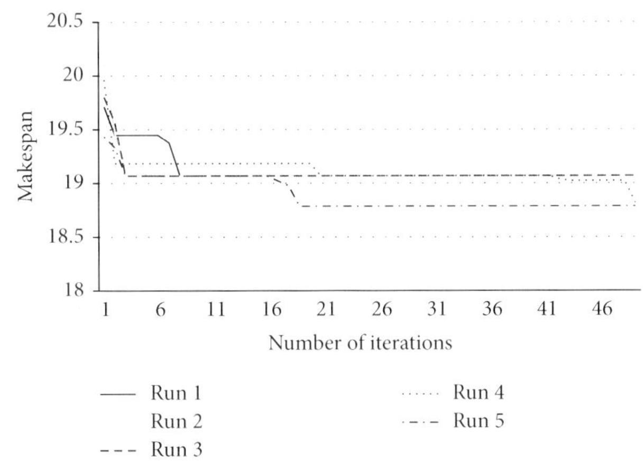

FIGURE 5: Makespan for all the 5 runs with 50 iterations.

TABLE 1: Average makespan.

Number of jobs	Number of resources = 5			Number of resources = 15		
	Min-Min	ACO	ABC	Min-Min	ACO	ABC
25	19.42	19.34	18.81	7.02	7.02	6.82
75	59.78	59.82	57.86	21.48	21.41	20.71
125	101.24	101.09	98.29	34.62	34.12	33.27
175	142.64	141.98	137.52	49.54	49.55	48.09

Simulations were also conducted by varying the number of jobs from 25 to 175 in increments of 25 and also increasing the number of resources from five to fifteen. The proposed ABC is compared with Min-Min scheduling and ACO based scheduling. Table 1 shows the average makespan obtained for different number of jobs and resources.

It is observed from the results that the makespan reduces significantly as the number of resources increases. The proposed ABC reduces makespan when compared to Min-Min scheduling and ACO scheduling in the ranges of

TABLE 2: Resource utilization.

Number of jobs	Number of resources = 5			Number of resources = 15		
	Min-Min	ACO	ABC	Min-Min	ACO	ABC
25	68.64	81.06	80.12	70.27	74.87	73.34
75	69.75	82.26	81.2	70.51	80.28	78.75
125	70.09	83.33	81.9	71.57	80.34	78.75
175	70.11	83.11	82.05	72.17	81.13	79.76

TABLE 3: Standard deviation (±).

Number of jobs	Number of resources = 5			Number of resources = 15		
	Min-Min	ACO	ABC	Min-Min	ACO	ABC
25	0.83	0.7	0.68	0.89	0.82	0.81
75	0.73	0.42	0.42	0.79	0.88	0.87
125	0.66	0.45	0.45	0.7	0.33	0.33
175	0.75	0.46	0.45	0.41	0.46	0.46

2.9% to 3.66% and 2.78% to 3.33%, respectively. Similarly, the proposed technique improves the makespan in the range of 2.89% to 3.98% compared to Min-Min scheduling and by 2.52% to 3.32% compared to ACO method when the number of resources is fifteen.

Table 2 shows the resource utilization.

From Table 2, it is seen that the resource utilization by proposed technique is higher. The proposed ABC improves resource utilization when compared to Min-Min scheduling in the range of 15.17% to 15.69% and by 1.16% to 1.73% when compared to ACO scheduling when the number of resources is 5. Table 3 shows the standard deviation obtained across five runs.

It is observed from Table 3 that the standard deviation for the proposed ABC is significantly lower than that of Min-Min scheduling justifying the stability of the proposed algorithm. The inherent advantages of the ABC algorithm such as the algorithm requiring fewer control parameters and good balance between local and global search processes produce better results as observed from the simulation results.

5. Conclusion

A sensor grid middleware has been designed to receive vital sign from the patients and monitor them continuously to check for abnormality. The scheduling component of this middleware is an imperative element which schedules the data to computational resource for executing in a SaaS. In this paper, we have adapted ABC scheduling algorithm which will efficiently schedule the data sets to computational resource to meet out the scope of the middleware successfully. Simulations are conducted with different number of jobs and resources. From the obtained simulations, it can be observed that proposed ABC algorithm performs better than ACO and Min-Min scheduling.

References

[1] I. Foster, C. Kesselman, and S. Tuecke, "The anatomy of the grid: enabling scalable virtual organizations," *International Journal of High Performance Computing Applications*, vol. 15, no. 3, pp. 200–222, 2001.

[2] I. Foster, C. Kesselman, J. Nick, and S. Tuecke, *The Physiology of the Grid: An Open Grid Services Architecture for Distributed Systems Integration*, Open Grid Service Infrastructure WG, Global Grid Forum, June 2002.

[3] I. F. Akyildiz, W. Su, Y. Sankarasubramaniam, and E. Cayirci, "Wireless sensor networks: a survey," *Computer Networks*, vol. 38, no. 4, pp. 393–422, 2002.

[4] M. Gaynor, S. L. Moulton, M. Welsh, E. LaCombe, A. Rowan, and J. Wynne, "Integrating wireless sensor networks with the grid," *IEEE Internet Computing*, vol. 8, no. 4, pp. 32–39, 2004.

[5] B. L. Hock, M. T. Yong, P. Mukherjee, T. L. Vinh, F. W. Weng, and S. Simon, "Sensor grid: integration of wireless sensor networks and the grid," in *Proceedings of the IEEE Conference on Local Computer Networks—30th Anniversary (LCN '05)*, pp. 91–98, Sydney, Australia, November 2005.

[6] C.-K. Tham and R. Buyya, "Sensorgrid: integrating sensor networks and grid computing," *Computer Society of India (CSI) Communications*, vol. 29, no. 1, pp. 24–29, 2005.

[7] M. A. M. Mohamed and T. Vigneswari, "Sensor grid architecture for health care monitoring," in *Proceedings of the 99th Indian Science Congress*, vol. 3 - 7, Bhubaneswar, India, January 2012.

[8] T. Vigneswari and M. A. Maluk Mohamed, "Sensor grid middleware for health care monitoring," in *Proceedings of the International Conference on Advancements in Information Technology*, Hong Kong, June 2012.

[9] M. Ruda and H. Rudová, "Grid scheduling and monitoring," in *Proceedings of the 4th Annual Workshop of the UK Planning and Scheduling Special Interest Group (PLANSIG '05)*, pp. 98–99, City University, London, UK, 2005.

[10] A. Krenek, "C-GMA—capability-based grid monitoring architecture," Tech. Rep. 6/2005, CESNET, Prague, Czech Republic, 2005.

[11] T. L. Casavant and J. G. Kuhl, "A taxonomy of scheduling in general-purpose distributed computing systems," *IEEE Transactions on Software Engineering*, vol. 14, no. 2, pp. 141–154, 1988.

[12] F. Dong and S. K. Akl, "Scheduling algorithms for grid computing: state of the art and open problems," Tech. Rep. 2006-504, School of Computing, Queen's University, Kingston, Ontario, Canada, January 2006.

[13] D. Karaboga and B. Akay, "Artificial bee colony (ABC), harmony search and bees algorithms on numerical optimization," in *Proceedings of the Innovative Production Machines and Systems Virtual Conference*, 2009.

[14] D. Karaboga and B. Basturk, "On the performance of artificial bee colony (ABC) algorithm," *Applied Soft Computing*, vol. 8, no. 1, pp. 687–697, 2008.

[15] A. L. Bolaji, A. T. Khader, M. A. Al-Betar, and M. A. Awadallah, "Artificial bee colony algorithm, its variants and applications: a survey," *Journal of Theoretical and Applied Information Technology*, vol. 47, no. 2, pp. 434–459, 2013.

[16] R. Buyya, D. Abramson, J. Giddy, and H. Stockinger, "Economic models for resource management and scheduling in grid computing," *Concurrency and Computation: Practice and Experience*, vol. 14, no. 13–15, pp. 1507–1542, 2002.

[17] P. Martincová and M. Zábovský, "Comparison of simulated GRID scheduling algorithms," *Systemova Integrace*, vol. 4, pp. 69–75, 2007.

[18] F. Xhafa and A. Abraham, Eds., *Meta. for Sched. in Distri. Comp. Envi.*, SCI 146, Springer, Berlin, Germany, 2008.

[19] F. Dong and S. G. Akl, "PFAS: a resource-performance-fluctuation-aware workflow scheduling algorithm for grid computing," in *Proceedings of the 21st International Parallel and Distributed Processing Symposium (IPDPS '07)*, Long Beach, Calif, USA, March 2007.

[20] L. Zhang, Y. Chen, R. Sun, S. Jing, and B. Yang, "A task scheduling algorithm based on PSO for grid computing," *International Journal of Computational Intelligence Research*, vol. 4, no. 1, pp. 37–43, 2008.

[21] V. V. Korkhov, J. T. Moscicki, and V. V. Krzhizhanovskaya, "The user-level scheduling of divisible load parallel applications with resource selection and adaptive workload balancing on the grid," *IEEE Systems Journal*, vol. 3, no. 1, pp. 121–130, 2009.

[22] Y. Gao, H. Rong, and J. Z. Huang, "Adaptive grid job scheduling with genetic algorithms," *Future Generation Computer Systems*, vol. 21, no. 1, pp. 151–161, 2005.

[23] S. Fidanova and M. Durchova, "Ant algorithm for grid scheduling problem," in *Large-Scale Scientific Computing*, pp. 405–412, Springer, Berlin, Germany, 2006.

[24] S. Fidanova, "Simulated annealing for grid scheduling problem," in *Proceedings of the IEEE John Vincent Atanasoff International Symposium on Modern Computing (JVA '06)*, pp. 41–45, Sofia, Bulgaria, October 2006.

[25] W.-N. Chen and J. Zhang, "An ant colony optimization approach to a grid workflow scheduling problem with various QoS requirements," *IEEE Transactions on Systems, Man and Cybernetics Part C: Applications and Reviews*, vol. 39, no. 1, pp. 29–43, 2009.

[26] V. Di Martino and M. Mililotti, "Sub optimal scheduling in a grid using genetic algorithms," *Parallel Computing*, vol. 30, no. 5-6, pp. 553–565, 2004.

[27] R. Garg and A. K. Singh, "Enhancing the discrete particle swarm optimization based workflow grid scheduling using hierarchical structure," *International Journal of Computer Network and Information Security (IJCNIS)*, vol. 5, no. 6, pp. 18–26, 2013.

[28] S. S. Kim, J. H. Byeon, H. Liu, A. Abraham, and S. McLoone, "Optimal job scheduling in grid computing using efficient binary artificial bee colony optimization," *Soft Computing*, vol. 17, no. 5, pp. 867–882, 2013.

[29] L. M. Khanli, M. E. Far, and A. Ghaffari, "Reliable job scheduler using RFOH in grid computing," *Journal of Emerging Trends in Computing and Information Sciences*, vol. 1, no. 1, 2010.

[30] Z. Pooranian, M. Shojafar, J. H. Abawajy, and M. Singhal, "GLOA—a new job scheduling algorithm for grid computing," *International Journal of Artificial Intelligence and Interactive Multimedia*, vol. 2, no. 1, 2013.

[31] M. Karimi and H. Motameni, "Tasks scheduling in computational grid using a hybrid discrete particle swarm optimization," *International Journal of Grid and Distributed Computing*, vol. 6, no. 2, 2013.

[32] S. Mandloi and H. Gupta, "Adaptive job scheduling for computational grid based on ant colony optimization with genetic parameter selection," *International Journal of Advanced Computer Research*, vol. 3, no. 9, pp. 66–71, 2013.

[33] V. Selvi and R. Umarani, "Comparative study of GA and ABC for job scheduling," *International Journal of Soft Computing and Engineering (IJSCE)*, vol. 2, no. 6, pp. 2231–2307, 2013.

[34] W. M. Omar and A. Taleb-Bendiab, "E-health support services based on service-oriented architecture," *IT Professional*, vol. 8, no. 2, pp. 35–41, 2006.

[35] S. E. Middleton, M. Surridge, S. Benkner, and G. Engelbrecht, "Quality of service negotiation for commercial medical grid services," *Journal of Grid Computing*, vol. 5, no. 4, pp. 429–447, 2007.

[36] S. Kailasam, S. Kumar, and J. Dharanipragada, "Arogyasree: an enhanced grid-based approach to mobile telemedicine," *International Journal of Telemedicine and Applications*, vol. 2010, Article ID 536237, 11 pages, 2010.

[37] R. Kamal, M. A. Razzaque, and C. S. Hong, "Grid middleware for invivo sensor nodes," in *Proceedings of the International Conference on Information Networking (ICOIN '11)*, pp. 200–205, Barcelona, Spain, January 2011.

[38] M. S. Kiran and M. Gündüz, "A novel artificial bee colony-based algorithm for solving the numerical optimization problems," *International Journal of Innovative Computing, Information and Control*, vol. 8, no. 9, 2012.

[39] S. M. Saab, N. K. T. El-Omari, and H. O. Hussein, "Developing optimization algorithm using artificial bee colony system," *Computing and Communication Journal*, vol. 4, no. 3, pp. 391–396, 2009.

[40] E. Mezura-Montes, M. Damín-Araoz, and O. Cetina-Domíngez, "Smart flight and dynamic tolerances in the artificial bee colony for constrained optimization," in *Proceedings of the 6th IEEE Congress on Evolutionary Computation (CEC '10)*, pp. 1–8, Barcelona, Spain, July 2010.

[41] G. Yan and C. Li, "An effective refinement artificial bee colony optimization algorithm based on chaotic search and application for pid control tuning," *Journal of Computational Information Systems*, vol. 7, no. 9, pp. 3309–3316, 2011.

9

Smartphone Medical Applications for Women's Health: What Is the Evidence-Base and Feedback?

Emma Derbyshire and Darren Dancey

School of Healthcare Science, John Dalton East Building, Oxford Road, Manchester M1 5GD, UK

Correspondence should be addressed to Emma Derbyshire; e.derbyshire@mmu.ac.uk

Academic Editor: Trevor Russell

Background. Smartphone medical applications have a major role to play in women's health with their roles being very broad, ranging from improving health behaviours to undertaking personalised tests. *Objective(s)*. Using Medline, Web of Knowledge, and the PRISMA guidelines 15 randomized controlled trials (RCTs) were identified, with mobile interventions being tested on 1603 females, in relation to key aspects of health. Using a similar systematic approach an iPhone database search identified 47 applications (apps) developed to improve women's health. *Findings*. Ten RCTs used text messaging or app interventions to support weight loss, with significant improvements being observed in eight studies. For other aspects of women's health RCTs are needed to determine possible health benefits. iPhone store data analysis identified that a substantial number of women's health apps did not have star ratings or feedback comments (68 and 49 per cent, resp.), raising concerns about their validity. *Conclusion*. Peer-review systems, supporting statements of evidence, or certification standards would be beneficial in maintaining the quality and credibility of future health-focused apps. Patient groups should also ideally be involved in the development and testing of mobile medical apps.

1. Introduction

Women appear to be taking the lead when it comes to smartphone technology (ST) phone use, with 56 percent owning a smartphone compared with 51 percent men. This also translates when it comes to using health applications (apps) with around 9 percent women more likely to use these compared with 4 percent men [1]. One American survey studying over two thousand people ($n = 2020$) found that women tend to seek technology that keeps up with their busy lifestyles, with 51 percent owning some form of apple device and 93 percent women keeping their smartphone within arms' length [2].

It is also becoming clear that certain phases of the life cycle for, example, pregnancy, may also affect the level of ST phone usage. For example, one survey of 203 pregnant women found that 94 percent reported that ST had changed their life for better, with 65 percent reporting that they had downloaded pregnancy apps, with an average of three being downloaded during the gestation period [3]. In low- and middle-income countries smartphones also provide an excellent platform to support and improve the quality of healthcare systems for women [4].

There is also growing interest in harnessing smartphone apps to promote behaviour change. These provide a unique opportunity to help users stay healthy, while potentially playing a key role in helping to prevent disease onset [5, 6]. Generally speaking, common modifiable risk factors underlie most major chronic diseases and include tobacco use, unhealthy diets, and physical inactivity [7]. For women especially, rates of overweight and obesity are rising and reaching epidemic proportions, which has broad health implications, including a predisposition towards obesity in the next generation [8].

In terms of other health outcomes, estimated stroke prevalence among women aged 35 to 54 years has tripled over the past two decades, which appears to correlate with increased waist circumferences sizes [9]. Personalised medicine is thought to be one way to target women's obesity prevention, which could consider complex-risk factors such as sex-specific medical conditions and ST could be one approach in terms of helping to deliver this in the future [10].

Other noncommunicable diseases including cardiovascular disease (CVD), diabetes, and cancer have long been leading threats to human health (WHO, 2000) [11]. Looking at the latest statistics, CVD is a leading cause of mortality in women, with over half resulting from coronary artery disease and acute coronary syndromes [12]. Rates of diabetes are estimated to further rise by 2030 with demographic changes such as obesity, sedentary lifestyles, and ageing fuelling the rises in both obesity and diabetes [13]. For female-related cancers, worldwide it has been estimated that more than one million women are diagnosed with breast cancer annually, with more than 410,000 mortalities, indicating that new approaches for preventing and controlling breast cancer, especially in low resource settings in developing countries are still needed [14].

Other health conditions are also generally more prevalent in women. For example, depression prevalence amongst women is almost twice that of men with around 21.3 percent women reporting a lifestyle prevalence of major depressive disorder compared with 12.7 percent of men. Women in their child-bearing years appear to have the greatest risk, with genetic vulnerability, hormonal fluctuations, and psychosocial events such as stress, internalization coping style, and disadvantaged social status thought to affect this [15]. Osteoporosis is also common among postmenopausal women, which increases the risk of fractures, with hip and spine fractures, in particular, being associated with high morbidity and mortality [16].

Given the extent and associated healthcare costs of these conditions preventive health care has the potential to play a key role in reducing the prevalence of these conditions, with approaches such as mobile messaging and app usage offering a convenient and cost-effective way to reinforce desirable behaviours [17]. With the emergence of ST technology now evolving at an alarming pace, it has been anticipated that new software apps will soon be converting smartphones into biomedical devices that are anticipated to play a central role within healthcare systems, potentially turning phones into microscopes, ultrasound machines, or heart-rate monitors [18].

While some RCTs have investigated whether ST use can improve certain aspects of women's health, findings from these have not yet been evaluated systematically. In this paper, we set out to evaluate whether ST use is effective in terms of significantly improving aspects of women's health, including reductions in body weight and improved health awareness for chronic diseases, including diabetes, heart disease, breast cancer, and osteoporosis. The uses of health apps to improve diet quality, support mental, and maternal health are also reviewed. In the second part of this publication, an iPhone database search of health apps developed for women has been undertaken. Data in relation to their cost, star ratings, and user feedback was analysed.

2. Materials and Methods

A systematic literature review was conducted, according to the Preferred Reporting Items for Systematic Reviews and Meta-Analyses (PRISMA) guidelines [19] which were used to select the studies and as a guide to the weight placed on these, that is, in this case, only randomized controlled trials were included within the systematic review.

Table 1: Medline and Web of Knowledge search terms.

(1) Women AND Weight AND Cellular phone OR mobile phone OR smartphone OR smart phone OR iPhone OR android phone OR blackberry OR Windows mobile OR mobile medical apps.
(2) Women AND Diabetes AND Cellular phone OR mobile phone OR smartphone OR smart phone OR iPhone OR android phone OR blackberry OR Windows mobile OR mobile medical apps.
(3) Women AND Heart Disease AND Cellular phone OR mobile phone OR smartphone OR smart phone OR iPhone OR android phone OR blackberry OR Windows mobile OR mobile medical apps.
(4) Women AND Osteoporosis OR Bone Health AND Cellular phone OR mobile phone OR smartphone OR smart phone OR iPhone OR android phone OR blackberry OR Windows mobile OR mobile medical apps.
(5) Women AND Breast Cancer AND Cellular phone OR mobile phone OR smartphone OR smart phone OR iPhone OR android phone OR blackberry OR Windows mobile OR mobile medical apps.
(6) Women AND Nutrition OR Diet AND Cellular phone OR mobile phone OR smartphone OR smart phone OR iPhone OR android phone OR blackberry OR Windows mobile OR mobile medical apps.
(7) Women AND Depression OR Mental Health AND Cellular phone OR mobile phone OR smartphone OR smart phone OR iPhone OR android phone OR blackberry OR Windows mobile OR mobile medical apps.
(8) Women AND Pregnancy AND Cellular phone OR mobile phone OR smartphone OR smart phone OR iPhone OR android phone OR blackberry OR Windows mobile OR mobile medical apps.

2.1. Medline and Web of Knowledge Search. The following search strategy was used: Medline and Web of Knowledge databases were searched for English language, peer-reviewed human studies published between August 1983 and 2013 (Figure 1), with the last search run on August 22, 2013. As shown in Table 1 the search was limited to studies looking at "women" and "weight," "diabetes," "heart disease," "osteoporosis or bone health," "breast cancer," "nutrition or diet," "depression or mental health," and "pregnancy," combined with "cellular phone," "mobile phone," "smartphone or smart phone," "iPhone," "android phone," "blackberry," "Windows mobile," or "mobile medical apps".

For the identification of studies, the search protocol included the following stages: screening of identified papers; examination of the full text of potentially relevant studies; and application of the inclusion criteria to select the included studies. All reports were assessed by ED for suitability. For the study to be included in the main systematic review, the following characteristics were screened and inclusion criteria were applied: (a) studies should use mobile devices to improve aspects of women's health, (b) the intervention group should be compared with a controlled group, (c) the publication must be a randomized trial, (d) the

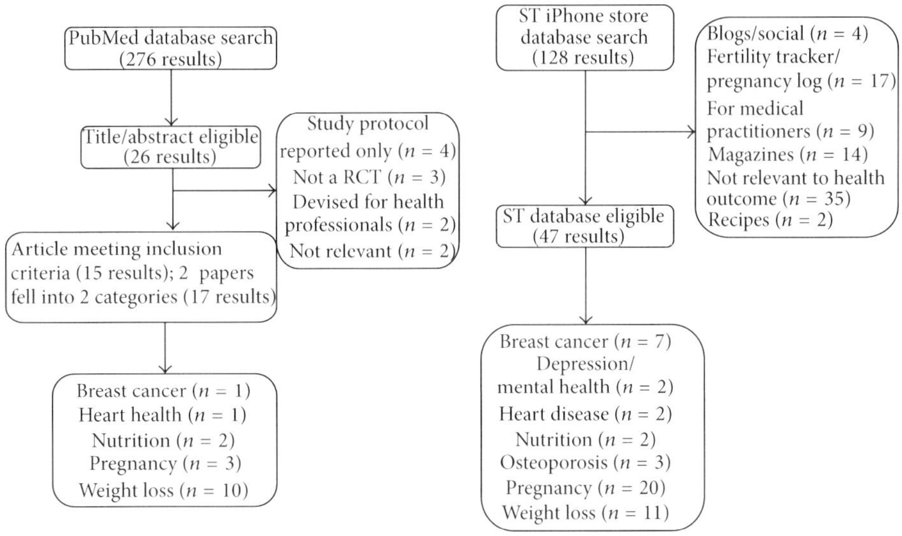

FIGURE 1: Methodology procedures for Medline, Web of Knowledge, and iPhone store database searches.

study was not a combined multi-intervention; and (e) access to the full text paper was available, either through Medline, Web of Knowledge or by contacting the author(s).

Papers were excluded if (1) they were a study protocol, (2) applications were for health professionals, (3) applications were appointment reminder systems, (4) the study did not include any measures of women's health or (5) intervention used computer-tracking systems rather than phone devices. The reference lists of scientific papers and reports were also hand searched by ED to identify relevant papers.

2.2. iPhone Store Search. The iPhone app store contains around 300,000 apps and it is growing [34]. A mobile iPhone database (application store) was searched with the same combination of terms used in the Medline search: "breast cancer," "depression/mental health," "diabetes management," "heart disease," "nutrition," "osteoporosis/bone health," "pregnancy," and "weight loss," combined with "women's health."

The search was limited to apps specifically developed for women's health, with the following being excluded: (1) apps for health magazines, (2) dictionary/medical term apps, (3) blogging/social apps, (4) apps developed for medical practitioners, (5) apps that did not relate to the specified health outcomes, or (6) apps that were games. In the case of pregnancy apps, those that were period/fertility trackers or pregnancy calendars were also excluded, as these did not relate directly to health.

All included apps had a central function that involved improving health/behaviour or preventing disease development. Once retrieved the ST apps were searched manually by ED for relevance. The last search was conducted on the 22 August 2013. Once relevant ST apps had been identified information in relation to their cost, star ratings and comments were collated. This data was extracted from the reviews section of each app and logged into an excel database for analysis.

3. Results

3.1. Medline Results. As shown in Figure 1, from our initial Medline search 276 articles were identified. A title and abstract review was undertaken, from which 26 articles were selected for detailed review, with 15 meeting the eligibility criteria (Table 2). Ten studies were found to investigate the use of ST health apps in relation to weight loss, while six studies focused on other aspects of women's health. No RCTs were found to study the effects of mobile messaging or app use in relation to markers of depression/mental health in women, diabetes, or bone health/osteoporosis.

From the 16 RCTs identified, ten studies have focused on the use of mobile short messaging services SMS/apps to assist with weight loss. Of these, two studies investigated the effects of SMS messages, received over a period of 12 months [30, 32]. One of the largest studies carried out by Shapiro et al., [30] recruited and randomized 111 overweight/obese females to receive either mobile text messages containing facts, tips, and motivational weight loss information or monthly newsletters. Results showed that adherence rates were good (60–69%), with strong compliers loosing significantly more weight at 6 ($P = 0.39$) and 12 months ($P = 0.23$) compared with those who were less adherent/did not follow the messages. A similar study by Haapala et al. randomized 96 overweight females to receive staggered instructions in relation to reducing food intake, with daily weight reporting and feedback over 12 months, or a control group (no intervention). After 12 months the experimental group had lost significantly more weight (4.5 kg) compared with the control group (1.1 kg) ($P = 0.006$) [32].

Table 2: Mobile medical applications and women's health.

Health outcome, publication, and location	Study population	Methods	Health application	Findings
Breast cancer				
Lakkis et al. [20] (2011), Lebanon	$n = 385$ females aged 40–75 years with a Health Insurance Plan	Prospective RCT. Randomized to two subgroups receiving SMS mobile phone texts: (1) to do a mammogram or (2) containing information about mammogram screening.	SMS tests either inviting women to do a mammogram or containing information about mammograms.	31% from group 1 and 32% from group 2 did a mammogram during the 6 months after intervention.
Heart health				
Park and Kim [21] (2012), Republic of Korea	$n = 67$ postmenopausal women	12-week RCT. Participants were asked to record their waist circumference and body weight, diet, and exercise levels using a weekly diary through the internet or by cellular phone.	Participants received weekly SMS/internet reminders about diet and exercise.	Systolic and diastolic blood pressure decreased by 6.5 and 4.6 mmHg in the intervention group. No significant changes were observed in the control group. Total cholesterol also reduced by 12.9 mg/dL in the intervention group but increased by 1.5 mg/dL in the control group.
Nutrition				
Mehran et al. [22] (2012), Iran	$n = 205$ females ≥ 18 yrs.	6-week RCT. Randomized to an intervention group that received text messages to enhance knowledge, attitudes, and practice concerning iron deficiency and iodized salt consumption.	The intervention group received daily text messages over 6 weeks. Urinary iodine concentration was measured at baseline and 8 weeks to see if there were any improvements.	Knowledge significantly improved by the end of the study ($P = 0.004$) but urinary iodine levels did not increased.
Norman et al. [23] (2013), USA	$n = 52$ overweight/obese adults, 80% female	4-month RCT. Randomized to intervention group receiving 2–5 weight management texts daily or a usual care comparison group.	Changes in fruit and vegetable intake and body weight were also measured.	Text messaging led to significant improvements in fruit and vegetable intake and eating behavior inventory scores.
Pregnancy				
Evans et al. [35] (2012), USA	$n = 123$, average age 27.6 years	RCT. Underserved pregnant women and new mothers were randomized to receive text messages to change their health, health beliefs, practices and behaviors to improve clinical outcomes, or to continue with usual health care.	Text4baby delivers text messages (https://text4baby.org/) to pregnant women and new mothers targeting underserved women facing health disparities.	There was an improvement of attitudes toward alcohol consumption from baseline to followup ($P = 0.029$).

Table 2: Continued.

Health outcome, publication, and location	Study population	Methods	Health application	Findings
Naughton et al. [24] (2012), UK	n = 207 pregnant mothers	11-week RCT. Women randomized to receive (1) a tailored self-help leaflet and 11-week tailored text messages or (2) a nontailored self-help leaflet.	11-weeks of tailored text messaging to quit smoking (MiQuit).	Those receiving the tailored text messages were more likely to set a quit date ($P = 0.04$) than controls.
Jareethum et al. [25] (2008), Thailand	n = 68 pregnant mothers	28-week RCT. Women randomized to receive prenatal support text messages sent from 28 weeks of pregnancy or a control group.	Two messages received per week from 28 weeks.	The confidence level was higher ($P = 0.001$) and anxiety level was lower ($P = 0.002$) amongst women receiving the text messages.
		Weight loss		
Brindal et al. [26] (2013), Australia	n = 58 overweight and obese women	8-week RCT. Allocated to a weight loss or control group.	With the support of an app the intervention group received information about meal replacement programme.	The weight loss difference between groups was not significant ($P = 0.08$) although women in the intervention reported a greater increase in positive mood ($P = 0.012$)
Carter et al. [27] (2013), UK	n = 128 overweight volunteers, 33% females	6-month RCT. Randomized to a smartphone application or a website or paper diary weight loss intervention.	The app was used to self-monitor diet and activity and feedback was provided via weekly message.	Body mass index reductions after 6 months were the highest amongst the app users ($-1.6\ kg/m^2$), followed by the diary group ($-1.0\ kg/m^2$) and the website group ($-0.5\ kg/m^2$), indicating that this app was acceptable and feasible.
Donaldson et al. [28] (2013), UK	n = 23 overweight and obese females	12-week RCT. Randomized to receive tailored practitioner weight loss feedback or weight checks only (control).	Patients texted their weight loss progress to practitioners and received tailored feedback.	Body weight, BMI, and waist circumference all reduced significantly in the intervention compared with the control group.
Napolitano et al. [29] (2013), USA	n = 52 students (87% female)	8-week RCT. Randomized to (1) Facebook, (2) Facebook + text messaging, and personalised feedback (3) control group.	Messages were received over 8 weeks with weight loss measured at 4 and 8 weeks.	The Facebook + messaging group lost significantly more weight (-2.4 kg) after 8 weeks compared with the other branches.
Norman et al. [23] (2013), USA	n = 52 overweight/obese adults, 80% female	4-month RCT. Randomized to intervention group receiving 2–5 weight management texts daily or a usual care comparison group.	Changes in fruit and vegetable intake and body weight were also measured.	Text messaging led to significant improvements in body weight.
Park and Kim [21] (2012), Republic of Korea	n = 67 postmenopausal women	12-week RCT. Participants were asked to record their waist circumference and body weight, diet, and exercise levels using a weekly diary through the internet or by cellular phone.	Participants received weekly SMS/internet reminders about diet and exercise.	Waist circumference and body weight significantly decreased by 3.0 cm and 2.0 kg at 12 weeks compared with baseline. Increases were found in the control group.

Table 2: Continued.

Health outcome, publication, and location	Study population	Methods	Health application	Findings
Shapiro et al. [30] (2012), USA	n = 170 overweight and obese adults, 65% females	12-month RCT. Randomized to receive daily interactive and personally weight-relevant text messages or monthly e-newsletters.	Daily weight-relevant SMS and MMS received 4 times/day over 12 months.	Participants with greater adherence lost more weight 6 ($P = 0.39$) and 12 months ($P = 0.23$) than loss who were less adherent. Text messaging could be a useful adjunct to weight loss treatments.
Turner-McGrievy and Tate [31] (2011), USA	n = 96 overweight females	6-month RCT. Assigned to Podcast-only or Podcast + Mobile groups.	The Podcast + Mobile group uses a diet and physical activity monitoring app on the mobile devise and interacted with study counsellors using twitter.	Prompting and mobile communication via twitter did not enhance weight loss.
Haapala et al. [32] (2009), Finland	n = 125 overweight 22–44 year olds, 96 females	12-month RCT. Randomized to (1) use a mobile phone operated weight loss programme or (2) control	Participants received texts messages over 12 months and instructed on how to reduce food intake with daily weight reporting and tailored feedback.	After 12 months the experimental group had lost significantly more weight than the control ($P = 0.006$)
Patrick et al. [33] (2009), USA	n = 75 overweight men and women, 52% females	4-month RCT. Randomized to receive (1) printed materials about weight control, (3) MMS, and SMS messaging intervention.	Participants received personalised MMS and SMS messages were send 2–5 times per day.	The group receiving the messages lost more weight (−1.97 kg; $P = 0.02$) compared with the control group by the end of the study.

BMI: body mass index; MMS: multimedia messaging service; RCT: randomized controlled trial; SMS: short messaging service.

A further four studies considered the effects of ST use as part of weight loss interventions. Brindal et al. [26] developed an app to support users taking part in a meal replacement programme (MRP). Fifty-eight overweight/obese women were randomized to receive either the MRP support app or a static app (control) for 8 weeks. No statistically significant differences were observed in relation to levels of weight loss, although women in the intervention group reported a greater increase in mood ($P = 0.012$) compared with the control. It is possible that 8 weeks were not long enough for effects to be observed in this study. A longer RCT by Carter et al., [27] conducted over 6 months, randomized 42 females to three groups: (1) app group, (2) website use, or (3) paper diet/physical activities diaries. The app group was able to self-monitor the diet and physical activity levels, with weekly feedback being provided. Findings showed that body mass index reductions after 6 months were the highest amongst the app users ($-1.6\,kg/m^2$), followed by the diary group ($-1.0\,kg/m^2$) and the website group ($-0.5\,kg/m^2$), indicating that this app was acceptable and feasible.

Patrick et al. and Norman et al. also found that weight management texts sent 2–5 times per day, over 4 months led to significant reductions in body weight [23, 33] while other work has shown that self-monitoring of body weight, that is, texting weight regularly to practitioners, or logging body weight measurements into mobile devices can lead to, also led, to significant improvements in body weight/waist circumference measurements [21, 28].

Finally, two RCTs have investigated the effects of ST apps in combination with social media application such as Facebook or Twitter. For example, one study found that while the number of podcasts downloaded was significantly and moderately correlated with weight loss in both the Podcast ($r = -0.53$, $P < 0.001$) and Podcast + Mobile ($r = -0.46$, $P = 0.001$) groups, prompting and mobile communication via Twitter, and monitoring the app without feedback did not appear to enhance weight loss, possibly because the addition of Twitter and mobile monitoring became a distraction [31]. Napolitano et al. randomized 45 female overweight or obese college students to (1) receive weight loss advice either via Facebook, (2) through Facebook, text messaging, and personalized feedback or (3) no advice (control). While it is difficult to separate out the effects of the text messaging and personalized advice, this intervention group was found to loose significantly more weight (2.4 kg) over 8 weeks compared with the other groups [29].

Three studies have investigated the use of mobile text messaging in relation to changing health behaviors in pregnancy but RCTs using apps remain to be understudied. Naughton et al. found that tailor text messaging was more successful in terms of helping women quit smoking during pregnancy, when compared with traditional leaflets containing information [24]. Evans et al. as part of the Text4baby study found that there was an improvement towards alcohol consumption compared with baseline ($P = 0.029$), although further findings are yet to be published from this work [35]. Finally, Jareethum et al. randomized women to receive text messages over 28 weeks, offering general support to women during the prenatal period for example, on how to prepare for having their baby and introducing it to the home environment. This intervention was successful in that confidence levels were significantly higher ($P = 0.001$) and anxiety levels significantly lower ($P = 0.002$) among women receiving the intervention messages [25].

Two studies have investigated the use of mobile SMS messaging in relation to other aspects of women's health. One study randomized 385 women to receive either a general SMS invite to do a mammogram or an invite, combined with additional SMS information about the benefits of mammogram screening. The number of women undertaking a mammogram after the intervention was similar for both groups (31 and 32%). This is still considered to be quite low, which could be attributed to the fact that 26.4% of cell phone numbers were invalid [20]. Another study carried out in Iran where median urinary iodine concentrations have been found to decline (an indicator of iodine deficiency), randomized 205 females to an intervention group receiving daily text messages via their mobile phone for 6 weeks about iodine deficiency and the use of iodised salt or a control group. Levels of knowledge about the topic of iodine deficiency were significantly improved by the end of the study ($P = 0.004$), although this was not reflected by a change in urinary iodine levels [22]. It is possible that the dietary adjustments made were not sufficient to generate a measurable, physiological change. Two studies investigating the effects of mobile messaging on markers of body weight and also identified important secondary findings. Park and Kim found that systolic and diastolic blood pressure and total cholesterol declined in the weight loss group receiving text messages [21] while Norman et al. found that fruit and vegetable intakes significantly improved [23].

3.2. iPhone Database Results. From the iPhone database search, using similar key terms, 128 related health apps were retrieved. However, after evaluating these, only 47 met the specified inclusion criteria, from which data was extracted and analyzed, as shown in Figures 2 and 3.

Just under half (46.8 percent) of the apps meeting the inclusion criteria were free. Of the 53.2% that were paid for, their average price was £1.44, SD 1.17. Fifty-six percent of the apps were priced at 69 pence, with the most expensive costing £4.50. In terms of star ratings and feedback comments, a large proportion of the apps (68 and 49 percent, resp.) did not have these reported. For those that had been star rated, the average score, out of a possible five was 2.5, SD 2.9. Figures 1 and 2 show the cost and star ratings of apps according to the specified health categories. Clearly, larger and more complete datasets are needed but preliminary analysis indicates that pregnancy apps are generally priced higher, yet appear to have lower star ratings.

For apps where comments were present, an anonymized table of commentaries is included in Table 3. Most of these indicate that users are in favor of apps that are of easy to use, contain new information, and are motivational. Areas in need of improvement appear to be the quality of graphics, speed of downloads, for example, graphs, compatibility with

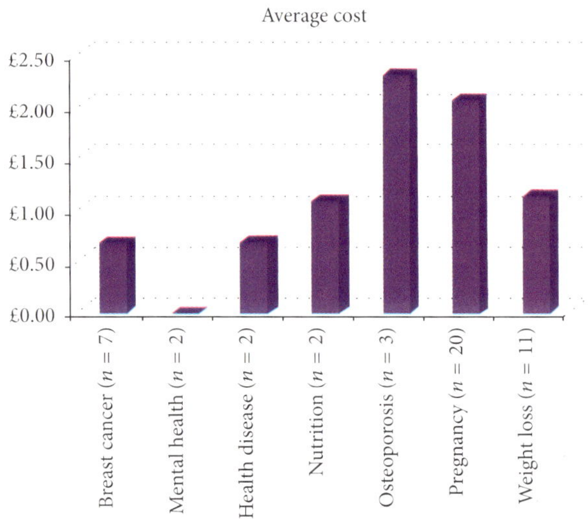

FIGURE 2: Average cost of women's health apps from the iPhone store. Note: mental health apps were both free.

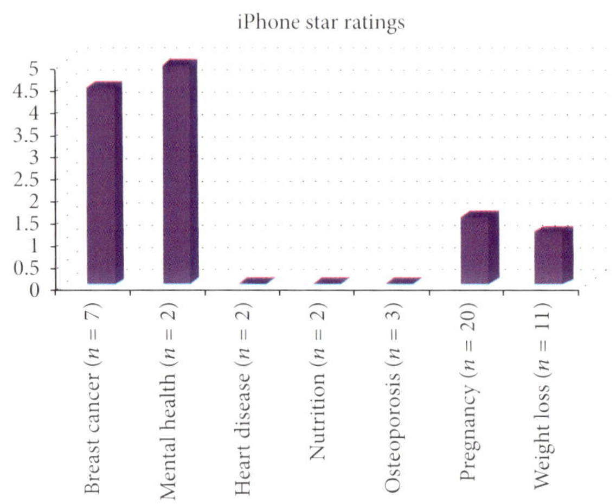

FIGURE 3: Average star ratings. Note: star ratings were not recorded for the heart disease, nutrition, or osteoporosis apps.

other devices, ability to transfer data on to new versions, and certification/affiliation with credible organisations.

TABLE 3: Examples of commentaries from women's health apps.

Overall positive comments	Room for improvement
Easy to use.	Data could not be transferred into new versions.
Great for keeping motivated and focused.	It did not tell me anything new.
Information was easy to digest.	Graphs did not download.
Information was very helpful.	Information was out of date.
Makes my life easier.	Information was slow to download.
	More zoom would be useful.
	Needs extra graphics.
	Not certified/sure who developed it.
	Not compatible with iPad.

4. Discussion

Overall, smartphone technology appears to hold great promise in the future in terms of helping to deliver health behaviour changes [36]. However, the present paper has identified some key areas for consideration. Firstly, in terms of published evidence, while their appears to be several studies investigating the effects of mobile messaging in relation to aspects of women's health, comparatively few studies have tested the efficacy of mobile medical apps.

Given the rise in the number of medical mobile applications there is a clear need to support these with a strong, scientific evidence-base, to ensure they deliver the desired benefits; otherwise, once in the public domain this could impact on user safety. In particular, one review of diabetes apps, downloaded through the iPhone store found that most of these lacked evidence in relation to clinical efficacy, concluding that they would not integrate well within the health care delivery system [37]. Equally, while these hold great potential in terms of improving clinical practice, possible dangers associated with their use have yet to be identified. For example, breaches of patient confidentiality, conflicts of interest, and apps with unclear or inaccurate clinical decisions/outputs could all have negative implications for patient care [38]. Peer-reviewing of medical applications, along with provisional testing by relevant patient groups, could be one way forward [39]. However, until further reaching and testing are undertaken, while the use of medical apps may be appealing, their clinical efficacy is less clear [40].

We have now also reached the era of personalised medicine and nutrition [41]. Given this, it is concerning to see that few apps have been developed with a view to accounting adequately for lifestyle and genetic factors, for example, family history, or tailored specifically to aspects of women's (and men's) health. Of the applications developed in relation to improving aspects of women's health, pregnancy and weight loss appeared to have the strongest presence within the iPhone app store. While these appear to be supported with some level of scientific evidence in the form of RCTs, given the number of apps for pregnancy available through the app store, this is something that should continue to be encouraged.

We identified that 68 and 49 percent of the women's health apps reviewed did not have any star ratings or feedback comments. Evidence from this review and related articles clearly indicates that users are increasingly concerned about whether apps come from are reputable and legitimate sources. One review concluded that smartphone apps developed by experts are generally considered to be more preferable than those from unknown or less reputable sources [6].

It should also be considered that some training may be needed to help users get the most out of ST applications. While adolescents have a tendency to pick up the applications quickly, there is evidence that older adults may be less efficient and that ST applications should ideally be age-specific [42]. It is also clear that adherence in terms of daily use of the ST intervention should also be considered in future studies, as shown in the weight loss interventions described [22, 30]. Further work is also needed to determine "how long" users are likely to comply with the mobile health intervention; that is, what is the maximum number of weeks [6].

Finally, in terms of specific health outcomes, eight studies found that mobile medical applications helped to support weight loss [21, 23, 27–30, 32, 33]. However, it should be considered that the frequency of messages delivered may have had some effect on this [30]. Equally, the downloading of other health apps, alongside the one being tested may skew results [26]. While one published RCTs tested the effects of a nutritional (iodine) SMS intervention on markers of health (urinary iodine concentrations) dietary changes made were probably not substantial enough to generate an effect [22]. Consequently, future studies testing the effects of supplement compliance of fortified food consumption are warranted, in relation to app use and markers of nutritional well-being.

5. Conclusions

Overall the number of mobile medical applications developed specifically for aspects of women's health is rising but there is much yet to be done. Clearly more gender-specific, personalised apps are needed, for example, for mental health issues and heart disease. Given the small number of RCTs published for key areas of women's health, clearly further studies are warranted, particularly in relation to embedding and using apps in health care settings. Based on the feedback analysis, women are looking for apps that are easy to use, motivational, and, most importantly of all, trustworthy and evidence-based.

Points of Relevance

(i) Fifteen RCTs appear to have tested the efficacy of smartphone apps/SMS in relation to improving key aspects of women's health.

(ii) Forty-seven apps were available through the iPhone store and developed with the intention of improving women's health.

(iii) A large proportion of the iPhone apps (68 and 49%, resp.) did not have star ratings or feedback comments, respectively.

(iv) Female users are looking to use credible apps, ideally developed by experts.

(v) A stronger evidence-base is needed, to support the development of future mobile medical applications and to determine their clinical efficacy.

References

[1] Oglivy Action, *Women Taking the Lead When It Comes to Mobile*, 2013, http://www.guardian.co.uk/media-network/media-network-blog/2012/aug/06/women-lead-mobile-technology-retail.

[2] Arbitron & Edison Research, *Mums and Media*, 2013, http://www.slideshare.net/webby2001/moms-and-media-2012.

[3] P. Petrie, *Pregnancy and the Changing World of Technology*, 2013, http://corporate.mumsviews.co.uk/about.php.

[4] M. J. Rotheram-Borus, M. Tomlinson, D. Swendeman, A. Lee, and E. Jones, "Standardized functions for smartphone applications: examples from maternal and child health," *International Journal of Telemedicine and Applications*, vol. 2012, Article ID 973237, 16 pages, 2012.

[5] K. Wac, "Smartphone as a personal, pervasive health informatics services platform: literature review," *Yearbook of Medical Informatics*, vol. 7, no. 1, pp. 83–93, 2012.

[6] L. Dennison, L. Morrison, G. Conway, and L. Yardley, "Opportunities and challenges for smartphone applications in supporting health behavior change: qualitative study," *Journal of Medical Internet Research*, vol. 15, no. 4, article e86, 2013.

[7] World Health Organisation, "Preventing chronic diseases: a vital investment," Chronic Disease Report, 2013, http://www.who.int/chp/chronic_disease_report/full_report.pdf.

[8] S. L. Gortmaker, B. A. Swinburn, D. Levy et al., "Changing the future of obesity: science, policy, and action," *The Lancet*, vol. 378, no. 9793, pp. 838–847, 2011.

[9] A. Towfighi, L. Zheng, and B. Ovbiagele, "Weight of the obesity epidemic: rising stroke rates among middle-aged women in the United States," *Stroke*, vol. 41, no. 7, pp. 1371–1375, 2010.

[10] N. Yang, G. S. Ginsburg, and L. A. Simmons, "Personalized medicine in women's obesity prevention and treatment: implications for research, policy and practice," *Obesity Reviews*, vol. 14, no. 2, pp. 145–161, 2013.

[11] World Health Organisation, "2008–2013 action plan for the global strategy for the prevention and control on noncommunicable diseases," Action Plan, 2013, http://whqlibdoc.who.int/publications/2009/9789241597418_eng.pdf.

[12] K. A. Bybee and T. L. Stevens, "Matters of the heart: cardiovascular disease in U.S. women," *Missouri Medicine*, vol. 110, no. 1, pp. 65–70, 2013.

[13] J. E. Shaw, R. A. Sicree, and P. Z. Zimmet, "Global estimates of the prevalence of diabetes for 2010 and 2030," *Diabetes Research and Clinical Practice*, vol. 87, no. 1, pp. 4–14, 2010.

[14] S. S. Coughlin and D. U. Ekwueme, "Breast cancer as a global health concern," *Cancer Epidemiology*, vol. 33, no. 5, pp. 315–318, 2009.

[15] R. E. Noble, "Depression in women," *Metabolism*, vol. 54, no. 5, pp. 49–52, 2005.

[16] North American Menopause Society, "Management of osteoporosis in postmenopausal women: 2010 position statement of The North American Menopause Society," *Menopause*, vol. 17, no. 1, pp. 25–54, 2010.

[17] V. Vodopivec-Jamsek, T. de Jongh, I. Gurol-Urganci, R. Atun, and J. Car, "Mobile phone messaging for preventive health care," *The Cochrane Database of Systematic Reviews*, vol. 2012, Article ID CD007457, 2012.

[18] L. Mertz, "Ultrasound? Fetal monitoring? Spectrometer? There's an app for that!: biomedical smart phone apps are taking healthcare by storm," *IEEE Pulse*, vol. 3, no. 2, pp. 16–21, 2012.

[19] D. Moher, A. Liberati, J. Tetzlaff, and D. G. Altman, "Preferred reporting items for systematic reviews and meta-analyses: the PRISMA statement," *BMJ*, vol. 339, article b2535, 2009.

[20] N. A. Lakkis, A. M. Atfeh, Y. R. EL-Zein, D. M. Mahmassani, and G. N. Hamadeh, "The effect of two types of sms-texts on the uptake of screening mammogram: a randomized controlled trial," *Preventive Medicine*, vol. 53, no. 4-5, pp. 325–327, 2011.

[21] M.-J. Park and H.-S. Kim, "Evaluation of mobile phone and Internet intervention on waist circumference and blood pressure in post-menopausal women with abdominal obesity,"

International Journal of Medical Informatics, vol. 81, no. 6, pp. 388–394, 2012.

[22] L. Mehran, P. Nazeri, H. Delshad, P. Mirmiran, Y. Mehrabi, and F. Azizi, "Does a text messaging intervention improve knowledge, attitudes and practice regarding iodine deficiency and iodized salt consumption?" *Public Health Nutrition*, vol. 15, no. 12, pp. 2320–2325, 2012.

[23] G. J. Norman, J. K. Kolodziejczyk, M. A. Adams, K. Patrick, and S. J. Marshall, "Fruit and vegetable intake and eating behaviors mediate the effect of a randomized text-message based weight loss program," *Preventive Medicine*, vol. 56, pp. 3–7, 2013.

[24] F. Naughton, A. T. Prevost, H. Gilbert, and S. Sutton, "Randomized controlled trial evaluation of a tailored leaflet and SMS text message self-help intervention for pregnant smokers (MiQuit)," *Nicotine & Tobacco Research*, vol. 14, no. 5, pp. 569–577, 2012.

[25] R. Jareethum, V. Titapant, C. Tienthai, S. Viboonchart, P. Chuenwattana, and J. Chatchainoppakhun, "Satisfaction of healthy pregnant women receiving short message service via mobile phone for prenatal support: a randomized controlled trial," *Journal of the Medical Association of Thailand*, vol. 91, no. 4, pp. 458–463, 2008.

[26] E. Brindal, G. Hendrie, J. Freyne, M. Coombe, S. Berkovsky, and M. Noakes, "Design and pilot results of a mobile phone weight-loss application for women starting a meal replacement programme," *Journal of Telemedicine and Telecare*, 2013.

[27] M. C. Carter, V. J. Burley, C. Nykjaer, and J. E. Cade, "Adherence to a smartphone application for weight loss compared to website and paper diary: pilot randomized controlled trial," *Journal of Medical Internet Research*, vol. 15, no. 4, article e32, 2013.

[28] E. L. Donaldson and M. Morris, "A text message based weight management intervention for overweight adults," *Journal of Human Nutrition and Dietetics*, 2013.

[29] M. S. Napolitano, G. G. Bennett, A. K. Ives, and G. D. Foster, "Using Facebook and text messaging to deliver a weight loss program to college students," *Obesity Reviews*, vol. 21, pp. 25–31, 2013.

[30] J. R. Shapiro, T. Koro, N. Doran, N. S et al., "Text4Diet: a randomized controlled study using text messaging for weight loss behaviors," *Preventive Medicine*, vol. 55, no. 5, pp. 412–417, 2012.

[31] G. Turner-McGrievy and D. Tate, "Tweets, apps, and pods: results of the 6-month mobile pounds off digitally (Mobile POD) randomized weight-loss intervention among adults," *Journal of Medical Internet Research*, vol. 13, no. 4, article e120, 2011.

[32] I. Haapala, N. C. Barengo, S. Biggs, L. Surakka, and P. Manninen, "Weight loss by mobile phone: a 1-year effectiveness study," *Public Health Nutrition*, vol. 12, no. 12, pp. 2382–2391, 2009.

[33] K. Patrick, F. Raab, M. A. Adams et al., "A text message-based intervention for weight loss: randomized controlled trial," *Journal of Medical Internet Research*, vol. 11, no. 1, article e1, 2009.

[34] P. C. Mag, *Apple App Store Tops 300,000 Apps*, 2013, http://www.pcmag.com/article2/0,2817,2373169,00.asp.

[35] W. D. Evans, J. L. Wallace, and J. Snider, "Pilot evaluation of the text4baby mobile health program," *BMC Public Health*, vol. 12, no. 1031, 2012.

[36] L. Hebden, A. Cook, H. P. van der Ploeg, and M. Allman-Farinelli, "Development of smartphone applications for nutrition and physical activity behavior change," *JMIR Research Protocols*, vol. 1, no. 2, article e9, 2012.

[37] D. S. Eng and L. M. Lee, "The promise and peril of mobile health applications for diabetes and endocrinology," *Pediatric Diabetes*, vol. 14, no. 4, pp. 231–238, 2013.

[38] A. W. Buijink, B. J. Visser, and L. Marshall, "Medical apps for smartphones: lack of evidence undermines quality and safety," *Evidence-Based Medicine*, vol. 18, pp. 90–92, 2013.

[39] B. J. Visser and A. W. G. Buijink, "Need to peer-review medical applications for smart phones," *Journal of Telemedicine and Telecare*, vol. 18, no. 2, article 124, 2012.

[40] G. R. Zanni, "Medical apps worth having," *The Consultant Pharmacist*, vol. 28, pp. 322–324, 2013.

[41] M. J. Gibney and M. C. Walsh, "The future direction of personalised nutrition: my diet, my phenotype, my genes," *The Proceedings of the Nutrition Society*, vol. 72, no. 2, pp. 219–225, 2013.

[42] B. L. Daugherty, T. E. Schap, R. Ettienne-Gittens et al., "Novel technologies for assessing dietary intake: evaluating the usability of a mobile telephone food record among adults and adolescents," *Journal of Medical Internet Research*, vol. 14, no. 2, article e58, 2012.

10

An ICT-Based Diabetes Management System Tested for Health Care Delivery

Claude Takenga,[1] Rolf-Dietrich Berndt,[1] Olivier Musongya,[2] Joël Kitero,[2] Remi Katoke,[2] Kakule Molo,[2] Basile Kazingufu,[3] Malikwisha Meni,[3] Mambo Vikandy,[3] and Henri Takenga[4]

[1] *Infokom GmbH, 17034 Neubrandenburg, Germany*
[2] *Health Department, Baptist Church in Central Africa (CBCA), Goma, Democratic Republic of Congo*
[3] *Ruwenzori State University (UOR), Butembo, Democratic Republic of Congo*
[4] *Provincial Health Division (DPS), Ministry of Health, North Kivu, Goma, Democratic Republic of Congo*

Correspondence should be addressed to Claude Takenga; ctakenga@infokom.de

Academic Editor: Cristiana Larizza

The demand for new healthcare services is growing rapidly. Improving accessibility of the African population to diabetes care seems to be a big challenge in most countries where the number of care centers and medical staff is reduced. Information and communication technologies (ICT) have great potential to address some of these challenges faced by several countries in providing accessible, cost-effective, and high-quality health care services. This paper presents the Mobil Diab system which is a telemedical approach proposed for the management of long-term diseases. The system applies modern mobile and web technologies which overcome geographical barriers, and increase access to health care services. The idea of the system is to involve patients in the therapy process and motivate them for an active participation. For validation of the system in African context, a trial was conducted in the Democratic Republic of Congo. 40 Subjects with diabetes divided randomly into control and intervention groups were included in the test. Results show that Mobil Diab is suitable for African countries and presents a number of benefits for the population and public health care system. It improves clinical management and delivery of diabetes care services by enhancing access, quality, motivation, reassurance, efficiency, and cost-effectiveness.

1. Introduction

The number of people with diabetes is increasing due to population growth, aging, urbanization, and increasing prevalence of obesity and physical inactivity [1]. Diabetes is associated with huge human and economic costs. Predictions show that the number of people with diabetes worldwide will double in the next generation. In [2] the quality of diabetes management in five countries with advanced economies (Australia, Canada, New Zealand, USA, and UK) has been analysed. Yearly costs (e.g., 132 Billions USD in the USA) and deaths due to diabetes (e.g., 143 308 people in the USA) are reported in that paper. In face of such a disastrous situation, nations have intensified their efforts to struggle with diabetes.

Improving accessibility of the African population to diabetes care seems to be a big challenge in most of African countries such as the Democratic Republic of Congo (DRC), a country which is four times bigger than France and where the number of care centers is reduced. DRC has 71 million inhabitants. Around 7% of the population in the capital city Kinshasa is affected by diabetes [3]. This situation is similar in other African countries. Most of diabetic patients in the DRC do not control regularly their glucose values, occasional checks are the only executed options.

What are the factors which are responsible for deficiency in the successful management of diabetes in Africa? A number of obstacles make the detection, prevention, monitoring, and treatment of diabetes difficult in most African countries [4].

The first group of difficulties is related to the health facilities which are not sufficient to cope with the scale of the problem. Prevention and education are not sufficiently promoted, although they should be given high priority. There are not enough medical specialists and the few existing focus their work in big cities without addressing the needs of rural populations. Therefore, patients from rural areas are forced to spend money and time travelling long and expensive journeys to access diabetes care. Another point, the priority of health politics in several African countries is oriented on the management of transmissible diseases such as HIV and not to chronic diseases like diabetes and high blood pressure.

The second group of difficulties is related to patients themselves. It is impossible for the majority of the population to afford the cost of the diabetes medication in particular insulin. Due to life condition, patients are unable to control a proper diet, especially when the family eats by hand in the same dish. Limited resources push the population to focus on high calorie foods rich in fat, sugar, and salt.

The third group of difficulties is related to the socio-cultural context which has a considerable weight in Africa. Africans have difficulty accepting the concept of chronic illnesses requiring lifelong treatment, so when diabetes is well balanced, patients often stop the treatment thinking the disease is cured. This then causes a relapse in the following days. Moreover, patients do not find it useful to carry out regular glucose checks although this is necessary for the adaptation of the insulin therapy. The next point deals with the fact that the struggle against obesity faces the belief that being fat is a sign of wealth, good health, and beauty. According to the African tradition, women beauty is proportional to weight. Weight loss, even if it is wanted, raises suspicion of possible HIV infection in the continent. Some religions create obstacles to the diabetes management in Africa. Fasting in churches and during Ramadan is another source of poor glucose control. The last obstacle is caused by traditional medicine which plays a key role in many African countries. This practice is often dangerous when it advices diabetes patients to stop effective treatments and use empirical drugs which have the advantage of being cheap.

Information and communication technologies have great potential to address some of the challenges faced by the public health care. A number of literature have been oriented on the exploitation of mobile devices for completing traditional therapy [5, 6]; other works have been focused on the architectural issues of a telemedicine intervention [7, 8].

A significant number of telemedical products in the area of diabetes management have been developed in the last decade. This is justified by the fact that recent studies have depicted a very critical situation; over 10% of the United States population over the age of 20 has diabetes. This number has been predicted to increase significantly in the future. As a result, diabetes is now ranked amongst the ten first leading causes of death. This situation motivates special attention towards both prevention and better diabetes treatment.

A web-based system for monitoring patients with type 2 diabetes is presented in [9]. In that system weight, blood sugar, and blood pressure are recorded using an application implemented on the mobile phone. In [10] Bayer's GLUCKOFACT DELUXE Software is described. The software recognizes the Bayer glucose meter connected to the personal computer and stores automatically the data in a database. The visualization of the recorded data is well organized. However, that software is not extended for online applications. This obliges the patient to regularly visit his doctor or to use another system in order to send the recorded data. A more advanced diabetic management system is presented in [11]. The software helps in tracking daily diabetic data; it has a simple interface for data entry and uses different devices for entering data (Windows-PC, Android phones, Windows mobile phones, iPhones, and Java phones). It has been proved in [12, 13] that telemedicine is a suited instrument to support health care providers in the effective management and prevention of diabetes complications.

Solution to the four listed main difficulties in properly addressing diabetes in Africa can be solved by providing a cost-effective telemedical system and a suitable educational program in order to increase the population awareness. This is the focus of this paper, in which we propose and validate an innovative mobile health application. The system manages a secure collection, processing, storage, and sharing of diabetes-related data and thus reduces the frequency of physical consultations to the treating physician. The system enables the organization of health information through a structured gathering of all relevant diabetes data in one central place enabling only access of authorized medical staff. The system helps improve the quality of service in the care process of diabetes by benefiting from rapid advances in mobile, web, and communication technologies. The system also provides educational programs in order to increase awareness on diabetes. We strongly believe that the outcome of this work will contribute toward the establishment of a model for diabetes management in countries where access to diabetes care is limited and number of medical care personnel is reduced due to high personnel costs. The diabetes management system Mobil Diab, presented in this paper, can serve as a complete hospital management system which supports several hospitals, each hospital having its own medical staff and patients and every clinician coaching a group of patients assigned to him. Moreover, since e-health systems store sensitive data and should have a proper security and privacy framework and mechanisms, this paper extends the state-of-the art by presenting a system which enables a secure data access, communication, and storage. Investigation of the impact of using this system Mobil Diab in assisting the therapy and treatment of diabetes is the major focus of this paper.

2. Materials and Methods

2.1. Mobil Diab System and Benefits. Mobil Diab system is an innovative solution for the assistance and care of diabetes patients. It enables diabetes patients to manage their self-control data around the clock using their mobile devices (Android, iPhone, and iPads) and/or web-based applications. Medical care personnel access patients' data through a protected web portal. The diabetes module is embedded on the telemedical platform. The platform is responsible for the following tasks: connection of web and mobile applications, user-hierarchical model (administration, hospital, doctor, and patient), access control of different user categories, and secure interface to hospital information systems.

The concept of the system aims at empowering patients to better manage their disease by allowing them to monitor their blood sugar trends over an extended period of time and draw some actionable conclusions. Acquired data are then sent using HTTP/HTTPS protocol to the central platform which ensures a secure storage and further processing of the information, Figure 1.

Mobil Diab guarantees a series of benefits for patients, health care staff, and public health system.

Benefits for the patients include, among others, unimpeded patient mobility, data input via smart phones and/or via web, regular self-control of diabetes-related data enables the right care to be administrated at the right time, potential to improve care process and quality of service, improvement in patient's motivation through their involvement in the therapy process, reduced check-up frequency to doctors, and use of mobile health technologies encourages diabetes patients to change their behavior/lifestyle and improve their health.

Benefits for the health care staff involve, among others, the following: complete and regular data input which is helpful for individual therapy plan, minimization of errors caused by lack of information about the disease history, improvement of the care process quality, getting specialist opinions, access to patients' data worldwide independent from time and location, and automatic alarm message in case of critical data from a patient.

Benefits for the Health System include, among others, the following: delaying and reducing diabetes complications, minimizing hospitalization rates due to diabetes complications, reducing death rates from diabetes, speeding up the transition of patients from hospitals to their own homes which leads to a reduction in costs, and enabling the organization of health information through a structured gathering of all relevant data in one central place.

The system helps to easy track patterns and trends in diabetes management process, helps in taking right treatment decisions and lead to a better glucose control, is suitable for self-care, home care, family physicians, clinics, and hospitals, presents statistics that cover everything doctors and patients need, allows risk monitoring with automated alarm message to care provider and trusted person, preserves mobility through the use of Apps and web technologies, and acquires a highly secured database platform with end-to end encryption and data are worldwide available in all major languages.

2.2. Mobile Application of Mobil Diab. The mobile application Mobil Diab has an intuitive user interface which is self-explained. You can choose the action you wish to perform as shown on the screenshot of Figure 2. Results are also represented in different ways as samples are shown in Figure 3. Data are automatically synchronized in background with the online system so that medical care providers receive these data in real time.

To record diabetes-related data, patients are presented with intuitive screens and they can enter data. These data may include, amongst others, the blood glucose measurement, insulin intake, sport done with duration, blood pressure measurements, and body weight and size. Data acquisition can also take place automatically from glucose meters supporting the IEEE 11073 Personal Health Data Standards. Data synchronization is done automatically and in two directions.

Therapy plans, instructions, and recommendations sent by the doctor from the doctor portal are received directly in the mobile application. For patients without smartphones (Mobil Diab app), they can still get these doctors' feedbacks in the protected patients' portal, through their email address or as sms if this service was activated.

2.3. Web-Based Applications of Mobil Diab. The web structure of the system is conceived in order to serve as a complete hospital management system. Four web-based portals are integrated to the system and hosted from the central platform. They are designed for four different types of users: patients, doctors, hospital administrators, and system administrator.

Figure 4 is a section of the screenshot of the doctor portal. The graphic shows the glucose measurements of one day, amount of carbohydrate taken (blue color facing up), and units of insulin injected (purple color facing down). Clinicians have a structured and understandable view of patients' data. Clear graphical representation of trends and statistics enables clinicians to make appropriate decisions on therapy adjustment. The tool helps medical staff save their times while providing high quality service to diabetes patients.

Doctors can receive messages from their patients directly in this portal. For emergency cases, an SMS is automatically generated and sent to the treating physician, to alert him to check the critical situation in the portal and be able to give direct instructions to the patient.

2.4. Architecture of the Telemedical Platform. The patent-protected platform illustrated by Figure 5 has been developed to help bridge the gap between health and mobility. Diverse healthcare modules have been implemented and other are planned in order to meet a complete health care service package from diabetes, dermatology, stress, fitness, and long-term health conditions up to the assisted-living for senior. The platform helps consumers track health, wellness, and vital information using a highly secure infrastructure. It allows consumers to share information with their health care professionals and family. Mobility is guaranteed by integrating mobile Apps and web-based applications. Moreover, interfaces to hospital information systems and practice management software are supported. In this work, the diabetes module was further developed, updated, tested, and validated. The four-layer architecture of the platform enables users to securely share sensitive information. Using different devices, such as smartphones and computers, users can access functionalities of applications supported by the core of the platform through the communication layer.

Security is a general requirement in modern computing environments, but in e-health systems security is an imperative requirement because those systems handle very sensitive

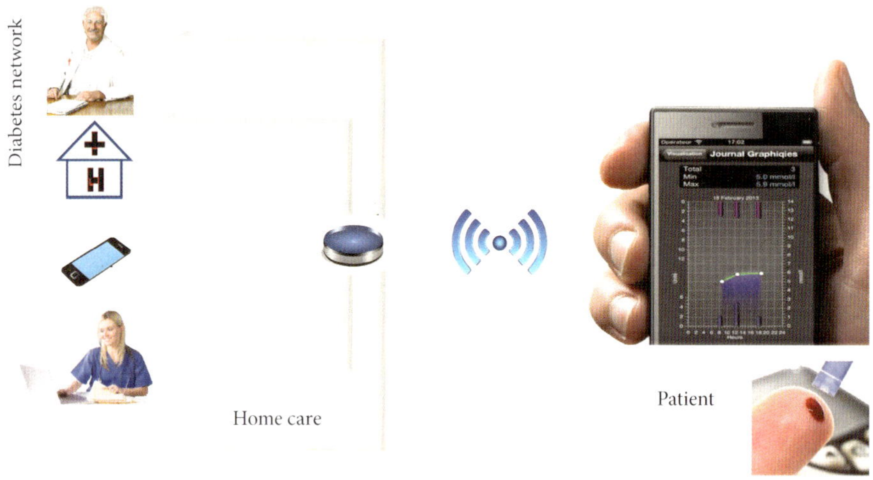

Figure 1: Mobil Diab system components.

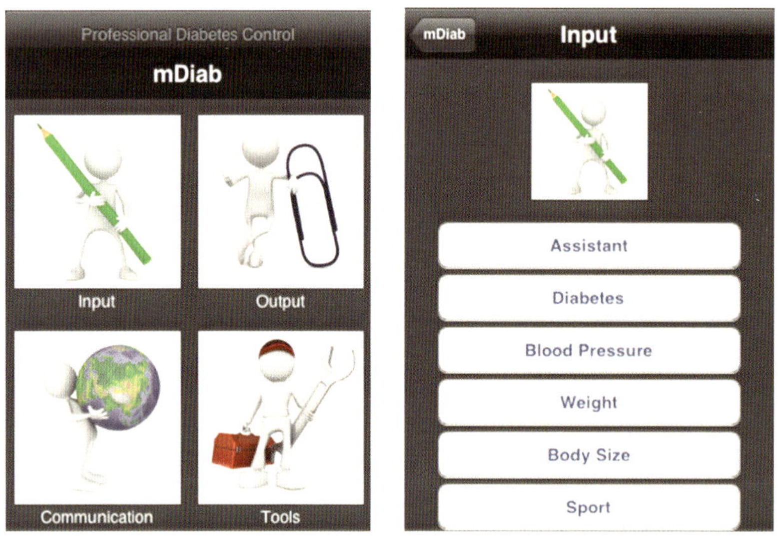

(a) (b)

Figure 2: Mobil Diab mobile application: screenshots of the main screen and the input choices.

data like medical and personal data. The platform acquires features enabling the following.

(i) Authentication: methods and mechanisms which allow an entity to prove its identity to a remote end.

(ii) Authorization: access control mechanisms and the ability of an entity to access shared resources.

(iii) Data integrity: mechanisms which ensure that when there is an interchange of data between two peer entities, the received data and the original ones are the same, and that no intermediate alteration has occurred.

(iv) Data confidentiality: it assures that stored or transmitted data are well protected from possible disclosure. A mean used to achieve data confidentiality is through cryptographic mechanisms.

(v) Privacy: it can be defined as an entity's ability to control how, when, and to what extent personal information about the entity will be communicated to third parties.

(vi) Secure data communication and storage.

(vii) Data availability: data can be accessed by authorized users independently from time and location.

Our proposed architecture addresses authentication and authorization issues, since each user is classified to a category that defines what he/she has access to. Moreover, data confidentiality is achieved through cryptographic mechanisms. Medical data and personal data are encoded and stored in separate data bases. All data are encrypted using the symmetric encryption method AES (Advanced Encryption

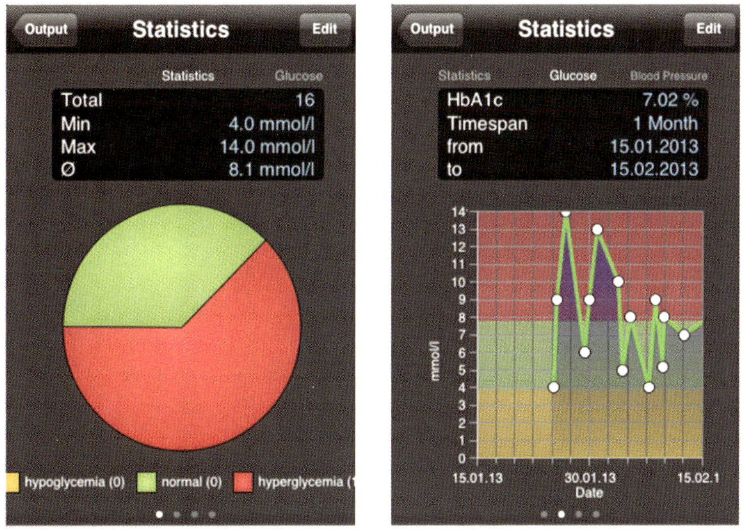

(a) (b)

Figure 3: Mobil Diab mobile application: output screens and blood glucose graph.

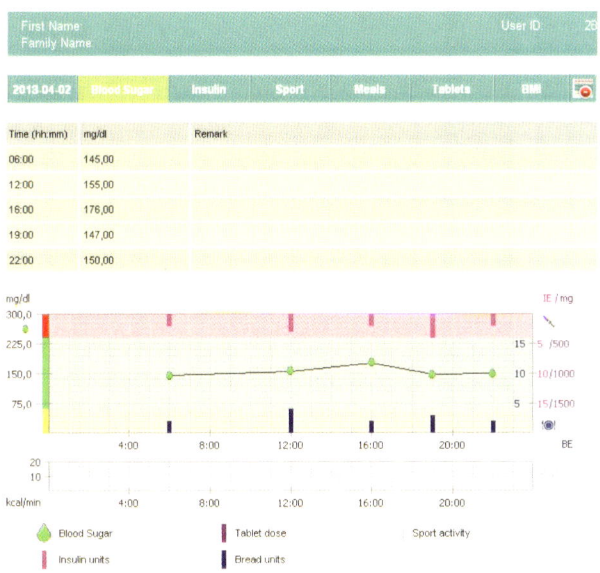

Figure 4: Mobil Diab web application: doctors' portal and glucose day graph.

Standard). For the protection of user's privacy, an implemented mechanism allows different groups of users to have access to different types of medical data.

The platform is composed of several modules, each one supporting its group of tasks. This structure makes the support of new services easier. The integration sublayer is responsible for formatting data in a needed standard. This extends the interoperability capability with other third-party systems. Some of the supported standards include HL7, CDA, WSDL, and XML. This platform was also presented in [14–16].

2.5. Experimental Settings and Recruitment Criteria. In order to test the effectiveness of the diabetes management system Mobil Diab in the context of African health care system, a trial was conducted in two cities in the eastern part of the Democratic Republic of Congo (Goma and Butembo). Patients diagnosed with type 2 diabetes and aged between 35 and 75 years were recruited randomly. A total of 40 patients were included in the trial phase. For classification and evaluation purpose, the cohort was divided into a control group (conventional therapy without the use of telemedicine system) and an intervention group (treatment with the use of telemedicine system Mobil Diab). To verify the comparability of the two groups, Table 3 shows that the control and intervention groups in terms of anthropometric data and metabolic control parameter are almost the same at the beginning of the trial: the mean age for the intervention group is 53.3 years with a standard deviation of 10.7 years and for the control group is 53.35 years with a standard deviation of 9.59 years. The mean HbA1c value for the whole intervention group before the trial was 8.67% and for the control group was 8.59%. The trial was conducted for a period of two months. During this trial period, medical staff of four local hospitals belonging to the health department of the Baptist Community in Central Africa (CBCA) accessed the system and coached the patients based on the analysis of the sent data.

At the end of the trial each participant had to fill a questionnaire evaluating the system Mobil Diab based on the three following metrics: usability and design, efficiency and therapy satisfaction, and acceptance and appreciations. Questions for patients were as follows.

(i) Q1: How often could you successfully use the system?

(ii) Q2: How easy was it for you to cope with the application?

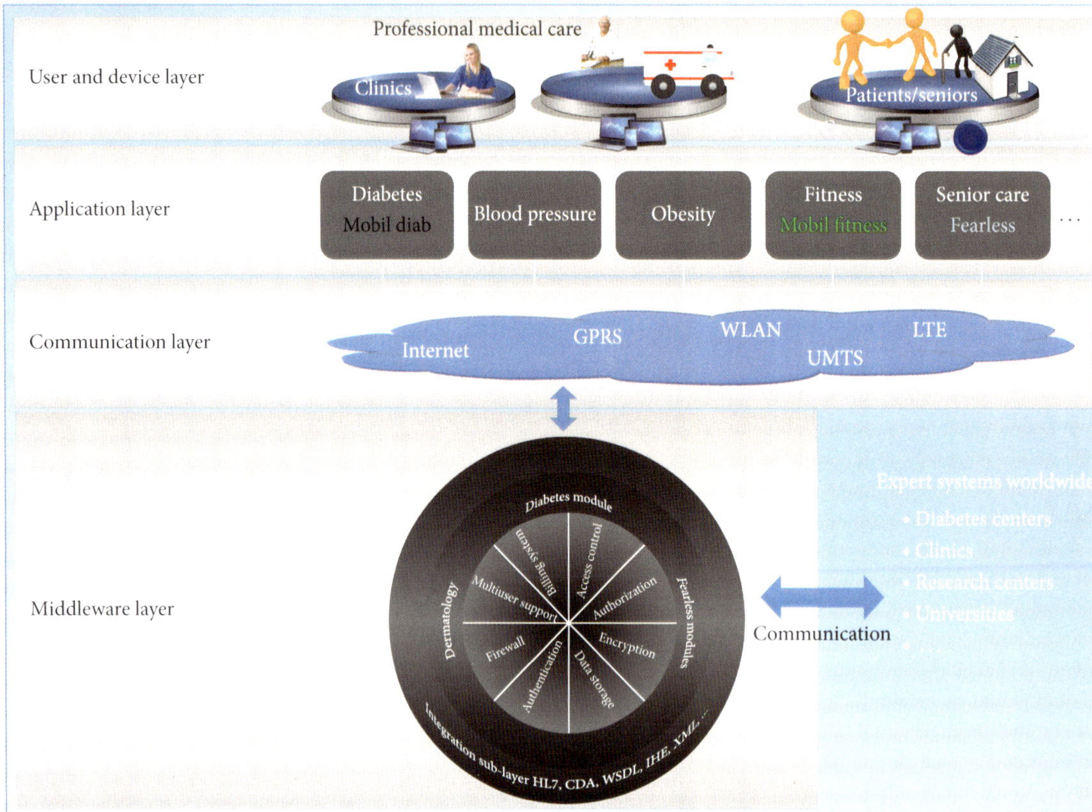

FIGURE 5: Architecture of the telemedical Platform.

(iii) Q3: How do you evaluate the input options and design of the application?

(iv) Q4: How do you evaluate the output options and visualization possibilities?

(v) Q5: How do you evaluate the design of the application?

(vi) Q6: Do you find Mobil Diab as a tool which motivates you in the control of your blood glucose levels?

(vii) Q7: Did feedbacks (messages and therapy) from doctors help in the diabetes management process?

(viii) Q11: Would you wish to continue using Mobil Diab for managing your diabetes?

(ix) Q12: Would you recommend the system to other users?

Each medical care personnel had to evaluate the system by answering the following questions.

(i) Q1: How difficult was it for you to use the doctor web application to interact with your patients?

(ii) Q2: How do you evaluate the design of the doctor portal?

(iii) Q3: How often could you successfully use the system?

(iv) Q4: How do you evaluate the representation of diabetes data in the portal?

(v) Q5: How do you evaluate the monthly representation of patient's data on graph?

(vi) Q6: How do you evaluate the feature for report generation?

(vii) Q7: How do you appreciate the page summarizing all important patient's data at glance?

(viii) Q8: Is the provided information in portal enough for improving the therapy adaptation?

(ix) Q12: Would you wish to continue using Mobil Diab for coaching your diabetes patients?

(x) Q13: Would you recommend the system to other medical care personnel?

A 10-point scale from 1 to 10 was used for questionnaire, with higher scores representing a better evaluation of the system based on the given question. Patients and medical care staff provided their evaluations as presented in Tables 1 and 2. Moreover, based on the analysis of patients' data collected during the trial period, the improvements in clinical outcome could be evaluated. Two metrics were used for this purpose: the mean amplitude of glycemic excursions (characterized by the mean blood glucose and its standard deviation) and the glycated hemoglobin (HbA1c), as Table 3 presents the results.

Before the trial could start, some settings, adaptations, and tests were made. All the involved partners (patients, medical care providers, support teams, administrators, internet and telephone providers, developers, and policy makers)

TABLE 1: Evaluation of usability, efficiency, and acceptance of Mobil Diab by patients.

Evaluation of MobilDiab by patients									
Subjects (patients)	Q1 (points)	Q2 (points)	Q3 (points)	Q4 (points)	Q5 (points)	Q6 (points)	Q7 (points)	Q11 (points)	Q12 (points)
P1	8	9	10	10	9	10	10	10	10
P2	7	5	8	7	5	8	7	8	7
P3	5	3	5	10	5	10	10	10	10
P4	8	8	8	9	6	10	7	10	10
P5	3	4	4	3	6	5	3	5	5
P6	10	10	7	8	10	10	10	10	10
P7	8	7	5	6	9	10	7	10	10
P8	4	4	8	2	4	10	7	10	10
P9	6	5	10	7	8	10	10	10	7
P10	7	8	9	9	8	9	8	9	10
P11	4	5	5	6	3	6	4	5	6
P12	6	7	7	8	10	8	4	9	7
P13	1	5	5	5	5	5	4	6	7
P14	5	6	7	8	8	10	8	10	10
P15	8	9	8	7	8	10	1	10	10
P16	9	10	8	8	8	10	10	10	10
P17	7	8	9	7	6	10	5	10	10
P18	9	10	7	9	8	10	8	9	10
P19	3	5	7	7	8	5	4	5	5
P20	6	6	6	7	8	7	4	8	8
Sum	**124**	**134**	**143**	**143**	**142**	**173**	**131**	**174**	**172**
Average for each question	**6.2**	**6.7**	**7.15**	**7.15**	**7.1**	**8.65**	**6.55**	**8.7**	**8.6**
			Usability and design			Efficiency and therapy satisfaction		Acceptance and appreciations	
Average (max. 10 points)			**7**			**7.43**		**8.65**	

TABLE 2: Evaluation of usability, efficiency, and acceptance of Mobil Diab by the medical staff.

Evaluation of Mobil Diab by the medical staff										
Doctors	Q1 (points)	Q2 (points)	Q3 (points)	Q4 (points)	Q5 (points)	Q6 (points)	Q7 (points)	Q8 (points)	Q12 (points)	Q13 (points)
D1	8	8	7	9	8	8	8	9	9	10
D2	9	7	6	7	7	8	8	5	8	8
D3	7	8	7	8	7	7	8	8	9	7
D4	9	8	2	7	7	8	8	8	7	8
D5	8	8	10	6	5	9	9	5	10	10
D6	6	8	9	9	6	6	7	7	9	9
D7	7	6	3	6	6	7	5	5	8	9
D8	7	7	5	7	6	8	7	8	9	10
Average for each question	**7.63**	**7.5**	**6.12**	**7.37**	**6.5**	**7.62**	**7.5**	**6.87**	**8.63**	**8.87**
	Usability and design				Efficiency and therapy satisfaction				Acceptance and appreciations	
Average (max. 10 points)	**7.56**				**7**				**8.75**	

TABLE 3: Evaluation of the impact of the use of Mobil Diab on the clinical results: intervention group versus control group.

(a) Intervention group: clinical results, changes in the quality of metabolic control after 60 days trial, and mean HbA1C for the intervention group before the beginning of the study which was 8.67%

Patients (sex, age)	Mean BG (mg/dL) day1–day60	Standard deviation (mg/dL)	HbA1C (%) day1–day60
P1 (M, 54)	208.2	91.9	8.8
P2 (F, 38)			
P3 (M, 52)	95.3	1.5	5.4
P4 (M, 58)	76.3	4.0	4.8
P5 (F, 60)	108.8	32.6	5.8
P6 (M, 48)	128.4	44.5	6.4
P7 (M, 55)	303.7	84.4	11.7
P8 (F, 49)			
P9 (M, 48)	130.0	38.4	6.4
P10 (M, 62)	141.4	48.0	6.8
P11 (M, 51)	180.1	15.8	7.9
P12 (M, 56)	134.2	38.0	6.6
P13 (M, 57)			
P14 (M, 43)	111.5	11.1	5.9
P15 (M, 60)	132.7	32.6	6.5
P16 (M, 58)	128.8	30.3	6.4
P17 (M, 50)	157.4	30.0	7.3
P18 (F, 35)	111	10.9	5.9
P19 (M, 70)	108	14.5	5.8
P20 (M, 62)	116.3	31.8	6.0
53.3 Mean age, St. deviation 10.7	143.5 Mean blood Glucose	33.0 Mean BG St. deviation	**6.89** Mean HbA1C at the end

(b) Control group: clinical results, changes in the quality of metabolic control after 60 days trial, and mean HbA1C for the control group before the beginning of the study which was 8.59%

Patients (sex and age)	Mean BG (mg/dL) day1–day60	Standard deviation (mg/dL)	HbA1C (%) day1–day60
Pc1 (M, 43)	261.8	44.2	10.4
Pc2 (M, 55)	187.2		8.2
Pc3 (M, 60)	174	48.2	7.8
Pc4 (F, 37)	227.8	33.2	9.4
Pc5 (M, 48)			
Pc6 (M, 67)	175.7	17.7	7.8
Pc7 (F, 40)	159	29.5	7.3
Pc8 (M, 42)	202.9		8.6
Pc9 (M, 57)	299.5	101.4	11.5
Pc10 (F, 53)			
Pc11 (M, 59)			
Pc12 (M, 66)			

(b) Continued.

Patients (sex and age)	Mean BG (mg/dL) day1–day60	Standard deviation (mg/dL)	HbA1C (%) day1–day60
Pc13 (M, 54)	163.2	35.1	7.4
Pc14 (M, 45)			
Pc15 (F, 58)	269.4	80.6	10.6
Pc16 (M, 61)	184.2	68.4	8.1
Pc17 (M, 75)	181.3	71.8	8.0
Pc18 (F, 49)			
Pc19 (F, 52)	180.4	12.6	8
Pc20 (F, 46)	160	40	7.3
53.35 Mean age, St. deviation 9.59	201.9 Mean blood glucose	48.6 Mean BG St. deviation	**8.6** Mean HbA1C at the end

(St. deviation: standard deviation, mean BG: mean blood glucose values).

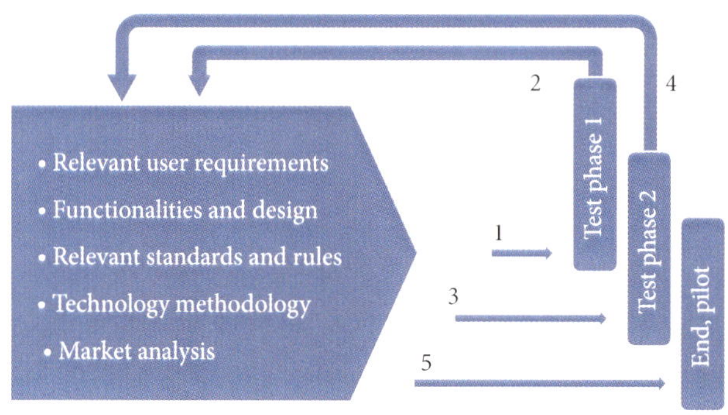

FIGURE 6: Flow of the trial process.

worked closely together during the development and adaptation process of the system. Figure 6 illustrates the flow of the trial. For each test stage, user requirements, functionalities and design, relevant standards and rules, and methodology and market analysis were discussed with all the involved players. Analysis of feedbacks from each stage constituted important input for the following stage. At the end, final modifications were made to obtain the final pilot ready for use in a larger scale.

Through collaboration with the local university, the Ruwenzori State University in Butembo, Democratic Republic of Congo, both its faculty of medicine and faculty of applied sciences will keep on conducting research in order to contribute to the adaptation of the system to meet other local specific needs.

3. Results and Discussion

Table 1 summarizes results of the questionnaire evaluating Mobil Diab by patients. Each question was evaluated based on a 10-point-scale from 1 to 10 point with high scores reflecting positive feedback from the user. Three metrics were considered for evaluation: usability and design, efficiency and therapy satisfaction, and acceptance and appreciations.

Score regarding usability and design was the average score for questions 1, 2, 3, 4, and 5 and resulted in a mean value of 7 points out of ten. This score is the average from all patients of the intervention group. Score for efficiency and therapy satisfaction was the average score for questions 6 and 7 and resulted in a mean value of 7.43 points out of ten. At last, score related to acceptance and appreciations was averaged from questions 11 and 12 and resulted in a mean value of 8.65 points out of ten. These results reflect an overall positive feedback of the patients about the system.

Table 2 represents the evaluation from the medical staff involved in the study. These include four medical doctors, two nurses, and two nutritionists. Score regarding usability and design was the average score for questions 1 and 2 and resulted in a mean value of 7.56 points out of ten. This score is the average from all medical care personnel. Score for efficiency and therapy satisfaction was the average score for questions 3, 4, 5, 6, 7, and 8 and resulted in a mean value of 7 points out of ten. Acceptance and appreciations score was averaged from questions 12 and 13 and resulted in a mean value of 8.75 points out of ten. These results reflect an overall positive feedback of the patients about the system.

The randomization of all the 40 patients in control and intervention group was successful. Both groups are statistically comparable in terms of relevant diabetes therapy.

Table 3 shows the impact of using Mobil Diab on the clinical results. Two metrics were used to assess the improvement in the quality of metabolic control: the mean amplitude of glycemic excursions (characterized from the mean BG and its standard deviation) and the mean HbA1c of each group. We should notice that the mean amplitude of glycemic excursions is the measure of diabetic instability, or a characteristic of blood glucose behavior and the HbA1c is the standard measure of average glycemic control predicting diabetes complications in type 1 and type2.

The approximate mapping between HbA1c values given in percentage (%) and mean BG (estimated average glucose) measurements was calculated using the following equation [17]:

$$\text{HbA1c } [\%] = \frac{(\text{mean BG } [\text{mg/dL}] + 86)}{33.3}. \quad (1)$$

Positive results have been noticed at the end of the trial, this is particularly evident in a significant improvement in the mean HbA1c values for the intervention group. The mean HbA1c for that group was 8.67% before the start of the trial and could be reduced to 6.89% at the end. This value of 1.78% in the improvement of HbA1c indicates that the risk of diabetes complications has been reduced or postponed, thus leading to cost savings.

Moreover, an important improvement could be noticed in the mean amplitude of glycemic excursions. This is shown in Table 3 by an important reduction of the glucose variability (characterized by the standard deviation of the mean BG). The mean BG standard deviation was 48.6 mg/mL for the control group whereas; this could be reduced to 33 mg/dL for the intervention group at the end of the trial.

Patients found the system as a helpful tool, since it helped them increase their motivation for regular glycemic control, motivated them to fix some goals or targets values for blood glucose control for the future, and helped them to control their meal since they could access easily the database containing the amount of carbohydrate for each meal and portion they were taking. Medical care personnel listed such benefits as follows: the system allowed them to coach several patients at the same time and at a distance, and modernization of health care system allowed them to get rich and useful data through a secure system. The amelioration in the clinical results is due to these above listed benefits provided by the system.

However, some disadvantages such as costs for internet connection and time needed for getting used to the application were the preoccupation of both categories of the users. Wishes from both categories of the subjects included to the trial (medical staff and patients) for the amelioration of the system were collected and included the following:

(i) Extend the drug list and meal database in the application to include all local foods, and applied drugs, since some of them were missing

(ii) More sensitizing activities and training sessions about the system to patients and medical staff

(iii) Include the support of the glucose measuring device kit in the model

(iv) Create a framework for sport activities for patients

4. Conclusions

An IT-enabled diabetes management with fully integrated provider-patient system has been presented in this paper. Results from the trial conducted in two eastern cities of the Democratic Republic of Congo have proved how the system Mobil Diab is suited not only for developed countries but also for communities traditionally underserved, those in remote or rural areas with few health services and staff. This population can access diabetes care using Mobil Diab, because the system overcomes distance and time barriers between health-care providers and patients.

The use of Mobil Diab showed improvement of clinical outcomes of the patients from the intervention group involved in the conducted trial. This has been demonstrated from the amelioration of both the HbA1c (from 8.67% to 6.89%) and the mean amplitude of glycemic excursions which is characterized from both the mean blood glucose and its standard deviation. The decrease of the blood glucose fluctuations is demonstrated from results of the mean blood glucose standard deviation from the intervention group compared to the control group at the end of the study (33.0 mg/mL instead of 48.6 mg/mL). This proves how the use of the system could help patients stabilize better their glucose values.

Positive evaluations of the system from patients and medical staff have been presented based on three metrics: usability and design, efficiency and therapy satisfaction, and acceptance and appreciations. The obtained scores are 7 points and greater out of the 10 maximum points.

The model developed from the conducted pilot in the Democratic Republic of Congo can be extended and applied for other countries in order to enhance awareness on the diabetes management in the continent and to improve the quality of service in the care process.

Acknowledgments

This paper is based on a trial conducted in the Democratic Republic of Congo in the frame of cooperation between Infokom GmbH, a German IT Company, and CBCA, Baptist Community in Central Africa. The project was partially supported by the United Evangelical Mission in Germany and some members of the CBCA, to whom authors express their gratitude.

References

[1] S. Wild, G. Roglic, and A. Green, "Global prevalence of diabetes," *Journal Diabetes Care*, vol. 27, no. 5, pp. 1047–1053, 2005.

[2] D. Si, R. Bailie, Z. Wang, and T. Weeramanthri, "Comparison of diabetes management in five countries for general and indigenous populations: an internet-based review," *BMC Health Services Research*, vol. 10, article 169, 2010.

[3] Report of Home Office UK Border Agency, Country of origin Information Report Democratic Republic of Congo, January 2009.

[4] C. Jaffiol, "The burden of diabetes in Africa: a major public health problem," *Bulletin de l'Academie Nationale de Medecine*, vol. 196, no. 6, pp. 1239–1254, 2011.

[5] G. Lanzola, D. Capozzi, G. D'Annunzio, P. Ferrari, R. Bellazzi, and C. Larizza, "Going mobile with a multiaccess service for the management of diabetic patients," *Journal of Diabetes Science and Technology*, vol. 1, no. 5, pp. 730–737, 2007.

[6] X. Liang, Q. Wang, X. Yang et al., "Effect of mobile phone intervention for diabetes on glycaemic control: a meta-analysis," *Diabetic Medicine*, vol. 28, no. 4, pp. 455–463, 2011.

[7] D. Capozzi and G. Lanzola, "Utilizing information technologies for lifelong monitoring in diabetes patients," *Journal of Diabetes Science and Technology*, vol. 5, no. 1, pp. 55–62, 2011.

[8] G. Lanzola, D. Capozzi, N. Serina, L. Magni, and R. Bellazzi, "Bringing the artificial pancreas home: telemedicine aspects," *Journal of Diabetes Science and Technology*, vol. 5, no. 6, pp. 1381–1386, 2011.

[9] R. Harper, P. Nicholf, M. McTear, J. Wallace, L. Black, and P. Kearney, "Automated phone capture of diabetes patients readings with consultant monitoring via the web," in *Proceedings of the 15th IEEE International Conference and Workshops on the Engineering of Computer-Based Systems (ECBS '08)*, pp. 219–226, Belfast, UK, April 2008.

[10] Diabetes Management Software, "Bayer's GLUCKOFACTS DELUXE Software," 2013, http://www.bayerdiabetes.com/sections/ourproducts/software.aspx.

[11] SiDiary—Diabetes Management Software, http://www.sinovo.de/.

[12] G. Charpentier, *Diabeo: Improving Diabetes Care with an Innovative Web and Mobile Telemedicine Solution*, Health Executive Summit, Paris, France, 2010.

[13] R. Bellazzi, "Telemedicine and diabetes management: current challenges and future research directions," *Journal of Diabetes Science and Technology*, vol. 2, pp. 98–104, 2008.

[14] R. D. Berndt, M. C. Takenga, S. Kuehn, P. Preik, D. Dubbermann, and M. Juenger, "Development of a mobile teledermatology system," *Telemedicine and e-Health*, vol. 18, no. 9, pp. 668–673, 2012.

[15] M. C. Takenga, R. Berndt, S. Kuehn et al., "Stress and fitness monitoring embedded on a modern telematics platform," *Telemedicine and e-Health*, vol. 18, no. 5, pp. 371–376, 2012.

[16] R.-D. Berndt, M. C. Takenga, S. Kuehn, P. Preik, G. Sommer, and S. Berndt, "SaaS-platform for mobile health applications," in *Proceedings of the 9th International Multi-Conference on Systems, Signals and Devices (SSD '12)*, pp. 1–4, Chemniz, Germany, March 2012.

[17] C. L. Rohlfing, H. M. Wiedmeyer, R. R. Little, J. D. England, A. Tennill, and D. E. Goldstein, "Defining the relationship between plasma glucose and HbA1c: analysis of glucose profiles and HbA1c in the diabetes control and complications trial," *Diabetes Care*, vol. 25, no. 2, pp. 275–278, 2002.

11

Patients' Experiences with Specialist Care via Video Consultation in Primary Healthcare in Rural Areas

Annette M. Johansson, Inger Lindberg, and Siv Söderberg

Division of Nursing, Department of Health Science, Luleå University of Technology, 971 87 Luleå, Sweden

Correspondence should be addressed to Annette M. Johansson; annette.johansson@ltu.se

Academic Editor: Max E. Stachura

Introduction. Video consultation (VC) can improve access to specialist care, especially for individuals who live in rural areas that are long distances from specialist clinics. *Aim*. The aim of this study was to describe patients' experiences with specialist care via VC encounters. *Method*. Interviews were conducted with 26 patients who had participated in a VC encounter. The data were analysed using thematic content analysis. *Result*. The analysis resulted in two themes. The theme "confident with the technology" was constructed from the categories "possibilities and obstacles in using VC encounters" and "advantages and disadvantages of the technology." The theme "personal satisfaction with the VC encounters" was constructed from the categories "support from the healthcare personnel," "perceived security," and "satisfaction with the specialist consultation." *Conclusion*. The patients who did not think that the VC was the best care still considered that the visit was adequate because they did not have to travel. An important finding was that the patients' perceived even short distances to specialty care as expensive journeys because many patients had low incomes. Among the patients who had more than one VC, the second encounter was perceived as safer. Additionally, good communication was essential for the patient's perception of security during the VC encounter.

1. Introduction

Video consultation (VC) can improve access to specialist care, especially for individuals who live in rural areas [1, 2]. Video consultation is a specialised type of telemedicine that uses technology to provide real-time visual and audio patient assessment at a distance [3]. This system permits a direct interaction between the patient and healthcare personnel because they are separated by space, not time [4]. In this method of meeting, the specialist physician changes the location of care by connecting patients and specialist physicians virtually instead of through the conventional face-to-face contact. Video consultation improves the quality of care and benefits the healthcare organisation [1]. The virtual meeting can provide opportunities to gain access to relevant expertise, without the significance of geographic distance. Video consultation offers opportunities to disseminate and receive knowledge so that misunderstandings can be avoided and/or solved immediately [5]. It is also an opportunity to enhance the local service provision, provides more rapid specialist assessment, and reinforces general practitioners' (GPs) clinical assessments and increases access to and support from the specialist physician [6]. In VC encounters between diabetes patients and endocrinologists, Fatehi et al. [2] found that the specialist physicians mostly were confident with their own recommendations. A lack of physical exam was not considered a limiting factor, and if necessary, the GP could perform the physical examination.

Traveling to healthcare centres is often difficult for individuals with poor health, disabilities, and/or low income. This difficulty can be amplified if the individual has chronic problems that require regular visits to specialist care. If the individual has a disability, the individual may need an escort and/or special transportation, which increases the cost for both the individual and the healthcare system. Visiting a healthcare provider for children is much more expensive because of the need for an accompanying individual [7]. Providing services directly to patients who live in the areas beyond the usual service boundaries are beneficial for hospitals and saves money because of the reduced travel costs [6].

Table 1: Overview of savings in time, costs, and environmental impact calculated in 10 VC.

Healthcare centre	A	B	C	D	E	Total
Distance[1]	440 km	46 km	260 km	310 km	136 km	1192 km
Travel time[1]	5 h 30 min	45 min	3 h 30 min	4 h 30 min	2 h	14 h 15 min
Number of visits	10	10	10	10	10	10
Number off km ($n = 10$)	4400 km	460 km	2600 km	3100 km	1360 km	11920 km
Saved journey ($n = 10$) time	55 h	7 h 30 min	35 h	45 h	20 h	162 h 30 min
Travel ($n = 10$) allowance[2]	4400 SEK	4600 SEK	2600 SEK	3100 SEK	1360 SEK	16 060 SEK
Patient petrol expenses/journey[3] ($n = 10$)	792 SEK (7920 SEK)	83 SEK (828 SEK)	468 SEK (4680 SEK)	558 SEK (5580 SEK)	245 SEK (2448 SEK)	2 146 SEK (21 456 SEK)
Carbon dioxide kg ($n = 10$ journeys)	612 kg[5] 588 kg[6]	64 kg[5] 61 kg[6]	362 kg[5] 347 kg[6]	431 kg[5] 414 kg[6]	189 kg[5] 182 kg[6]	1658 kg[5] 1592 kg[6]

[1] Back and forth.
[2] County Council provides compensation of 10 SEK/10 km if traveling by own car.
[3] Calculated on patient expenses 18 SEK/10 km (the County Council give 10 SEK in travel allowance).
[4] Gasoline.
[5] Diesel.

Video consultation in real time allows the simultaneous and rapid exchange of information, which is advantageous if the conversations are complex or of an urgent nature, whether it is a patient consultation or a case discussion [7]. Because of the need for visual assessment in skin examinations, VC can be a valuable tool in the diagnosis and management of dermatologic diseases, especially in rural areas located long distances from specialist care [4]. An accurate and comprehensive medical history can easily be communicated via VC, but if there are circumstances that require a physical examination for a successful assessment, VC may be less suited. Therefore, collaboration and confidence in the assessment by an individual qualified to perform and report the findings are most likely important components for VC success [3].

Agha et al. 2009 [8] suggested that the use of the latest technology can be translated into "quality care" for some patients. Additionally, the attention from two healthcare professionals may promote a patient's confidence [9]. To build trust and patient satisfaction with care, it is important that the patient has confidence in the healthcare provider's clinical skills [8]. There is a continuing need for larger studies of telemedicine that use controlled interventions and telemedicine innovations that involve complex processes and an ongoing collaboration. As the field is rapidly evolving, new knowledge is constantly needed. Understanding the patients' experiences from a qualitative perspective is an area of great interest [10]. Therefore, this study focused on the patients' experiences with specialist care via VC.

1.1. Context. This study was performed in northern Sweden. The county of Norrbotten is the largest county in Sweden; it covers one-quarter of the country's total land area but has fewer than 250,000 inhabitants, that is, 2.6% of the Swedish population. Most inhabitants live within a few miles of the largest city in the county, and the central hospital is situated close to the largest city; the rest of the county is sparsely populated [11]. This study area was chosen because the County Council of Norrbotten was planning to implement the use of VC encounters for specialist care in all health centres in the county. Five primary healthcare (PHC) centres reported that they were interested in participating in the study. The patient came to their PHC centre and together with the GP they had encounter with the specialist physician via video consultation.

The distance to the nearest hospital was between 23 kilometres and 220 kilometres ($m = 119$ kilometres). Table 1 shows the estimated cost/savings (based on ten VC) for the patient, the County Council [12], and also the environment [13]. It is not taken into account that in the winter there can be many delays due to snow and unploughed roads and this means that it is not certain that the patient will make it to be the specialist appointment in time.

2. Aim of the Study

The aim of this study was to describe patients' experiences with specialist care via VC encounters.

3. Methods

3.1. Design. A qualitative design and thematic content analysis were chosen to achieve the aim of the study.

3.2. The Intervention: Video Consultation. Healthcare personnel at each PHC centre were given information about the study. They were also given education on the equipment and how to perform video consultation. The technology consisted of a desktop speaker, a microphone, a Logitech camera, and Polycom CMA desktop videoconferencing software. A pilot test was performed in order to train the healthcare personnel to become secure in how the technology worked.

3.3. Participants and Procedure. Twenty-six patients were interviewed, including 11 men and 15 women between 18 and 83 years of age (Md = 63, $m = 59$) (Table 2).

Table 2: Demographic data.

Gender male (n = 11)/age	Gender female (n = 15)/age
33–46–59–60–64–70–72–74–78–81–83	18-19–25–39–42–49–59–61–63–68–72-73–77–77–82

The following inclusion criteria for the participants were used: individuals who had participated in VC encounters at the PHC centre with a specialist (dermatologist $n = 1$ or specialist nurse $n = 1$ in heart disease) at the main hospital. The GP provided an information letter about the study and a letter of informed consent to the patient after the VC. The first author contacted the patients who agreed to participate by phone and established a time and place for the interview. Before the interview, the patient received verbal information about the study and the voluntary participation. The interviews were conducted at the PHC centre, in the patient's home or via phone.

3.4. Data Collection. Individual semistructured interviews were conducted with the patients. An interview guide was used and contained the following questions: "please tell me about your experience with the VC," "tell me what you think VC might mean for your future care," "please share your thoughts on specialist care via VC," "please tell me what opportunities and obstacles you can see with VC," "can you tell me which areas of care you think VC at a distance would be helpful for you," "please tell me how was your experienced about the support from the personnel and why it was good or bad," "what did you feel about the answers/advice you got from the specialist physician," "would you consider having VC alone in the room if the staff were available outside if needed," and "how long did you have to wait before the VC encounter." Clarifying questions were also used, for example, "can you give some examples," "how do you think now," "what do you think it would mean for you," and "what could have been done differently." The interviews were performed between June 2010 and December 2011, and they lasted between 10 and 30 minutes (md = 15 minutes), were audio taped, and later were transcribed verbatim.

3.5. Data Analysis. A qualitative thematic content analysis was used to analyse the interview texts. According to Baxter [14], thematic analysis is the most complex method because the researcher's interpretations are based on a holistic analysis. Themes are threads of meaning that emerge from the categories. The transcribed interview text was read through several times to obtain a sense of the whole. Then, units of analysis, including words, phrases, sentences, or whole text that corresponded with the aim of the study, were identified and encoded by content, for example, security, advantages, disadvantages, and so forth. The encoded units of analysis were sorted into categories based on the similarities or differences in content. The categories were then sorted into two themes with five categories (Table 3); a theme can be described as threads of meaning that appeared in categories after categories. The researches discussed the categories and themes in order to reach a common outcome. When the categorisation was finished, the units of analysis were reread and checked for the accuracy of their categorisation.

Table 3: Overview of themes and categories from the interviews (n = 27).

Theme	Categories
Confident with technology	Possibilities and obstacles in using VC encounters
	Advantages and disadvantages of the technology
Personal satisfaction with the VC encounters	Support from the healthcare personnel
	Perceived security
	Satisfaction with the specialist consultation

4. Results

The analysis revealed two themes with five categories. The themes and categories are presented and illustrated with quotations from the interviews.

4.1. Confident with Technology. The theme "confident with the technology" was constructed from the categories "possibilities and obstacles in using VC encounters" and "advantages and disadvantages of the technology."

4.1.1. Possibilities and Obstacles in Using VC Encounters. Participants described that the VC encounters were a good first step for meeting a specialist physician and receiving a diagnosis was possible from this encounter. Most participants considered there were few or no barriers in using VC, but some participants thought face-to-face encounters would be more appropriate than VC encounters in certain situations. Participants emphasised the importance of the VC equipment being placed in a room where no other individuals, other than the participants in the VC encounter, were present. The obstacles that the participants described were related to the physicians; for example, if the picture quality was poor, the specialist physician's ability to make a diagnosis was affected. Therefore, the participants thought a face-to-face meeting would be better;

> *It is not good that the computer is placed in a room where people often enter because someone forgot to press the "busy" key [Participant 15].*

Participants thought that a possible disadvantage of having VC encounters could be that the specialist physician could not experience the patient's problems the same way as they would when meeting face-to-face. Several participants described being disappointed in not having the choice to participate in a VC encounter because of the GP's reluctance to use the technology. The reason for this reluctance was that the GP had no experience with the VC equipment or was not interested. Some participants described that they have not had the opportunity of a VC encounter since it was ambulatory GPs at the PHC. Consequently, the patient booked a new appointment when their regular GP returned to work, so they could have a VC encounter instead of traveling a long distance for a specialist consultation. Another obstacle that the participants highlighted was that VC encounters were not possible at all the PHC centres. Some participants said that they wanted to have the opportunity for a VC encounters in the future, so that they would not have to drive to the hospital by themselves when they are older;

> *The thing that was bad was that the ambulatory physician did not want to deal with the video consultation, so we waited for our regular GP [Participant 20].*

4.1.2. Advantages and Disadvantages of the Technology. The majority of participants reported that they saw technology as a major advantage that saved resources;

> *I see it (technology) as a big plus and one that saves resources [Participant 25].*

Most participants that used VC encounters considered the picture and sound quality to be good. They were pleased that the specialist physician could see clearly despite the long distance. There were also participants that did not think that the technology worked well. The sound was described as a problem by a few of the elderly participants who had impaired hearing. They said that the participants should be able to hear the specialist physician and suggested that a headset could be provided. In some cases, the GP and the nurse had to explain what was said during the VC encounter because the participant could not hear what was said;

> *It had very bad sound, so the nurse and the doctor who was with me explained what she (specialist physician) said; they could provide better sound for older people [Participant 3].*

Some participants expressed that the VC encounters were slightly abnormal because the picture of the specialist physician was very small and was located at the bottom corner of the computer screen. They said that a larger picture would make it feel more like a face-to-face conversation. There were times when the participants could not see the computer screen because it was turned the wrong way, and they did not understand that they could request that the screen should be repositioned. A short cable to the camera also caused some patients to sit/lie in awkward positions to provide a good image of the problem;

> *It was a little awkward to get your feet up on the table because the camera cable was too short, but I managed to do it [Participant 26].*

Participants described that the nurse took care of the technology, and the GP informed the specialist physician about the participant's problem. This was not considered negative but was merely a statement of fact. Participants who participated in VC encounters described several areas of use for the technology. They considered the VC encounters as an opportunity to contact a specialist physician for a less severe disease or ailment that did not require hospitalisation. Some areas they described included external ailments and injuries, psychiatry, and various medical conditions, such as diabetes, heart disease, and medication adjustments. Participants expressed that the VC encounters should be used based on the patient's problem;

> *It depends entirely on what you have as an ailment; certain ailments cannot be dealt with via computer [Participant 5].*

4.2. Personal Satisfaction with the VC Encounters. The theme "personal satisfaction with the VC encounters" was constructed from the categories "support from the healthcare personnel," "perceived security," and "satisfaction with the specialist's advice."

4.2.1. Support from the Healthcare Personnel. Participants described that they were well supported by the personnel during the VC encounters. In general, a district nurse and a GP were present with the participant during the VC encounter. The GP was considered to provide support mainly by explaining the problem to the specialist physician, as the GP had access to dates and past medical history that could be difficult for the participant to remember. The support from the district nurse was primarily because she took care of the participant and explained what would happen during the VC encounter. None of the participants had thought about whether VC affected their privacy. VC encounter was seen as an opportunity to receive help with treatment and/or a diagnosis, even if they had to undress for the camera. Participants expressed that they would consider participating alone in the VC encounters with the specialist physician if the GP first responded to the specialist physician's questions and the participant was able to handle the camera as needed;

> *I do not see it as a hindrance to have to undress in front of the camera, but I see it as an opportunity to get help [Participant 17].*

Most participants described the VC encounters as different, but these encounters were not viewed negatively. They experienced the VC as a personal encounter, although the meeting occurred via a computer;

> *Of course it feels different when you're talking to a computer screen, but it was not negative [Participant 5].*

The VC encounter with the specialist physician was described in positive terms and was perceived as a three-part conversation. Some participants described that the VC encounters were similar to face-to-face meetings. However, some participants also expressed that the VC encounters felt strange or slightly artificial and were not the same as talking to a human. Participants also described that they considered that the specialist physician could see the entire individual in a different way during face-to-face meetings compared with the VC encounters. Although the patients had concerns about the VC encounters, they were considered positive experiences by the participants;

> *I thought it was quite personal anyway, even though we were not sitting in the same room but communicated via computer [Participant 7].*

4.2.2. Perceived Security. Participants expressed that they felt secure when they were allowed to choose for themselves whether to participate in the VC encounters or receive a referral;

> *I had to choose [to have a VC or not], and it's good that I, as a patient, get to choose [Participant 4].*

Participants who had tried VC encounters previously described that they felt safer the second time, as they had knowledge of the procedure. Participants were pleased to have the GP or specialist's statements repeated or explained immediately what they did not hear or understand. Participants felt secure during the VC encounters if the visit was performed at their own PHC centre in the presence of personnel they recognised and were familiar with. Participants that met the GP for the first time during the VC encounter described that they felt sidelined, as they had not previously met the GP at the PHC centre. However, security decreased if many individuals were present in the room during the VC encounter. Participants felt uncomfortable if their medical problem was located in an intimate place, even if they knew the GP well. In these situations, the participants preferred to be alone during the VC encounter. Participants described that having the opportunity to talk to a specialist physician made them feel content and secure, particularly when it was not possible to meet the same GP, due to a lack of permanent GPs at their PHC centre. Participants felt uncomfortable with the technology if they had to conduct the VC alone in a room. However, they would conduct the meeting alone if the personnel began the VC encounter and was then available outside. However, the participants expressed the importance of having personnel in the room for more severe diseases or if the patient so desired;

> *It felt good mentally when you got to talk to the specialist; we do not have our own GP, so we meet the same ambulatory physician just twice [Participant 6].*

4.2.3. Satisfaction with the Specialist Consultation. Most participants were very satisfied with the VC encounters and experienced that they were helped by the specialist physician's advice and diagnosis. They also considered they received answers to their questions, and they believe they would have received the same answer if they had met the specialist physician in person;

> *I do not think I would have any other help if I met with the specialist face-to-face [Participant 1].*

Participants who did not receive a diagnosis via the VC were pleased with the tests that were ordered by the specialist physician and that they would later be provided with answers. Participants felt that they would discover and treat their disease more quickly through the VC encounters. Participants experienced that VC encounters at the PHC centre meant increased access to specialist care. Video consultation was considered a smooth, easy, and positive method to receive specialist care. Participants were very satisfied with the short waiting time as VC encounter meant compared to waiting for a referral to a face-to-face meeting. The patients could wait up to several months for a face-to-face visit, whereas they only had to wait a few days before they could participate in the VC encounter with the specialist physician.

If the participant was not helped by the treatment regime suggested during the VC encounter, the GP recommended that the patient go to the specialist physician for a face-to-face visit instead of performing another VC encounter. Participants were worried about not being seen as a person because of the technology. Most participants were very pleased with the VC encounter and wanted to use it as needed for the same or other problems. They felt that, whatever the problem, having the specialist physician "come to the patient" via a VC encounter was better than the patient traveling to the specialist physician;

> *It does not matter what condition you have; it has to be smoother with VC than to transport people to the specialist physician [Participant 17].*

The greatest benefit that the participants experienced was that they did not have to travel an entire day to meet with the specialist physician. They said that they were pleased to not have to travel, even if the specialist physician was located nearby. Participants described the VC encounter as a financial gain if travel was considered expensive despite receiving travel grants. Participants expressed satisfaction with not having to take time off from work for a whole day;

> *It means a lot for future care to avoid taking time off from work for a whole day [Participant 20].*

They thought VC encounters would be beneficial in their future when they will have difficulty moving because of age and disorders. Video consultation encounters also allowed individuals to save time, and individuals considered that VC benefited the environment. Participants expressed great optimism in not having to need referrals for some specialist areas in the future;

> *For my future care, it [VC] means I will get faster help when I do not need a referral [Participant 18].*

They reported that if the diagnosis could not be made at the VC encounter, they considered it to be more quickly to go to a specialist physician for a face-to-face visit. Participants who had met the specialist physician face-to-face considered the follow-up meetings through VC encounters as advantageous. They also considered that VC encounters saved time for the GP.

5. Discussion

Patients described that VC encounter was a good first step for meeting a specialist physician and receiving a diagnosis. This finding is inconsistent with the study by Johansson et al.

[15] in which healthcare personnel considered that the first meeting with the specialist physician should be face-to-face. According to Harrison et al. [16], VC encounters can improve patient satisfaction by increasing access to healthcare and can be a tool to increase patient choice about where to have their specialist care. Whitten and Mair [17] described that patients found the new technology exciting. In our study, the majority of participants saw the technology as a major advantage that saved resources, and they considered that the picture and sound quality was adequate. Liu et al. [18] reported that both patients and physicians considered VC encounters as a good idea. In our study the participants with impaired hearing described that if there was problem in hearing, the GP or nurse explained what was said, so that was no problem for them.

In our study, the participants reported that they considered the specialist physician's ability to make a correct diagnosis affected if the picture was not sufficiently clear. In these situations, they considered that a face-to-face meeting would have been better. Gray et al. [7] found that the quality of the video picture and sound was critically important for efficient communication and patient acceptance of VC encounters. Furthermore, the participants described that they were well supported by the GP during the VC encounter. Harrison et al. [16] found that patients liked having their GP present during the VC encounters. Although the GP's role in the VC encounter was minor, the mere presence of the GP gave the patient confidence. In this study, the participants expressed that receiving an immediate explanation of what they did not hear or understand was helpful. According to Hjelm [19], our perception of what we see on the computer screen is influenced by our experience of watching TV; therefore, VC encounters might not be experienced as being real. This perception may cause elderly patients to not accept that the physicians can see and listen to them properly. Participants expressed that they would conduct the VC encounter alone, but because they felt uncertain about the technology, they wished to have healthcare personnel nearby. According to Johansson et al. [15], the healthcare personnel should be comfortable with the technology to ensure patient safety during VC encounters. Additionally, the assessments performed in VC must be clinically reliable and comparable to the usual methods used to deliver care. Incorrect diagnosis can lead to misstatements and possibly fatal consequences [7].

Most participants described the VC encounter as a positive experience and thought of the encounter as a three-part conversation. According to Liu et al. [18], appropriate communication between the physician and patient was important to develop a good relationship and to achieve a positive outcome for the patient. Participants described that the support from the GP during the VC encounter included the GP explaining the patient's medical history and the patient's current problem. Harrison et al. [16] reported that most patients liked that the GP and the specialist physician used medical terminology. They thought that this communication provided a better presentation of their problem compared with what they could have done by themselves. Liu et al. [18] reported that patients did not find any difference in satisfaction between face-to-face encounters and VC encounters. The only difference was the number of requests for repeated utterances; the repetition was much higher for VC encounters compared with face-to-face encounters [18, 20]. This result may have been affected by the patients having VC encounters and face-to-face meetings in the same day to compare VC versus face-to-face encounters.

The results show that the participants were satisfied with the specialist consultation via VC. The VC encounters reduced waiting time, enhanced access to specialist care, and reduced travel. This result concurs with several studies (e.g., [7, 18, 21]) that examined patient satisfaction with VC encounters. Participants described that meeting the specialist physician via VC was better than traveling a long distance. Harrison et al. [16] and Gordon [22] reported that patients appreciated the improved convenience and punctuality associated with VC encounters compared with the outpatient clinics. Mair and Whitten [21] also found that patients who had used VC encounters had the impression that the examinations were more thorough, and the benefits of VC were clear. However, patients experienced an emotional distance between themselves and the specialist. In this study, participants' experiences were consistent with the study performed by Liu et al. [18] in which a VC encounter was less time consuming than a face-to-face consultation. This finding is also consistent with Gordon [22], who found that receiving medical care via VC encounter was easier and that the patients did not think that they would have received better care if they had met the specialist physician face-to-face.

Limitation of the study may be that only two specialist areas were included. But it is questionable whether the outcome would have been different if more areas had been included, since the results were very uniform between the two specialities. The number of participants in this study can be considered as many given that it is a qualitative study and that is a strength of the study. Strength of the study is also that it extends over a long time.

6. Conclusion

A majority of the participants considered the VC encounter as a positive experience and thought of the encounter as a three-part conversation. Even for the patients who did not believe the VC encounter provided the best care, the patients still considered VC as a possible option because they did not have to travel. This shows that VC is a possible solution to increase accessibility to specialized care in rural areas. The patients who completed VC encounters more than once perceived the second encounter as safer. This finding may be because these participants had knowledge of how the meeting would proceed. Additionally, good communication was essential for the patient's perception of security during the VC encounter. Another important finding was that even short distances to the specialist physician were perceived as expensive, particularly because many patients had low incomes. Further research should be conducted to investigate whether district nurses responsible for the VC encounter can improve the access to specialist care in rural areas when regular GP is not available. There is also need for studies if VC can increase access to specialist care in other specialities. Also research about the economic and environmental factors need to be examined in larger scale to see the gains VC can provide.

Ethical Approval

The respondents were guaranteed confidentiality and an anonymous presentation of the results. The study was approved by the Regional Ethical Board (dnr. 2010-5-31).

Acknowledgments

This study was supported by the Department of Health Science and was funded by 2nd goal EU contributions through the e-Health Innovation Centre (EIC) at Luleå University of Technology, Luleå, Sweden. The authors thank the patients for participating in the interviews.

References

[1] A. Darkins, "Patient safety considerations in developing large telehealth networks," *Clinical Risk*, vol. 18, no. 3, pp. 90–94, 2012.

[2] F. Fatehi, L. C. Gray, and A. W. Russell, "Telemedicine for clinical management of diabetes a analysis of video consultations," *Journal of Telemedicine and Telecare*, vol. 19, no. 7, pp. 379–382, 2013.

[3] C. Kitamura, L. Zurawel-Balaura, and R. K. S. Wong, "How effective is video consultation in clinical oncology? A systematic review," *Current Oncology*, vol. 17, no. 3, pp. 17–27, 2010.

[4] E. M. Warshaw, Y. J. Hillman, N. L. Greer et al., "Teledermatology for diagnosis and management of skin conditions: A systematic review," *Journal of the American Academy of Dermatology*, vol. 64, no. 4, pp. 759–772, 2011.

[5] R. Taylor, "Use of the internet to optimise collaborative healthcare research," *Nursing Standard*, vol. 22, no. 38, pp. 35–38, 2008.

[6] J. J. Moffatt and D. S. Eley, "The reported benefits of telehealth for rural Australians," *Australian Health Review*, vol. 34, no. 3, pp. 276–281, 2010.

[7] I. C. Gray, N. R. Armfield, and A. C. Smith, "Telemedicine for wound care: current practice and future potential," *Wound Practice and Research*, vol. 18, no. 4, pp. 158–163, 2010.

[8] Z. Agha, R. M. Schapira, P. W. Laud, G. McNutt, and D. L. Roter, "Patient satisfaction with physician-patient communication during telemedicine," *Telemedicine and e-Health*, vol. 15, no. 9, pp. 830–839, 2009.

[9] E. A. Miller, "The technical and interpersonal aspects of telemedicine: effects on doctor-patient communication," *Journal of Telemedicine and Telecare*, vol. 9, no. 1, pp. 1–7, 2003.

[10] A. G. Ekeland, A. Bowes, and S. Flottorp, "Effectiveness of telemedicine: a systematic review of reviews," *International Journal of Medical Informatics*, vol. 79, no. 11, pp. 736–771, 2010.

[11] Central Statistics Office of Sweden, Demografisk rapport (Demographic report), 2013.

[12] http://www.nll.se/sv/Halsa-och-sjukvard/Sjukresor-avgifter-och-bidragl/Fardsatt/.

[13] https://www.Transportstyrelsen.se/sv/Press/Statistik-over-koldioxidutslapp/Stat.

[14] L. Baxter, "Content analysis," in *Studying Interpersonal Interaction*, B. M. Montgomery and S. Duck, Eds., The Guilford Press, New York, NY, USA, 1994.

[15] A. M. Johansson, I. Lindberg, and S. Söderberg, "The views of health-care personnel about video consultation prior to implementation in primary health care in rural areas," *Primary Health Care Research & Development*, vol. 15, no. 2, pp. 170–179, 2014.

[16] R. Harrison, A. MacFarlane, E. Murray, and P. Wallace, "Patients' perceptions of joint teleconsultations: a qualitative evaluation," *Health Expectations*, vol. 9, no. 1, pp. 81–90, 2006.

[17] P. S. Whitten and F. Mair, "Telemedicine and patient satisfaction: current status and future directions," *Telemedicine Journal and e-Health*, vol. 6, no. 4, pp. 417–423, 2000.

[18] X. Liu, Y. Sawada, T. Takizawa et al., "Doctor-patient communication: a comparison between telemedicine consultation and face-to-face consultation," *Internal Medicine*, vol. 46, no. 5, pp. 227–232, 2007.

[19] N. M. Hjelm, "Benefits and drawbacks of telemedicine," *Journal of Telemedicine and Telecare*, vol. 11, no. 2, pp. 60–70, 2005.

[20] Z. Agha, D. L. Roter, and R. M. Schapira, "An evaluation of patient-physician communication style during telemedicine consultations," *Journal of Medical Internet Research*, vol. 11, no. 3, p. e36, 2009.

[21] F. Mair and P. Whitten, "Systematic review of studies of patient satisfaction with telemedicine," *British Medical Journal*, vol. 320, no. 7248, pp. 1517–1520, 2000.

[22] J. Gordon, "Dermatologic assessment from a distance: the use of teledermatology in an outpatient chemotherapy infusion center," *Clinical Journal of Oncology Nursing*, vol. 16, no. 4, pp. 418–420, 2012.

12

Improving Perinatal Care in the Rural Regions Worldwide by Wireless Enabled Antepartum Fetal Monitoring: A Demonstration Project

Roberto Tapia-Conyer,[1] Shelley Lyford,[2] Rodrigo Saucedo,[1] Michael Casale,[2] Hector Gallardo,[1] Karen Becerra,[2] Jonathan Mack,[2] Ricardo Mujica,[1] Daniel Estrada,[2] Antonio Sanchez,[3] Ramon Sabido,[3] Carlos Meier,[2] and Joseph Smith[2]

[1]*Instituto Carlos Slim de la Salud, Insurgentes Sur 3500, 14060 Ciudad de México, DF, Mexico*
[2]*Gary and Mary West Health Institute, 10350 N Torrey Pines Road, La Jolla, CA 92037, USA*
[3]*Servicios de Salud de Yucatán, Calle 72, No. 463 Entre 53 y 55, Centro, 97000 Merida, YUC, Mexico*

Correspondence should be addressed to Joseph Smith; jmsmith@westhealth.org

Academic Editor: Carlos De Las Cuevas

Background. Fetal and neonatal morbidity and mortality are significant problems in developing countries; remote maternal-fetal monitoring offers promise in addressing this challenge. The Gary and Mary West Health Institute and the Instituto Carlos Slim de la Salud conducted a demonstration project of wirelessly enabled antepartum maternal-fetal monitoring in the state of Yucatán, Mexico, to assess whether there were any fundamental barriers preventing deployment and use. *Methods.* Following informed consent, high-risk pregnant women at 27–29 weeks of gestation at the Chemax primary clinic participated in remote maternal-fetal monitoring. Study participants were randomized to receive either prototype wireless monitoring or standard-of-care. Feasibility was evaluated by assessing technical aspects of performance, adherence to monitoring appointments, and response to recommendations. *Results.* Data were collected from 153 high-risk pregnant indigenous Mayan women receiving either remote monitoring ($n = 74$) or usual standard-of-care ($n = 79$). Remote monitoring resulted in markedly increased adherence (94.3% versus 45.1%). Health outcomes were not statistically different in the two groups. *Conclusions.* Remote maternal-fetal monitoring is feasible in resource-constrained environments and can improve maternal compliance for monitoring sessions. Improvement in maternal-fetal health outcomes requires integration of such technology into sociocultural context and addressing logistical challenges of access to appropriate emergency services.

1. Introduction

While most historical efforts to improve health outcomes in rural communities across the world have focused on prevention and treatment of infectious disease, in recent years attention has turned to noncommunicable disease, as well as maternal-child health (MCH). Within Mexico, the nationwide strategy *Equal Start in Life* was implemented in 2001 to enable pregnant women and families to access quality health services [1]. The *Equal Start in Life* program is focused on achieving universal coverage and equal quality care conditions to women during pregnancy, childbirth, and postpartum, as well as to children (boys and girls) from birth through two years of age. This program, which included mobile health units, increased roles of community healthcare workers (CHWs), enhanced family planning services, and made significant advances in regard to maternal and child mortality. In 2007, the Instituto Carlos Slim de la Salud (ICSS), part of the Carlos Slim Foundation, which was established to create sustainable health initiatives for Mexico and Latin America, developed the AMANECE model to improve MCH outcomes [2]. Like the *Equal Start in Life* program, the AMANECE model focuses on maternal and newborn care, and that operates in joint partnership with the federal government, state government public health facilities, and the private sector. Conceptually, AMANECE aims to improve MCH outcomes by creating networks of care that range from community-level health services to highly specialized hospitals; using technology to enhance clinical communication and decision making; and focusing on prevention and early detection of pregnancies, systematic assessment of health risks during prenatal care, and timely treatment of signs of alarm to either prevent the incidence or reduce the severity of obstetric complications. AMANECE strengthens these networks of care by deploying a number of innovations, including a traditional midwife kit containing low-cost medical instruments; AMANECEnet, a tablet-based program to help CHWs identify pregnant women and assess them in the community; SI-VA Amanece, a hybrid online-offline risk assessment platform to ensure high-quality prenatal care at the clinic; cloud software to facilitate referral to regional hospitals; and a hospital rapid response team to deploy a standardized obstetric emergency protocol. To date, the AMANECE program has made significant advances in MCH within Mexico and Latin America. With the aim of furthering achievement of the Millennium Development Goals, ICSS has partnered with the Ministry of Health of Mexico to create networks of care in 15 states in highly populated urban areas and marginalized rural communities; in addition, it has partnered with the Bill and Melinda Gates Foundation and the Government of Spain to implement MCH interventions in Central America.

In 2010 the ICSS and the Gary and Mary West Health Institute (WHI), a nonprofit medical research organization based in La Jolla, CA, collaborated to conduct a feasibility demonstration project of remote, wireless antepartum fetal monitoring for high-risk pregnant women. WHI was established to help bring forth solutions to increase access to, improve the quality of, and lower the cost of healthcare. For this deployment, WHI contributed the MiBebe fetal remote monitoring prototype kits (Figure 1) to a rural clinic in Chemax, YUC, which is part of the AMANECE network. The project, called Salud Maya, was established within the AMANECE network of Valladolid, YUC, México. With the deployment of Salud Maya, WHI and ICSS introduced a clinic-based electronic maternal-fetal monitoring prototype kit to improve broad clinical education and communication to and from Valladolid General Hospital.

Currently, prenatal care in the AMANECE network of care consists of paper-based medical records and a standard set of tests (urine markers, blood pressure, blood glucose, ultrasound testing, and select vaccinations). Typically, "low-risk" women are provided four prenatal visits (12, 20, 28, and 35 weeks of gestation) in a primary care clinic, after which they are referred to Valladolid General Hospital for near-term care and delivery. If the primary care physician (PCP) determines high-risk status during prenatal care, these women are referred to Valladolid, where an OB/GYN physician determines how frequently patients should come in for prenatal visits. The average distances women must travel to the Chemax clinic and Valladolid General Hospital are 1.2 km and 30.4 km, respectively. Due to the distance and cost of travel to Valladolid, many high-risk women do not comply

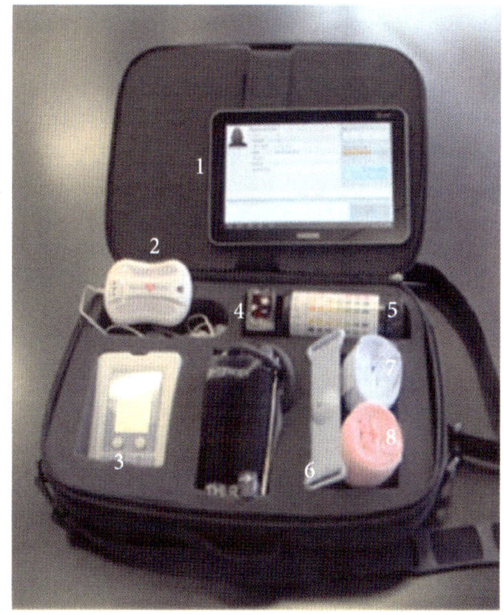

Figure 1: MiBebe fetal remote monitoring kit prototype technology with components as deployed in YUC, Mexico: (1) tablet/phone with fetal monitoring app; (2) fetal monitoring central unit; (3) FORA (blood pressure and glucometer); (4) pulse oximeter; (5) urine strips; (6) Toco; (7) elastic strap for central unit; (8) elastic strap for Toco.

with referrals to the hospital. Given the known benefits of fetal monitoring [3, 4], it is expected that providing pregnant women with increased access to monitoring will likely result in increased adherence to monitoring, thereby improving healthcare outcomes.

The present investigation focused on better understanding the feasibility of implementing a remote wireless antepartum fetal monitor prototype kit within rural Mexico through the Salud Maya project. We specifically addressed technical, infrastructural, and sociocultural challenges. It is important to note that, in performing this feasibility study, we also sought to address existing cultural, economic, and structural barriers to fetal monitoring.

2. Methods

2.1. Setting. The Salud Maya project was implemented in the jurisdiction of Valladolid, which encompasses the city of Valladolid and surrounding indigenous communities such as Chemax. Although most of the population speaks Spanish in the Chemax community, approximately 37% speak Mayan. The average yearly income in Chemax is less than US $1,000.00, and most of the population has an education at or below the eighth grade. Valladolid General Hospital, located in the city of Valladolid, is a 40-bed hospital that serves as a referral center from 5 urban and 13 rural clinics. As one of the referring rural clinics, the Chemax clinic serves the population southeast of Valladolid. The Chemax clinic is a primary care facility of ~180 square meters, containing four examination rooms staffed by a medical director, four PCPs, and eight community nurses. Prior to the project, the clinic had no phone or internet access. The standard care for fetal monitoring included a fetoscope and an obstetric tape measure.

Table 1: Salud Maya participant inclusion and exclusion criteria.

Inclusion (high-risk criteria)	Exclusion
<19 or >35 years old	<27 or >29 weeks of gestation
Three or more prior pregnancies	Twin pregnancy
Diabetes or gestational diabetes	Obstetric emergency or hemorrhage
Hypertension/preeclampsia or cardiomyopathy	Active labor
History of prior miscarriage	Epilepsy
Placenta previa	Dengue fever, influenza, or HIV
Kidney disease not requiring renal substitution therapy	Known allergies or hypersensitivities to plastics
Thyroid disease	History of a heart attack

The clinic also had a standard supply of nutritional packages for pregnant women.

2.2. Project Phases. The Salud Maya project consisted of two phases. Phase I included importing prototype kits into Mexico, setting up clinics where the AMANECE network had been created to deploy the project, performing on-site demonstration of prototype technology kit use, training and proficiency certification in maternal-fetal monitoring, establishing connectivity and electric power, and creating a fetal monitoring room within each clinic. We granted final study initiation certification to the clinics only after each trainee, under supervision of the MD field researcher, had passed the technical certification. The certification test required trainees to demonstrate an understanding of the system and proficiency in using it on actual participants. Test data were reviewed by a participating OB/GYN specialist, and clinic certification was granted only after each trainee demonstrated proficiency during at least ten consecutive monitoring sessions and a final independent submission was completed.

Phase II (Figure 3) included recruiting subjects and deploying the fetal monitoring intervention. To create social awareness and improve recruitment efforts, the project was introduced to the public health and medical community in Valladolid General Hospital, to the Chemax clinic, and to the state authorities. In addition, to increase awareness of the program, a vehicle driven around the Chemax community delivered a series of health announcements via a public announcement system. The clinic supported these efforts to raise awareness by conducting monthly pregnancy health fairs and support groups, both of which gave potential participant women the opportunity to talk with peers and traditional midwives. Participants at 27–29 weeks of pregnancy with evidence of one of the high-risk inclusion criteria and the absence of exclusion criteria (Table 1) were enrolled after providing a written informed consent. At the first appointment, all potential participants were encouraged to bring a family member who wished to attend and witness the informed consent process.

Table 2: Distribution of risk factors[a].

Risk factors	Study group ($n = 74$)	Standard of care ($n = 79$)
<19 or >35	31%	37%
>3 pregnancies	68%	75%
Gestational diabetes	3%	3%
HBP/preeclampsia	18%	13%
Miscarriage	30%	27%
Placenta previa	3%	3%

[a]No statistically significant differences were found between the risk factors in the two groups per a binomial test with alpha = 0.05.

2.3. Subject Description. Recruitment commenced on September 5, 2012, and ended on July 30, 2013, with a total of 172 enrolled women. Nineteen were excluded because they did not meet the inclusion criteria for maternal and gestational age, an obstetric event/delivery was not recorded, or they attended less than two visits. Following exclusion, there remained 153 eligible women who were randomly assigned to either the Salud Maya intervention ($n = 74$) or the standard care control group ($n = 79$). Table 2 provides relevant study subject demographic information. No demographic characteristics were significantly different between the two groups ($P > 0.05$).

Two Mayan-speaking nurses were selected as part of the Chemax clinical team to assist with clinical data collection and address the language barriers between physicians and patients. Patient communications were mainly provided in Mayan.

Women enrolled in the study group attended their scheduled visits at the Chemax primary clinic. During each fetal monitoring visit, nurses collected urine samples and measured height, weight, blood pressure, and blood glucose; the PCP measured fundal height and reviewed and assessed clinical data; nurses performed fetal monitoring for 30 minutes, after which all data were uploaded to the cloud, reviewed at the hospital, and recorded as reactive or nonreactive. Clinical management was determined by the hospital OB/GYN specialist. Participants in the study group typically received fetal monitoring at 1- to 2-week intervals. Women enrolled in the control group and who served as the baseline cohort were referred for fetal monitoring to Valladolid General Hospital where they received standard care.

2.4. Study Materials. The core of the WHI technology kits is the MiBebe fetal remote monitor prototype, which includes a fetal ultrasound heart monitor and a uterine tocodynamometer. The kit also contains tools to capture maternal blood pressure, blood glucose, and urinary protein values (Figure 1). Through a Bluetooth interface and Web access, the information is securely stored in the cloud and is available for reading at any hospital or remote location (Figure 2). Additional technical information on the prototype system and its architecture can be found in a separate publication [5].

2.5. Study Outcomes. The primary outcome of interest was adherence to antepartum clinic visits. To understand this, we

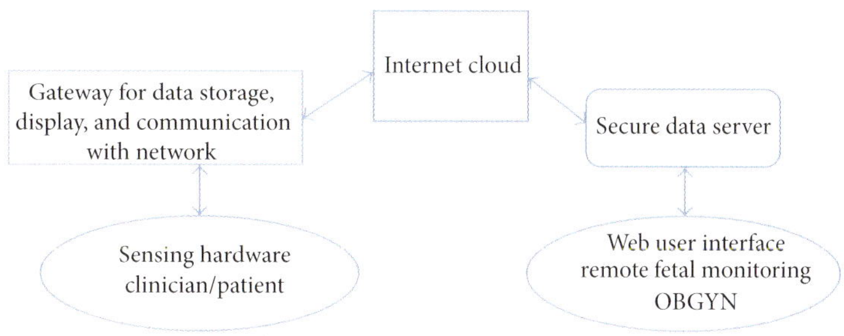

FIGURE 2: Remote maternal-fetal monitoring. Information is collected from the sensor hardware and uploaded to a secure cloud-based storage via Bluetooth. Data can then be accessed remotely by a clinician in a remote location.

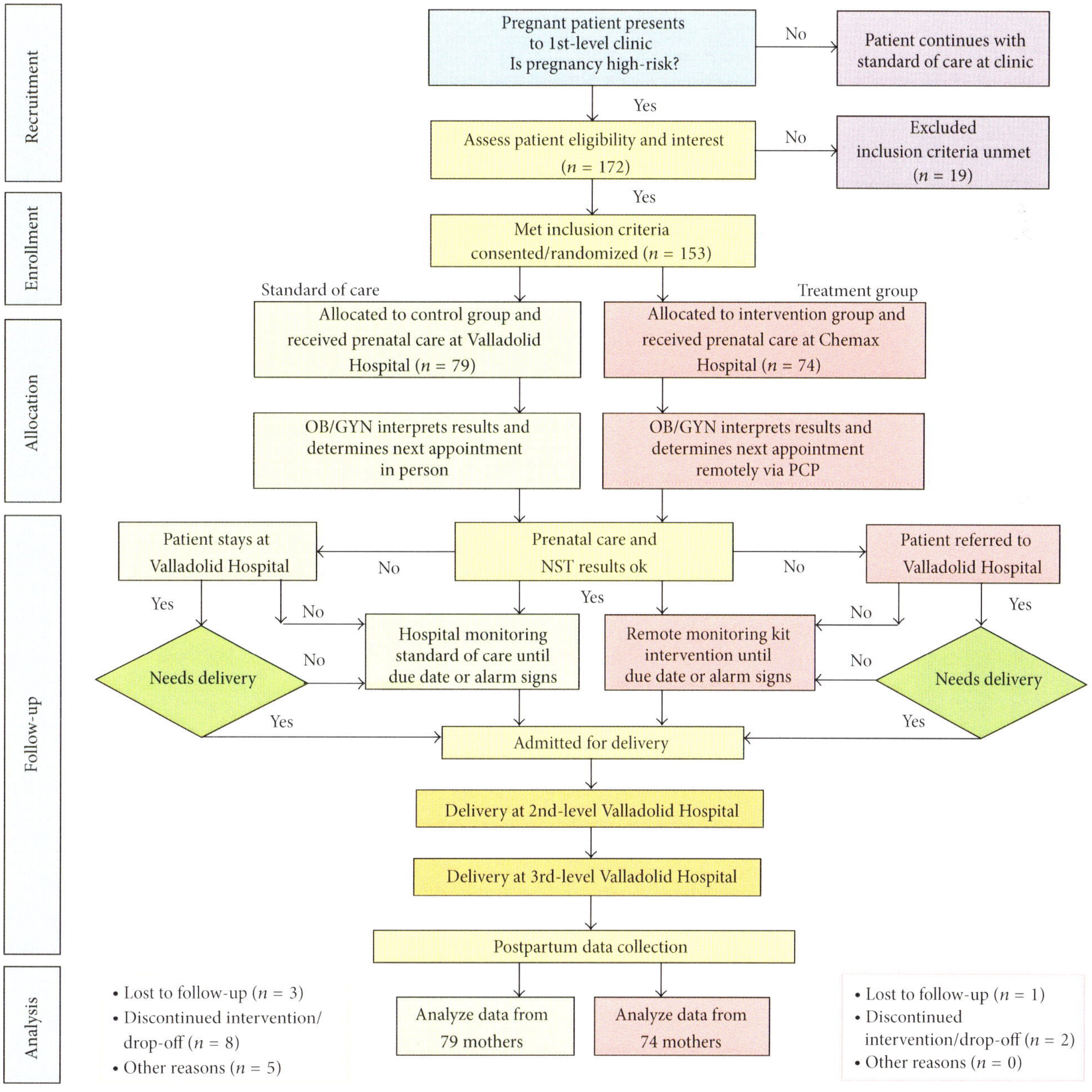

FIGURE 3: Flow chart illustrating the intervention process for participants.

Table 3: Inclusion criteria for the selection of informant subjects for the qualitative surveys.

Stakeholders	Criteria
Clinical staff	Must be a primary care physician or nurse at the 1st level of care working in a facility that belongs to the ICSS AMANECE Valladolid program, treating pregnant women Must have approved the Virtual Diploma in Maternal and Child Health, granted by the National Polytechnic Institute and provided through ICSS' PIEENSO platform
Pregnant women	High-risk pregnant women being cared for at Chemax Health Services facility and monitored with the fetal monitoring kit Age: women 19 years of age and more, who represent different moments of life and thus have different views on their pregnancies: teenagers (19 to 20 years), young adults (21 to 34 years), and older adults (35 to 45 years) Educational level: literature indicates that education, particularly a woman's schooling, is a great contributor to her and her family's health Health insurance: people's insurance, IMSS, ISSSTE, or no insurance; this variable is linked directly with pregnant women's access to healthcare services and the type of services they receive (service portability) Special population group: for instance, indigenous populations have particular cultural aspects that are not seen in other population groups
Husbands/partners of pregnant women and midwives	Related persons to the pregnant women who have influence on the healthcare access decisions (partners, husbands, or midwives)

compared the adherence rate for participants enrolled in the demonstration project to that of the baseline cohort.

In order to assess cultural/structural barriers that may impact program adoption, a follow-up questionnaire was established. The pregnant women, their husbands/partners, and traditional midwives as well as select health personnel who were in contact with the remote monitoring prototype kits were randomly sampled and queried regarding acceptability and satisfaction with the program. An independent bilingual team (Universidad de Oriente, Valladolid, YUC) conducted the interviews in either Spanish or Mayan (Tables 3, 4, and 5). Interviewers administered the questionnaire in open-ended face-to-face interviews conducted at the participant's home and video recorded.

In addition, during the project, the engineers and clinicians at WHI were responsive to all hardware and software potential errors via a bidirectional study feedback form. Potential errors were noted and recorded by individuals at the clinics via computer software spreadsheets that were stored locally and subsequently shared electronically with the team at WHI. The reported errors were classified as one of the following: (1) hardware, (2) software, (3) connectivity (cellular or webpage), or (4) other. Data errors were reviewed again later to assess the feasibility of the project.

Finally, clinical data were collected (1) upon enrollment, (2) during the monitoring sessions, and (3) after delivery. All clinical data collected are listed in Table 6. Economic impact questionnaires were independently administered to 30 pregnant mothers and their husbands/partners (data reported separately).

Since the primary aim of the present paper was to determine the overall feasibility of implementing the novel remote fetal monitoring system, we examined the results of each data type mentioned above to assess whether there were any fundamental barriers preventing the implementation of the Salud Maya demonstration project.

3. Results

3.1. Maternal and Infant Outcomes. Data analysis indicated no differences between individuals receiving the intervention and the control with respect to the proportion of deliveries at home versus hospital or in terms of term gestation, birth weights, or obstetric complications due to preeclampsia, eclampsia, hemorrhage, or sepsis (Table 7).

Adherence, the major outcome measure, was defined as attending scheduled fetal monitoring appointments, either through monitoring on-site at Chemax for the study group or through patient's referral to Valladolid Hospital for antepartum testing for the baseline cohort. Participants in the study group attended 481 of the 510 scheduled fetal monitoring appointments at Chemax, resulting in a compliance rate of 94.3%. Of remotely monitored participants, 40 study participants were referred to the hospital, based on observations from their remote monitoring, but only 17 complied, resulting in a referral compliance rate of 42.5%.

For the control group, the actual number of attended fetal monitoring appointments was 111. Out of a potential 246 recommended visits for antepartum monitoring to Valladolid General Hospital, this represents an approximate 45% adherence rate.

3.2. Interviews. Qualitative analysis of the interviews was performed to identify potential sociocultural barriers related to acceptance and adoption of the novel fetal monitoring kit demonstration project. Transcripts of the interviews conducted in Mayan were reviewed and the overarching themes extracted and analyzed. Among the pregnant women, the main perceived benefit of the program was the ability to hear the baby's heart, as they could infer the baby's health. Mayan women are generally very shy and reluctant to talk about themselves, so the fact that interviews were performed by an independent team may have limited the responses. Nonetheless, the Mayan pregnant women stated they were comfortable having a nurse perform the fetal monitoring session.

Table 4: Questionnaires for the informants (pregnant women and healthcare oersonnel).

Pregnant women: during pregnancy	Healthcare providers	Pregnant women: postpartum
Why did you accept the device?	Do you know how the device works, what is your opinion?	What do you think of the device that monitored your pregnancy?
How do you feel when you have the device on you?	Do you think the device is reliable?	Which do you think is more reliable: monitoring with the device or the directions from the midwife?
What have been some comments you have received from your relatives since you started using the device?	Do you think the operation of the device is complicated?	Did you trust the results of the device?
Have your expenses decreased with the use of the device?	Did you receive training prior to handling the device, how?	What do you think should improve the overall implementation of the device?
How much have you saved?	Have you had difficulties operating the device, which one?	What comments have you received from your family about the use of the prototype?
What do you do with the money you have saved?	How do you get organized to implement the device operation in pregnant patients?	Would you accept to use it again?
Do you understand the results that are shown in the device?	Did you observe any cultural inconvenience to use the device?	If it had any cost would you pay for it?
Would you recommend the use of this device to all pregnant women?	What have been the work flow changes in the process of caring for pregnant women during the consultation?	
Are there days that you have not come to receive the application of the device, why?	How do you think we can improve the implementation of this technology?	
What benefits do you think you get from this device?	List some basic features that you think are important to cover as health personnel that applies the device.	
Do you see any difficulty using the device?	Do you use some strategies to encourage participation from husband? Which?	
Would you use the device again in another pregnancy?		

Table 5: Questionnaires for husbands and midwives.

Husbands	Midwives
What do you think about the device your wife is using?	What have you heard of the device that is offered to pregnant women at risk?
Do you agree with this device that monitors the pregnancy of your wife? Why?	What do you think of the device?
What was your reaction when your wife first started using this device?	What do you think of the use of the device associated with the work you do?
How did you decide to use the device?	How often do pregnant women using the device visit you?
What did your wife tell you about the device?	Do you believe that pregnant women at risk feel safe and well cared for with the use of this device?
Have you seen any benefit in your economy with the use of the device?	What advantages have you observed from the device on your work as a midwife?
How often do you accompany your wife to the appointments?	What disadvantages does the use of the device bring to you?
What is your involvement during the consultation? Why?	Do you think there is any risk in using it?
What advantages do you think the device has?	Would you have liked to use the device?
What disadvantages do you think the device has?	Would you recommend the use of the device to all pregnant women?
	How is the care given to pregnant women at the clinic (nurses, physicians)?

Table 6: Information collected during regular monitoring sessions.

Baseline	Pregnancy	Postpartum
Obstetric information	Electronic database	Electronic database
Medical record	Medical record	Medical record
	Technical functionality for the remote monitoring kits	
Feedback form	Feedback form	Feedback form
	Feasibility (study group); economic impact (study group)	
Pregnant women survey	Pregnant women survey	Pregnant women survey
Husbands/partners survey	Husbands/partners survey	Husbands/partners survey
Midwives survey	Midwives survey	Midwives survey
Health personnel survey	Health personnel survey	Health personnel survey

Table 7: Place of delivery, obstetric complications, gestational age, and weight at birth[a].

	Study group ($n = 74$)	Standard of care ($n = 79$)
	Place of delivery	
Hospital	74%	77%
At home/midwife	26%	23%
	Obstetric complications	
Preeclampsia	11%	10%
Eclampsia	0%	3%
Hemorrhage	0%	0%
Sepsis	0%	0%
	Gestational age at birth	
28 to 35 weeks	4%	3%
36 to 37 weeks	12%	20%
37+ weeks	84%	77%
	Weight at birth	
Under 1000 gms	0%	0%
1000–1500 gms	0%	0%
1501–2500 gms	9%	6%
Over 2501 gms	91%	94%

[a]None of the differences between the two groups were statistically significant per a binomial test with alpha = 0.05.

Among the spouses/partners, the most common perception was the benefit of monitoring for the health of the baby. That they perceived the remote monitoring kit to be a positive intervention primarily in regard to infant health is not surprising, as Mayan indigenous communities have strong ties to the family, and looking after elder members and infants is among the most important values.

Midwives expressed a generally positive opinion of the monitoring but had little direct interaction with the monitoring process. This may be in part attributable to the method of deploying the RM kit, which was very sensitive to the midwives' hierarchy in the community. The Mayan population is very keen to follow and respect traditions, and thus the role of the traditional midwife is instrumental in monitoring the pregnancies at the household. Thus, both doctors and nurses involved them at the monitoring sessions to assure better acceptance. Among the health personnel, responses indicated confidence in the value of the remote monitoring to identify risk situations. They supported incorporating the service as standard care.

The Mayan population has a profound respect for traditional values and interventions and therefore does not often use modern technology. Pregnant women and especially traditional midwives were reluctant at first to use a new technology. Nonetheless, many participants reported that the attractive design of the fetal monitor and the bonding between the nurses (who were fluent in Mayan) and the pregnant women eased its adoption.

3.3. Hardware and Software System Reports. Over the duration of the study, there were a total of 52 reported potential errors with the hardware and software systems. All potential errors were recorded by the field team in YUC and entered into a local copy of a spreadsheet to which all field team members had access (in some instances, reported errors were due to improper usage rather than hardware or software failure. For example, in one instance, the field team believed the prototypes were not performing properly. However, it was confirmed that the placement of the prototypes was incorrect, signaling the potential need for improved training with the system). Of the 52 reports, 24 were related to hardware, 15 to software, and 3 to connectivity, with an additional 10 classified as other.

All reports were reviewed within WHI's Quality Management System to ensure that the reports were evaluated and mitigated. Over the course of the study, the only reports that were not remedied were those related to physical deficits in the casing of the fetal monitor units. Ultimately, new cases were made to replace the deficient ones so that the study could continue. No physical deficiencies in the units were reported after replacement of the casing.

4. Discussion

The results of this study demonstrate both the feasibility and challenges of using technological interventions to improve MCH in rural regions. This study demonstrated that it is possible to achieve remote wireless antenatal fetal monitoring in a resource-poor and educationally challenged environment with a culturally diverse population. Results indicated a significant reduction in the number of participants requiring referral to the regional hospital for antepartum surveillance and an improved local adherence to antepartum fetal monitoring, as compared to hospital monitoring referral.

Given the restrictions of the small sample, the distribution of risk factors between intervention and control groups was not significantly different (see Table 2). As regards health outcomes, while there was an observed difference in the rate of eclampsia (3% in the control group versus 0% in the intervention arm) and gestational age (84% being 37+ weeks in the intervention arm versus 77% in the control group), neither of these differences achieved statistical significance. It is appreciated that one of the goals of antenatal monitoring (fetal heart rate, blood pressure, and urine) in the developed world is to diagnose preeclampsia and deliver the baby before the mother gets eclampsia. Therefore, this difference of eclampsia rate needs to be further explored and/or validated in future studies.

4.1. Adherence. In regard to appointment adherence, it is notable that women in the study group needed to travel comparatively short walking distances to the clinic, whereas individuals receiving standard of care had to travel up to 2 hours by car (if transportation was available) to the hospital and endure average waiting times that totaled 6–8 hours. These differences likely explain the difference in appointment adherence between those in the demonstration project and those receiving standard of care.

It is worth noting that, of the 40 women in the study group that were referred to the hospital, only 17 adhered. This lack of adherence, likely explicable by a combination of travel requirements and cultural challenges (hesitancy for women to travel alone), greatly limited the opportunity for impact of this screening methodology. It is important to emphasize that sociocultural factors need to be addressed along with the introduction of technology—for instance, financial support or childcare support for the woman's existing children provided on the day of appointment or having transportation provided may address such barriers.

4.2. Deployment Learning. The remote fetal monitoring demonstration project provided an opportunity to address barriers to enhance prenatal care. The program increased the workload and complexity for the Chemax clinic staff, requiring recruitment of additional nurses and the need for ongoing training.

Despite initial evidence of staff technical proficiency in system use, there were challenges with implementation. Previous to the study, physicians and nurses in the primary clinic had not directly cared for women with high-risk pregnancies, as previously these cases had been referred to the hospital for services. Project implementation resulted in a better-prepared first level of care team that was able to collect and transmit information appropriately to the specialist and directly deliver instructions back from the OB/GYN specialist to the participants. This enabled the specialist to identify which participants needed additional support. To successfully implement this, additional clinical training was required, including the execution and interpretation of a non-stress test.

Additionally, the project plan required adjustment to accommodate the Chemax clinic medical director's workload. Initially, the director was required to oversee use of the remote monitoring prototype technology kits and execute clinical directions provided by the hospital's OB/GYN specialist. However, the medical director's workload did not facilitate completion in a timely manner. Accordingly, the protocol was modified such that a dedicated primary care physician (PCP) was responsible for the remote monitoring session and supervision of the project nursing team.

There were further barriers associated with lack of human resources at the hospital level, as the two trained hospital OB/GYN specialists already had an excessive patient load. The project established workflow where the specialist would allocate time between 12:00 and 2:00 p.m. daily to review all daily monitoring sessions from the Chemax clinic. In this manner, the PCP could expect to have the monitoring sessions reviewed and commented on by the specialist in the early afternoon each day.

Additionally, all the medical data sources required validation, as the hospital and clinic used different medical record formats. These issues were addressed with the implementation of a simplified electronic record methodology for data capture and storage, with unified criteria for capturing the data. This required an initial internal training of the field team to coordinate all existing databases.

The PCPs demonstrated competence in identifying high-risk pregnancy factors and reasons for referral to the hospital but lacked knowledge regarding assessment of fetal monitor tests. None of the nurses were experienced with smartphone use (an integral component of the prototype technology kits), so there were significant educational challenges in recording and transmitting results. For example, nurses would often not upload all of the antepartum monitoring sessions, discarding sessions that they deemed of poor quality, because they felt such submission would affect their perceived performance. ICSS spent significant time training the nurses not only in performing fetal monitoring sessions but in using a smartphone for both simple tasks (opening an application, sending a text message) and more technical ones (reviewing cellular network coverage, substituting the battery, and changing a password). Overall, survey results demonstrated a significant acceptance of the monitoring at the clinic.

Due to lack of available staff, we were unable to immediately obtain all the required data related to home births performed by traditional midwives. Typically, these data are collected when the home-delivering mother subsequently comes to the clinic to obtain the birth certificate and vaccination schedule. Furthermore, we had to rely on scarce community resources (volunteers) to track and locate participants who did not show up for appointments.

4.3. Infrastructure Issues. The main infrastructure barriers included the unreliable electricity service, which impacted both the phone system and charging of prototype unit batteries. This ultimately required the addition of two electricity stabilizers. Cellular network coverage variations affected data upload and communication. The environmental conditions were hotter and more humid than expected, requiring the addition of air conditioning in the clinic fetal monitoring room.

In addition, there were infrastructure barriers at the hospital level. Despite recent hospital construction, the hospital did not have telephone lines, internet service, or computers, and the cellular network had intermittent coverage. ICSS provided computer equipment and mobile 3G/GSM SIM cards with sufficient data capacity, which not only facilitated data upload but also resolved the communication problems between the two distant healthcare units via the Web-based platform, phone calls, and/or text messages.

4.4. Sociocultural Challenges. Among the main sociocultural challenges experienced during the project were the native Mayan language and cultural barriers between the physicians and participants. Most women spoke Mayan and thus developed a closer relationship with the nurses, who were Mayan speakers, thus limiting direct communication with the PCP. One limitation of the interviews was the length of time between study informed consent, birth, and the administration of the questionnaires, which in some instances exceeded 4 months. It is also important to note that there are recognized strong Mayan cultural values focused on the umbilicus and the heart, which are associated with the perception of health balance. Furthermore, the overall number of participants queried was limited.

4.5. Technical Challenges. Study results indicated that new prototype technology may suffer hardware and software issues during implementation, so it is important to have adequate reporting tools as well as clear protocols and mitigation procedures in place to guarantee safe and effective execution. These results also highlighted the value of ongoing education and the importance of project oversight. Nonetheless, the hardware and software issues found during the course of the project did not impede the monitoring sessions.

Other technical challenges were related to clinic staff introducing unexpected protocol changes, none of which were part of the original study protocol. For example, nurses used several previously donated technologies during monitoring sessions, including a pencil-like Doppler monitor. Nurses used the Doppler monitor to prelocate the fetus within the mother's abdomen and then placed the prototype technology central unit at this location. However, the location site indicated by this pencil-like monitor did not correlate with the optimal site for the central unit, resulting in the perception of inferior fetal monitoring sensitivity from the prototype system.

Another deviation involved the use of a small pair of electrically powered audio speakers instead of the kit-provided headphones. Clinical staff introduced the speakers so that the nurses, mother, and family could all hear the baby's heart beat during the 30-minute recorded monitoring session. The audio speakers enabled a closer connection between the clinical staff, the mother, and her family; however, this deviation affected the ultrasound signal quality. This problem was identified after the nurses and field coordinator reported a decline in fetal monitoring system performance.

Software challenges included smartphones receiving text messages and calls during monitoring sessions, as well as participants installing applications not related to the study, which interfered with the clinical software application. Staff members were subsequently retrained on smartphone operation, and a single cell phone was assigned to the clinic for all phone communication. For this deployment, the system was used with a 3G cellular connection to upload the recorded data to the Internet where it was available to specialists in any of the remote sites. 3G coverage was intermittent, necessitating that sessions be stored in a system queue; the reception problems were more common during cloudy or rainy days or peak cell use hours. To remedy this situation, the project initiated a double login from the clinicians to assure the queued data would be appropriately uploaded once a proper signal was available.

The initial system design required each user to have a unique login ID and password. However, after several weeks of using the system, the clinical staff requested modification of the access case so all users could have the same login ID and password. The access was thus modified, but an unforeseen consequence occurred, resulting in looping of data uploads and duplicated copies of recordings. WHI engineers ultimately rewrote the software code to remedy this issue, and no impact on data occurred.

5. Conclusions

This study evaluated the feasibility and challenges of deploying a specially designed wireless, remote prototype technology system for antenatal fetal monitoring in a culturally diverse, resource-poor, and educationally challenged remote setting. Although there were many infrastructure, technical, and sociocultural challenges, this study nonetheless readily demonstrated that such prototype technology can be successfully adopted for use in a rural, resource-poor environment. Moreover, we observed more than twice as much adherence to antenatal monitoring for participants in the demonstration project as compared to the standard of care. However, differences in health outcomes were not observed, potentially due to cultural and logistical barriers that prevented women from accessing care at the hospital following diagnosis.

In regard to acceptability, pregnant participants, their husbands and/or partners, and midwives were receptive to the use of the prototype technology kits, as the study group maintained a high compliance of attendance to the Chemax clinic throughout the study. Both primary care staff and OB/GYN specialists supported the system's use and preferred it to the existing process of referrals to the hospital. The clinicians' rapid acceptance of the technology and their resourcefulness in following up with remote communications facilitated the study workflow. The technology facilitated the specialist being given advanced notification of any potentially concerning situation. However, as acknowledged above, the women did not always have readily available transportation for travel between the clinic and hospital, which may have limited their referral attendance.

In summary, this project demonstrates significant successes of an MCH intervention program and points to structural, educational, and cultural features that need to be addressed to assure more effective widespread dissemination in developing countries.

Ethical Approval

The project was established with approval of Servicios de Salud de Yucatán (SSY) research protocol no. SSY/DG/0097/2011 and the Federal Commission for the Protection against Sanitary Risks (COFEPRIS for its Spanish acronym) no. 123300115D0288. All participants provided written, informed consent. All study prototype technology was tested at the Gary and Mary West Health Institute in La Jolla, CA.

Acknowledgments

The Instituto Carlos Slim de la Salud and the Gary and Mary West Health Institute thank the collaboration of the Servicios de Salud de Yucatán and Universidad de Oriente for their contributions and support in conducting this project. The authors would also like to thank Dr. Kelly Harkey and his research team at Scripps Memorial Hospital in La Jolla, CA, and former WHI collaborators Jonathan Mack RN, Ph.D.; Sharon Harkey CNM, MSN; and Robert Matthews Ph.D. for their valuable contributions to the success of this project. The authors are grateful to the entire Gary and Mary West Health Institute team that worked tirelessly to conceptualize, create, and test the prototype systems and to the entire Instituto Carlos Slim de la Salud team that supported the deployment of the Salud Maya project in the community.

References

[1] J. Sepúlveda, F. Bustreo, R. Tapia et al., "Improvement of child survival in Mexico: the diagonal approach," *The Lancet*, vol. 368, no. 9551, pp. 2017–2027, 2006.

[2] AMANECE, *Salud maternal atencion del embarazo, parto y puerperio: Guía comunitaria*, Instituto Carlos Slim de la Salud, Mexico City, Mexico, 2011.

[3] C. R. Graves, "Antepartum fetal surveillance and timing of delivery in the pregnancy complicated by diabetes mellitus," *Clinical Obstetrics and Gynecology*, vol. 50, no. 4, pp. 1007–1013, 2007.

[4] E. P. Schneider, J. Milton Hutson, and R. H. Petrie, "An assessment of the first decade's experience with antepartum fetal heart rate testing," *The American Journal of Perinatology*, vol. 5, no. 2, pp. 134–141, 1988.

[5] M. Roham, E. Saldivar, S. Raghavan, M. Zurcher, J. Mack, and M. Mehregany, "A mobile wearable wireless fetal heart monitoring system," in *Proceedings of the 5th International Symposium on Medical Information and Communication Technology (ISMICT '11)*, pp. 135–138, March 2011.

13

Development of a Wearable-Sensor-Based Fall Detection System

Falin Wu,[1] Hengyang Zhao,[1] Yan Zhao,[1] and Haibo Zhong[2]

[1]*School of Instrumentation Science and Optoelectronics Engineering, Beihang University, Beijing 100191, China*
[2]*Space Star Technology Co., Ltd., Beijing 100086, China*

Correspondence should be addressed to Hengyang Zhao; hengyang178@163.com

Academic Editor: Fei Hu

Fall detection is a major challenge in the public healthcare domain, especially for the elderly as the decline of their physical fitness, and timely and reliable surveillance is necessary to mitigate the negative effects of falls. This paper develops a novel fall detection system based on a wearable device. The system monitors the movements of human body, recognizes a fall from normal daily activities by an effective quaternion algorithm, and automatically sends request for help to the caregivers with the patient's location.

1. Introduction

Falls of the elderly always lead to serious health issues as the decline of their physical fitness [1]. Fracture is the most common injury in fall of an elderly and there is also a certain possibility to get coma, brain trauma, and paralysis. At most fall situations, the fall process is the main source of injury because of the high impact. But sometimes the late medical salvage may worsen the situation [2]. That means the faster the salvage comes, the less risk the elderly will face.

Progress of technology brings more possibilities to help us protect the elderly. Low power consumption components make it possible to realize wearable monitoring device. MEMS (microelectro mechanical systems) sensors have simplified the design and implementation of sensor system. Location based service (LBS) makes it more convenient to locate the elderly in health monitoring. Beside these, mobile computing makes remote health monitoring easier to realize.

Several kinds of fall detection methods have been developed or applied in our life [3]. One of them is computer vision based method. Cameras are distributed at limited space to offer pictures or videos of human activities to implement fall detection algorithm. External supports such as motion sensors could be used to enhance computer vision based fall detection method [4], and a data fusion algorithm can operate the validation and correlation among the two subsystems to raise robust performance of fall detection. These computer based methods work effectively in indoor environment, but they are hard to realize in outdoor environment as the deployment of cameras is always limited.

Motion sensor-based method is also commonly used. Accelerometer and gyroscope could provide linear and angular motion information directly. Sensor measurements or their proper fusion could be used to distinguish a real fall. There are several kinds of detection methods which differ in constitution of motion sensors and detection algorithms. The first kind of detection method is using an accelerometer. A single triaxial accelerometer can provide object's accelerations in three directions which include the influence of gravity. A coordinate will be built when the accelerometer is fixed on human's body. The influence of gravity or dynamic acceleration is available by using a low pass filter or a high pass filter [5]. Some kinds of angular movement information can also be calculated based on the relationship between acceleration components and their vector sum [6]. The second kind of detection method is based on both accelerometer and gyroscope [7]. Gyroscope can offer angular velocity and the accelerometer could offer linear motion information. The third kind of detection method also uses a magnetometer. A triaxial magnetometer can detect magnetic strength in three directions, and it can also provide angular motion information in the horizontal plane. But the environment magnetic field may disturb the geomagnetic field which reduces the reliability of the magnetometer outputs, for instance, in

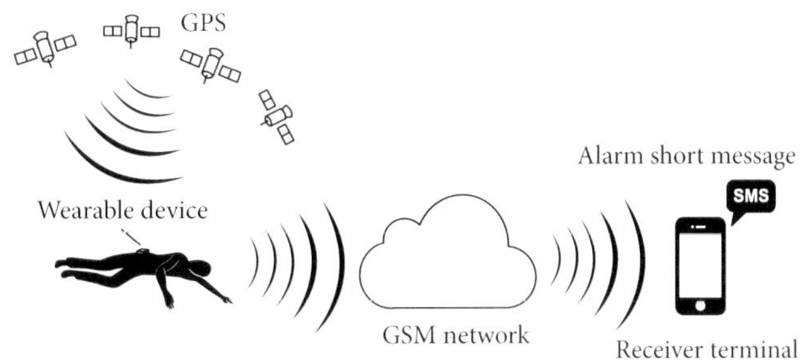

FIGURE 1: System architecture.

some steel structure architecture or near some objects with strong electromagnetism. As angular information can also be extracted from accelerometer measurements, a state space filter such as the Kalman filter is a commonly used technique to combine angular motion information [8]. Beside these, sensors such as barometer can also assist pure motion sensors at human gait recognition [9].

But, in fact, using more sensors means more power consumption, and it is a challenge to design a proper algorithm to fuse different kinds of sensors. A single triaxial accelerometer is quite enough for human fall detection as sufficient information could be extracted from its measurements. Besides this, the accelerometer coordinate does not have to be fixed if only the magnitude of sum vector is needed [10], and that is quite convenient for wearable application. In this paper, a fall detection system based on a wearable device is developed. The hardware and software realization of the device is mainly based on a single triaxial accelerometer and GPS/GSM module. The device uses an efficient fall detection algorithm with less resource and power consumption, which means that it is a proper design for outdoor application.

2. System Design

The architecture of the developed system is described in Figure 1. A wearable device is placed on human's waist. The system can detect the elderly's falling by acceleration analysis. Then it will get the elderly's geographic position and send fall alarm short message to caregivers. So the elderly who has fallen can get timely help to minimize the negative influence.

3. Fall Detection Algorithm

3.1. Overview. Choice of recognition feature has decisive significance to successful fall detection. Information like linear movements (e.g., displacement, velocity, and acceleration) and angular movements (e.g., angle, angular velocity, and angular acceleration) could be obtained directly or indirectly. Beside these, frequency domain parameters could be extracted from basic sensor measurements by techniques such as FFT and wavelet [11, 12]. For single triaxial accelerometer application, accelerations and derived angular parameters could be used as recognition features.

Fall detection algorithm design is based on the choice of recognition features. According to the recognition feature, fall detection algorithms are classified as threshold based and machine learning based. For threshold based method, threshold of recognition feature is set by the designer before application which makes the algorithm have rapid response and less resource consumption [13]. But the choice of threshold needs both rigorous schemes and adequate experiments. For machine learning based design, the classification of fall and normal activities is available with the assistance of technologies such as support vector machine (SVM) and neural network [14, 15]. Machine learning assistance may enhance system robustness to some extent, but its algorithm design is always high computing resource consumed which limits its application in wearable device. As the compact wearable device requires low power consumption and a single triaxial accelerometer could provide effective information, threshold based fall detection algorithm will be used in this system.

3.2. Algorithm Design. Algorithm used in this fall alarm system is based on thresholds of sum acceleration and rotation angle information. When a real fall happens, collision between human's body and ground will produce obvious peak value at the sum acceleration **a** which has magnitude as

$$|\mathbf{a}| = \sqrt{a_x^{\,2} + a_y^{\,2} + a_z^{\,2}}, \quad (1)$$

where a_x, a_y, and a_z present accelerometer measurements of three axes. The system uses the sum acceleration as the first step to distinguish high intensity movements from others. But normal motions such as jumping or sitting also produce peak values, which mean that additional detection features are required.

The second feature used here is an angle calculated based on acceleration measurements. As human's motion has low acceleration, it is feasible to get gravity component in each axis by using a low pass filter. If gravity components could be separated before and after human's fall, then it is possible to calculate the rotation angle of accelerometer coordinate in 3D space, which is also equivalent to the rotation angle of gravity vector relative to fixed coordinate. Coordinate constructed by the accelerometer and the gravity vector is shown in Figure 2. The rotation of gravity vector in fixed coordinate is shown in Figure 3.

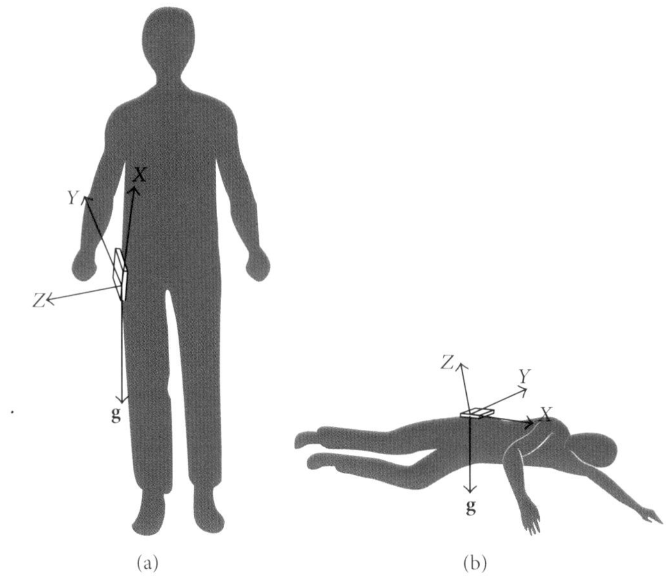

FIGURE 2: Coordinate and gravity before and after falling. (a) Before falling. (b) After falling.

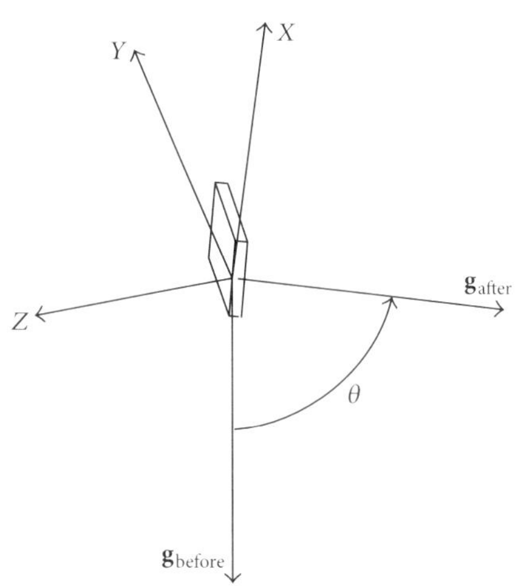

FIGURE 3: Rotation of gravity relative to fixed coordinate.

Quaternion is an effective tool to describe rotation movement in human's gait change which also includes falling [16]. A quaternion could be described as

$$\mathbf{Q} = q_0 + q_1 \cdot \bar{i} + q_2 \cdot \bar{j} + q_3 \cdot \bar{k} \tag{2}$$

which has magnitude as

$$\|\mathbf{Q}\| = \sqrt{{q_0}^2 + {q_1}^2 + {q_2}^2 + {q_3}^2}. \tag{3}$$

Unit quaternion which has magnitude $\|\mathbf{Q}\| = 1$ can be described as

$$\mathbf{Q} = \cos\frac{\theta}{2} + \sin\frac{\theta}{2} \cdot q_x \cdot \bar{i} + \sin\frac{\theta}{2} \cdot q_y \cdot \bar{j} + \sin\frac{\theta}{2} \cdot q_z \cdot \bar{k}. \tag{4}$$

As shown in Figure 3, rotation angle of $\mathbf{Q}$ equals θ. The rotation axis is orthogonal to the rotation plane and its direction is in accordance with right hand screw rule. q_x, q_y, and q_z are three components of the unit vector which describes the orientation of the quaternion at the fixed coordinate.

Besides rotation movement, quaternion can also describe a vector in 3D space, such as the gravity vector $\mathbf{g}$ which could be described as a quaternion

$$\mathbf{g} = 0 + g_x \cdot \bar{i} + g_y \cdot \bar{j} + g_z \cdot \bar{k}. \tag{5}$$

g_x, g_y, and g_z are three components of $\mathbf{g}$ which has quaternion magnitude as

$$\|\mathbf{g}\| = \sqrt{g_x^2 + g_y^2 + g_z^2} = g. \tag{6}$$

A unit quaternion $\mathbf{Q}$ is used to describe human's falling movement, which can also be divided into three rotation quaternions $\mathbf{Q}_1$, $\mathbf{Q}_2$, and $\mathbf{Q}_3$ to simplify the calculation as shown in Figure 4.

With the help of gravity vector information before and after human's falling movement as shown in Figure 3, these three separated quaternions are all available.

$\mathbf{Q}_1$ could be expressed as

$$\mathbf{Q}_1 = \cos\frac{\theta_1}{2} + \sin\frac{\theta_1}{2}\sin\alpha \cdot \bar{i} + \sin\frac{\theta_1}{2}\cos\alpha \cdot \bar{j} \tag{7}$$

which has rotation angle and rotation axis information as

$$\begin{aligned} \theta_1 &= \arctan\frac{g_{\text{before},z}}{\sqrt{g_{\text{before},x}^2 + g_{\text{before},y}^2}}, \\ \sin\alpha &= \frac{-g_{\text{before},y}}{\sqrt{g_{\text{before},x}^2 + g_{\text{before},y}^2}}, \\ \cos\alpha &= \frac{g_{\text{before},x}}{\sqrt{g_{\text{before},x}^2 + g_{\text{before},y}^2}}. \end{aligned} \tag{8}$$

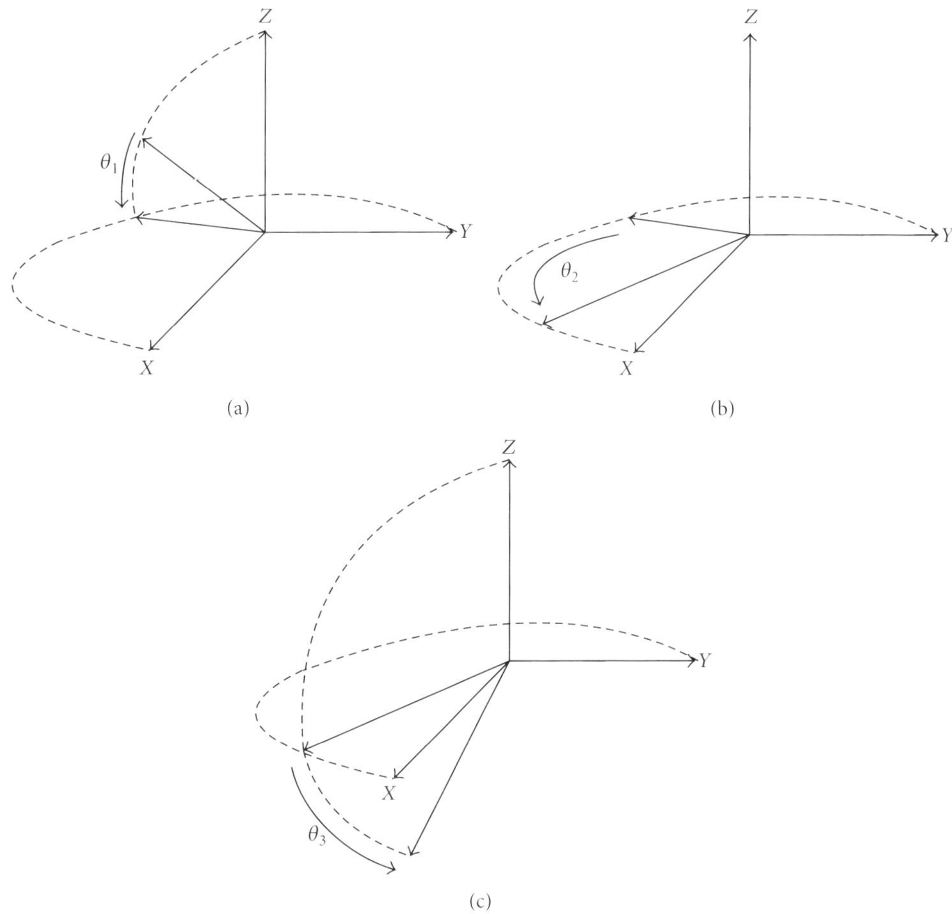

FIGURE 4: Decomposition of fall rotation quaternion $\mathbf{Q}$. (a) Quaternion $\mathbf{Q}_1$. (b) Quaternion $\mathbf{Q}_2$. (c) Quaternion $\mathbf{Q}_3$.

Quaternion $\mathbf{Q}_2$ can be calculated as

$$\mathbf{Q}_2 = \cos\frac{\theta_2}{2} + \sin\frac{\theta_2}{2}\cdot\bar{k} \tag{9}$$

which has rotation angle as

$$\theta_2 = \arctan 2\frac{g_{\text{after},y}}{g_{\text{after},x}} - \arctan 2\frac{g_{\text{before},y}}{g_{\text{before},x}}. \tag{10}$$

Quaternion $\mathbf{Q}_3$ is

$$\mathbf{Q}_3 = \cos\frac{\theta_3}{2} + \sin\frac{\theta_3}{2}\sin\beta\cdot\bar{i} + \sin\frac{\theta_3}{2}\cos\beta\cdot\bar{j} \tag{11}$$

with rotation angle and rotation axis information as

$$\begin{aligned}\theta_3 &= -\arctan\frac{g_{\text{after},z}}{\sqrt{g_{\text{after},x}^2 + g_{\text{after},y}^2}},\\ \sin\beta &= \frac{-g_{\text{after},y}}{\sqrt{g_{\text{after},x}^2 + g_{\text{after},y}^2}},\\ \cos\beta &= \frac{g_{\text{after},x}}{\sqrt{g_{\text{after},x}^2 + g_{\text{after},y}^2}}.\end{aligned} \tag{12}$$

Then the rotation of the fall movement can be expressed by quaternion multiplication as

$$\begin{aligned}\mathbf{g}_{\text{after}} &= \mathbf{Q}\otimes\mathbf{g}_{\text{before}}\otimes\mathbf{Q}^*\\ &= \mathbf{Q}_3\otimes\mathbf{Q}_2\otimes\mathbf{Q}_1\otimes\mathbf{g}_{\text{before}}\otimes\mathbf{Q}_1^*\otimes\mathbf{Q}_2^*\otimes\mathbf{Q}_3^*,\end{aligned} \tag{13}$$

where $\mathbf{Q}^* = q_0 - q_1\cdot\bar{i} - q_2\cdot\bar{j} - q_3\cdot\bar{k}$ is the conjugate quaternion of $\mathbf{Q}$. Quaternion algebra is normally implemented based on basic matrix algebra [17]. Quaternion multiplication used above could be realized by matrix multiplication as

$$\begin{aligned}\mathbf{Q}\otimes\mathbf{g}_{\text{before}} &= \mathbf{M}(\mathbf{Q})\begin{bmatrix}0\\ g_{\text{before},x}\\ g_{\text{before},y}\\ g_{\text{before},z}\end{bmatrix}\\ &= \begin{bmatrix}q_0 & -q_1 & -q_2 & -q_3\\ q_1 & q_0 & -q_3 & q_2\\ q_2 & q_3 & q_0 & -q_1\\ q_3 & -q_2 & q_1 & q_0\end{bmatrix}\begin{bmatrix}0\\ g_{\text{before},x}\\ g_{\text{before},y}\\ g_{\text{before},z}\end{bmatrix}.\end{aligned} \tag{14}$$

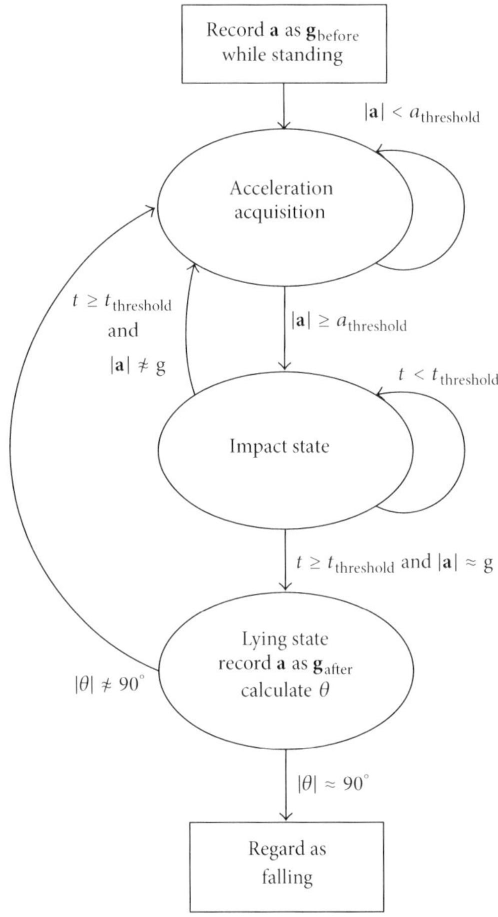

Figure 5: Fall detection algorithm state machine.

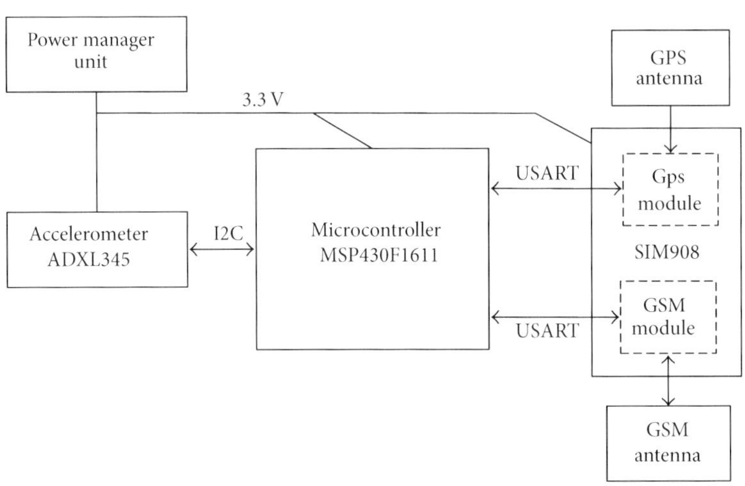

Figure 6: Basic hardware structure.

The whole rotation quaternion can also be decomposed as

$$\begin{aligned}\mathbf{Q} &= \mathbf{Q}_3 \otimes \mathbf{Q}_2 \otimes \mathbf{Q}_1 \\ &= \mathbf{M}(\mathbf{Q}_3)\,\mathbf{M}(\mathbf{Q}_2)\,\mathbf{Q}_1.\end{aligned} \quad (15)$$

$\mathbf{Q}_1$, $\mathbf{Q}_2$, and $\mathbf{Q}_3$ are all available based on gravity information before and after the falling movement. At last, it is possible to get four elements of quaternion $\mathbf{Q}$ by the equation above and the rotation angle θ could be calculated as

$$\theta = 2 \cdot \arctan\left(\frac{\sqrt{{q_1}^2 + {q_2}^2 + {q_3}^2}}{q_0}\right). \quad (16)$$

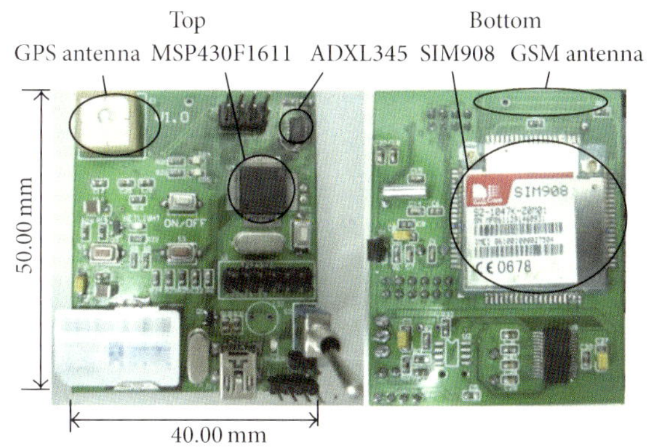

FIGURE 7: PCB board prototype.

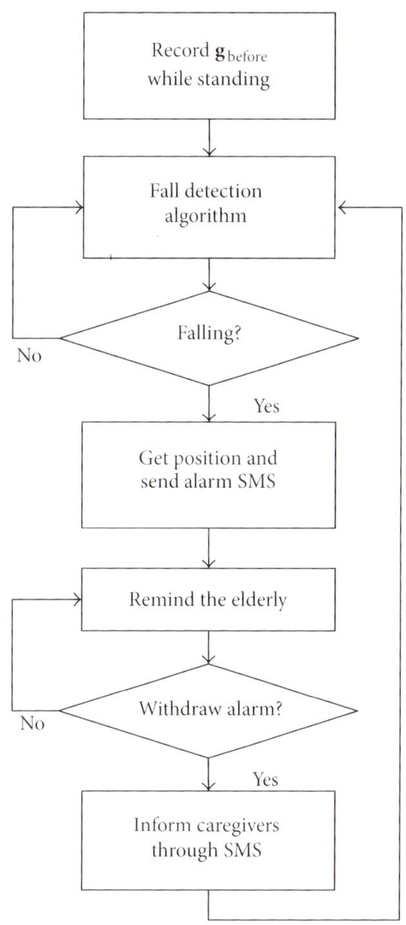

FIGURE 8: System software flow diagram.

When an object is falling, magnitude of θ will approach 90° which is also a character different from most normal activities. So it could be used as the second detection feature beside sum acceleration.

The flow chart of the proposed algorithm is depicted in Figure 5.

The wearable device will be mounted on human's waist at first to reflect the motion of human body closely [18], and the device will record $\mathbf{g}_{\text{before}}$ while the elderly is standing still. There is no special requirement of the device orientation but only keep stationary during the wear. $a_{\text{threshold}}$ means the threshold of sum acceleration magnitude and $t_{\text{threshold}}$ means the threshold of oscillation time duration after the break of $a_{\text{threshold}}$.

When measurements in three different axes have been acquired, the sum acceleration $|\mathbf{a}|$ will be calculated. When a real fall happens, sum acceleration will reach peak value of $|\mathbf{a}| \geq a_{\text{threshold}}$. In a real falling, the fluctuation of acceleration

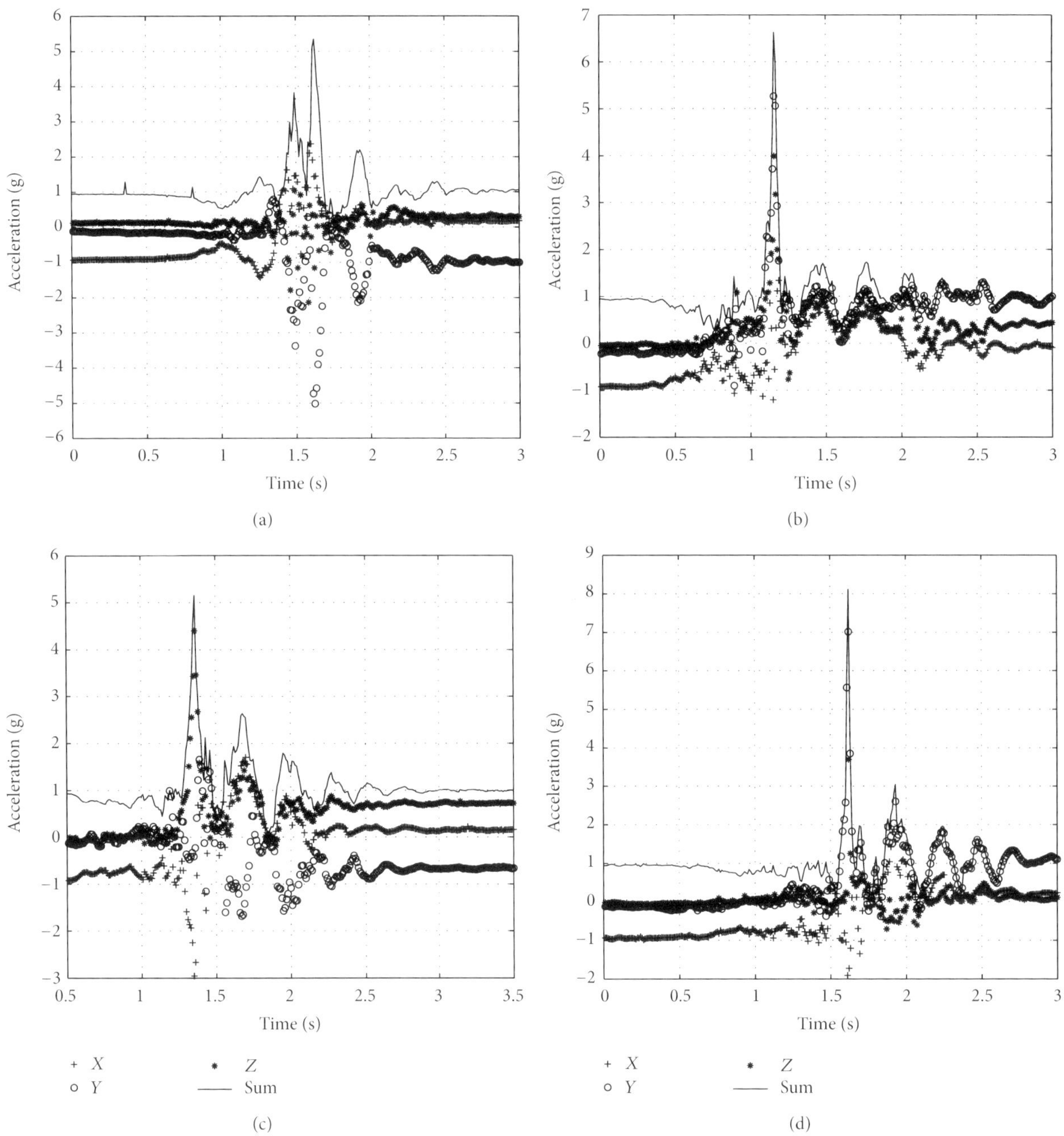

FIGURE 9: Acceleration waveforms during fall. (a) Forward fall. (b) Backward fall. (c) Leftward fall. (d) Rightward fall.

will stop in time duration $t_{\text{threshold}}$ and then the sum acceleration is $|\mathbf{a}| \approx g$ as the elderly will lie on the ground. Then the acceleration $\mathbf{a}$ is recorded as $\mathbf{g}_{\text{after}}$. Quaternion rotation θ will be calculated based on information $\mathbf{g}_{\text{before}}$ and $\mathbf{g}_{\text{after}}$. At last, the system will consider it as a fall if the rotation angle $|\theta| \approx 90^{\circ}$.

4. Implementation

4.1. Hardware. ADI's digital triaxial accelerometer ADXL345 is the motion sensor used in this system. The GPS service and GSM communication function are integrated in SIMCom's SIM908 module. TI's 16 bits MCU MSP430F1611 is used to control the whole system and imply the detection algorithm [19].

The measurement range of accelerometer could be set at ±2 g, ±4 g, ±8 g, or ±16 g, and the maximal sampling rate is 3.2 kHz. As human's activities are normally at low frequency bands [20], 100 Hz is a proper sampling rate for human fall detection. There is an inner digital filter in ADXL345 which could weaken noise and reduce the burden of digital signal processing in MCU to some extent. The measurements will be sent through IIC (interintegrated circuit) bus communication between the sensor and the MCU.

SIM908 can offer GPS and GSM service on serial port communication with MCU, and it can also work in low power mode.

Each hardware component of the wearable device is working under low voltage and the detection algorithm does not need complex calculation resource, so the power consumption of the whole device is quite low. A 1200 mAh, 3.7 V polymer lithium battery is quite enough to provide the need of the wearable device for a couple of days.

Hardware structure of the detection device is shown in Figure 6, and the PCB board prototype is shown in Figure 7.

4.2. Software. The software design of the system can be divided into two parts. One of them is the software design in wearable device, and the other is in the caregiver's handset.

4.2.1. Wearable Device. Flow diagram of the wearable device software is shown in Figure 8.

After initialization of the system, $\mathbf{g}_{\text{before}}$ would be extracted from acceleration measurements by using a low pass filter when the elderly is standing. After that, the fall detection algorithm will be applied. If a fall has been detected, the wearable device will locate the user and send alarm short message to caregivers immediately. Then the device will remind the elderly through vibration. If the user withdraws the alarm by pressing a button manually, the device will get back to fall detection state and a short message will be sent to inform the caregivers.

4.2.2. Caregiver's Handset. There is a URL (universal resource locator) which links to a web map in the alarm short message. The fall location information will be highlighted on a web map when the caregiver opens this link.

5. System Test

System test of the fall detection system has been conducted based on the system design described above.

5.1. Wearable Device and Fall Detection Algorithm. The sampling rate of accelerometer is set at 100 Hz and the measurement range is ±16 g with a maximum precision of 4 mg. MCU will read raw measurements from sensor's inner FIFO and apply the detection algorithm.

The test objects are three different volunteers at the ages of 23, 42, and 60, respectively. Based on analysis of these volunteers' experiment data, $a_{\text{threshold}}$ and $t_{\text{threshold}}$ are set as 2 g and 2 s, respectively. In order to get $\mathbf{g}$ when standing and lying after the fall, sum acceleration $\mathbf{a}$ which has magnitude between $(1-0.3)$ g and $(1+0.3)$ g will be considered as $\mathbf{g}_{\text{before}}$ and $\mathbf{g}_{\text{after}}$. Considering that the tilt of the ground or the lying posture of the elderly may affect the rotation angle, rotation angle θ between $(90-30)^\circ$ and $(90+30)^\circ$ will infer that the elderly has fallen.

System test contains five kinds of activities of daily living (i.e., walking, jumping, squatting, sitting, and resting) and four kinds of fallings (i.e., forward, backward, leftward, and rightward).

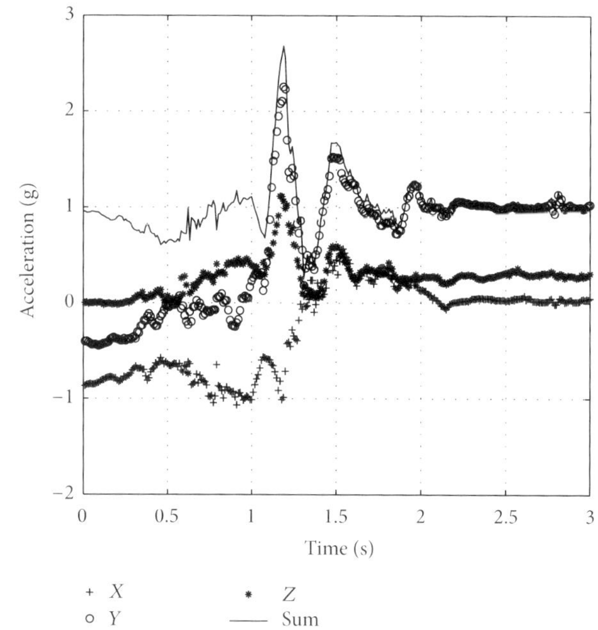

FIGURE 10: Resting.

TABLE 1: Test results for four kinds of falling and five kinds of ADL.

Motion type	Alarm times/test times	
	Proposed design	Acceleration threshold based design
Forward fall	60/60	59/60
Backward fall	56/60	54/60
Leftward fall	58/60	52/60
Rightward fall	59/60	55/60
Walking	0/60	4/60
Jumping	0/60	11/60
Squatting	0/60	0/60
Sitting	0/60	9/60
Resting	5/60	10/60

Each kind of motion has been repeated 20 times on each volunteer, and the detection results of the proposed algorithm and an acceleration threshold based algorithm [13] are listed in Table 1.

The sensitivity and specificity [21, 22] of the proposed system can be got from the test data in Table 1. Sensitivity of the proposed algorithm is 97.1%, and the specificity is 98.3%. Test results of acceleration threshold based algorithm show lower sensitivity and specificity at 91.6% and 88.7%, respectively.

Figure 9 shows the accelerations in different kinds of fallings which all trigger the fall alarm correctly and the corresponding rotation angles are 91.9°, −100.5°, 104.7°, and −114.1°.

Figure 10 shows acceleration during activity of lying down and resting which has rotation angle of −117.0° and similar

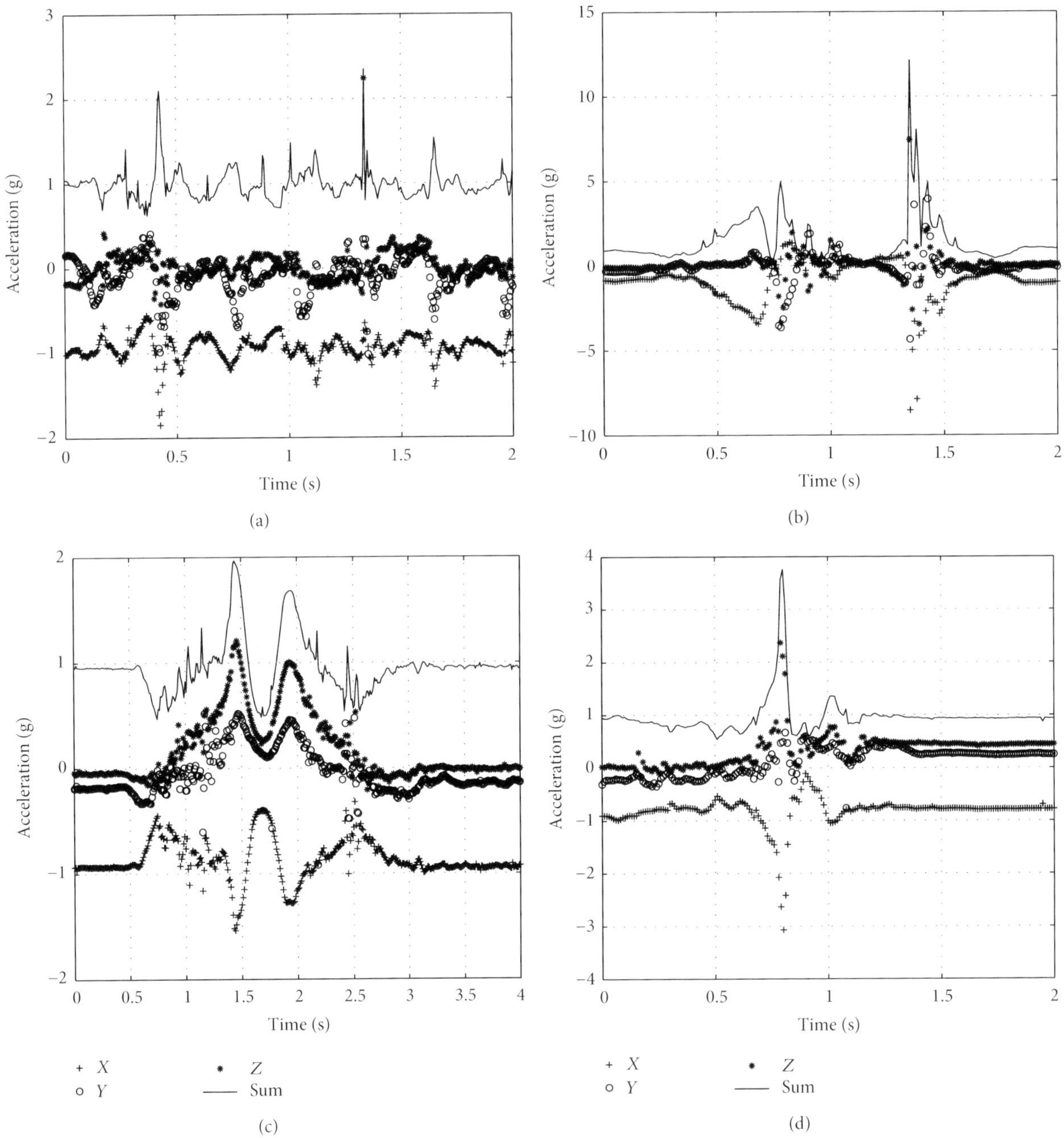

FIGURE 11: Acceleration waveform during ADL. (a) Walking. (b) Jumping. (c) Squatting. (d) Sitting.

waveform to falling [23], but the peak acceleration is much lower. Fall alarm has not been triggered yet at this situation.

Figure 11 shows acceleration during other ADL tests. They all do not have rotation about 90°; even some of the peak values are quite high, so the fall alarm has not been triggered.

5.2. Location Based Service. Alarm receiving function on caregiver's handset has also been tested. An alarm SMS (short message service) containing a map URL has been received by the handset as shown in Figure 12 when a fall has been detected. Clicking the URL will open a map in Web browser on which the fall location will be displayed accurately as shown in Figure 13.

6. Conclusion

This paper developed a fall detection system based on a single triaxial accelerometer based wearable device. There is no special requirement of the device's mounting orientation because the algorithm does not claim the axes of accelerometer to be fixed strictly. The system has low power consumed hardware design and highly efficient algorithm which could extend the service time of the wearable device. Both the hardware and software designs are suitable for wearable and outdoor application.

As normal activity of resting also has similar rotation as falling, it may trigger fall alarm when the body hits

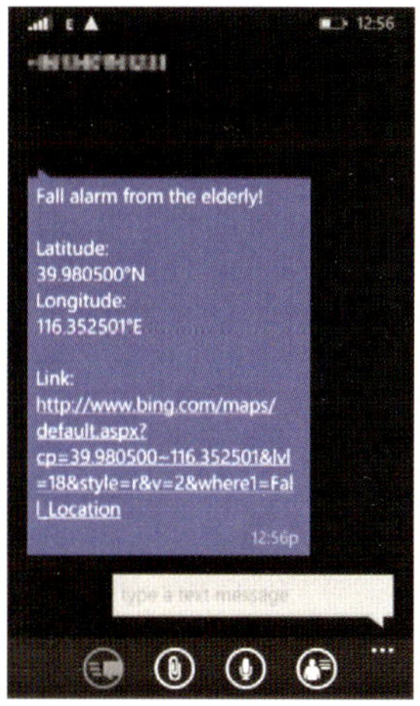

FIGURE 12: Fall alarm SMS which contains fall location URL.

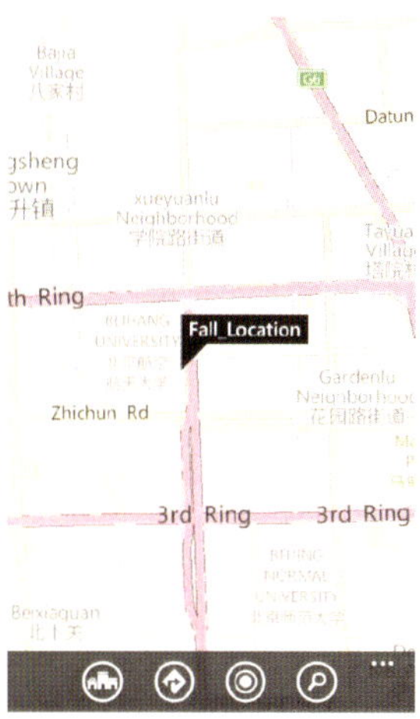

FIGURE 13: Fall location displayed on a Web map.

ground heavily. So the choice of $a_{\text{threshold}}$ is quite important to distinguish falling from heavily lying activity. Sufficient sample number collected from subjects with different age and gender will improve the reliability and robustness of the threshold. Beside these, technologies such as SVM and neural network are considerable to seek out a proper classification method based on the features used in this system.

Acknowledgments

The research is partially supported by the Open Research Fund of the Academy of Satellite Application under Grant no. 2014_CXJJ-DH_07, the Scientific Research Foundation for the Returned Overseas Chinese Scholars, State Education Ministry, and the Specialized Research Fund for the Doctoral Program of High Education, China.

References

[1] M. K. Karlsson, H. Magnusson, T. von Schewelov, and B. E. Rosengren, "Prevention of falls in the elderly—a review," *Osteoporosis International*, vol. 24, no. 3, pp. 747–762, 2013.

[2] T. Shany, S. J. Redmond, M. R. Narayanan, and N. H. Lovell, "Sensors-based wearable systems for monitoring of human movement and falls," *IEEE Sensors Journal*, vol. 12, no. 3, pp. 658–670, 2012.

[3] M. Mubashir, L. Shao, and L. Seed, "A survey on fall detection: principles and approaches," *Neurocomputing*, vol. 100, pp. 144–152, 2013.

[4] M. Grassi, A. Lombardi, G. Rescio et al., "An integrated system for people fall-detection with data fusion capabilities based on 3D ToF camera and wireless accelerometer," in *Proceedings of the 9th IEEE Sensors Conference (SENSORS '10)*, pp. 1016–1019, Kona, Hawaii, USA, November 2010.

[5] A. K. Bourke, K. O'Donovan, A. Clifford et al., "Optimum gravity vector and vertical acceleration estimation using a tri-axial accelerometer for falls and normal activities," in *Annual International Conference of the IEEE Engineering in Medicine and Biology Society (EMBC '11)*, pp. 7896–7899, Boston, Mass, USA, 2011.

[6] G. Anania, A. Tognetti, N. Carbonaro et al., "Development of a novel algorithm for human fall detection using wearable sensors," in *Proceedings of the IEEE Sensors*, pp. 1336–1339, IEEE, Lecce, Italy, October 2009.

[7] L. Qiang, J. A. Stankovic, M. A. Hanson, A. T. Barth, J. Lach, and G. Zhou, "Accurate, fast fall detection using gyroscopes and accelerometer-derived posture information," in *Proceedings of the 6th International Workshop on Wearable and Implantable Body Sensor Networks (BSN '09)*, pp. 138–143, Berkeley, Calif, USA, June 2009.

[8] S. Sabatelli, M. Galgani, L. Fanucci, and A. Rocchi, "A double-stage kalman filter for orientation tracking with an integrated processor in 9-D IMU," *IEEE Transactions on Instrumentation and Measurement*, vol. 62, no. 3, pp. 590–598, 2013.

[9] F. Bianchi, S. J. Redmond, M. R. Narayanan, S. Cerutti, and N. H. Lovell, "Barometric pressure and triaxial accelerometry-based falls event detection," *IEEE Transactions on Neural Systems and Rehabilitation Engineering*, vol. 18, no. 6, pp. 619–627, 2010.

[10] S.-L. Hsieh, K.-R. Chen, C.-L. Yeh et al., "An unfixed-position smartphone-based fall detection scheme," in *Proceedings of the IEEE International Conference on Systems, Man and Cybernetics (SMC '14)*, pp. 2077–2081, San Diego, Calif, USA, 2014.

[11] S. D. Bersch, C. M. J. Chislett, D. Azzi, R. Kusainov, and J. S. Briggs, "Activity detection using frequency analysis and off-the-shelf devices: fall detection from accelerometer data," in *Proceedings of the 5th International Conference on Pervasive Computing Technologies for Healthcare and Workshops (PervasiveHealth '11)*, pp. 362–365, Dublin, Ireland, May 2011.

[12] A. H. Khandoker, D. Lai, R. K. Begg, and M. Palaniswami, "A wavelet-based approach for screening falls risk in the elderly using support vector machines," in *Proceedings of the 4th International Conference on Intelligent Sensing and Information Processing (ICISIP '06)*, pp. 184–189, Bangalore, India, December 2006.

[13] A. K. Bourke, J. V. O'Brien, and G. M. Lyons, "Evaluation of a threshold-based tri-axial accelerometer fall detection algorithm," *Gait and Posture*, vol. 26, no. 2, pp. 194–199, 2007.

[14] T. Zhang, J. Wang, L. Xu et al., "fall detection by wearable sensor and one-class SVM algorithm," in *Intelligent Computing in Signal Processing and Pattern Recognition: International Conference on Intelligent Computing, ICIC 2006 Kunming, China, August 16–19, 2006*, vol. 345 of *Lecture Notes in Control and Information Sciences*, pp. 858–863, Springer, Berlin, Germany, 2006.

[15] S. Abbate, M. Avvenuti, F. Bonatesta, G. Cola, P. Corsini, and A. Vecchio, "A smartphone-based fall detection system," *Pervasive and Mobile Computing*, vol. 8, no. 6, pp. 883–899, 2012.

[16] A. M. Sabatini, "Quaternion-based strap-down integration method for applications of inertial sensing to gait analysis," *Medical and Biological Engineering and Computing*, vol. 43, no. 1, pp. 94–101, 2005.

[17] J. Vince, *Quaternions for Computer Graphics*, Springer, London, UK, 2011.

[18] J. Chen, K. Karric, D. Chang et al., "Wearable sensors for reliable fall detection," in *Proceedings of the 27th Annual International Conference of the Engineering in Medicine and Biology Society (EMBS '05)*, pp. 3551–3554, Shanghai, China, 2005.

[19] F. Wu, C. Hu, H. Zhao, and Y. Zhao, "Development of a fall alarm system based on multi-sensor integration," in *Proceedings of the 25th International Technical Meeting of the Satellite Division of the Institute of Navigation (ION GNSS '12)*, pp. 3805–3813, Nashville, Tenn, USA, September 2012.

[20] C. V. C. Bouten, K. T. M. Koekkoek, M. Verduin, R. Kodde, and J. D. Janssen, "A triaxial accelerometer and portable data processing unit for the assessment of daily physical activity," *IEEE Transactions on Biomedical Engineering*, vol. 44, no. 3, pp. 136–147, 1997.

[21] M. Kangas, I. Vikman, J. Wiklander, P. Lindgren, L. Nyberg, and T. Jämsä, "Sensitivity and specificity of fall detection in people aged 40 years and over," *Gait & Posture*, vol. 29, no. 4, pp. 571–574, 2009.

[22] P. Jantaraprim, P. Phukpattaranont, C. Limsakul, and B. Wongkittisuksa, "Evaluation of fall detection for the elderly on a variety of subject groups," in *Proceedings of the 3rd International Convention on Rehabilitation Engineering & Assistive Technology (ICREATE '09)*, pp. 1–4, Singapore, April 2009.

[23] S. Abbate, M. Avvenuti, G. Cola et al., "Recognition of false alarms in fall detection systems," in *Consumer Communications and Networking Conference (CCNC '11)*, pp. 23–28, Las Vegas, Nev, USA, 2011.

14

Health-Related Quality of Life of Rural Clients Seeking Telepsychology Services

Kevin R. Tarlow,[1] Carly E. McCord,[2] Timothy R. Elliott,[1] and Daniel F. Brossart[1]

[1] *Educational Psychology, Texas A&M University, College Station, TX 77843, USA*

[2] *School of Public Health, Texas A&M Health Science Center, 8441 Highway 47, Clinical Building 1, Suite 1300, Bryan, TX 77807, USA*

Correspondence should be addressed to Carly E. McCord; cmccord@sph.tamhsc.edu

Academic Editor: Malcolm Clarke

Sixty million US residents live in rural areas, but health policies and interventions developed from an urban mindset often fail to address the significant barriers to health experienced by these local communities. Telepsychology, or psychological services delivered by distance via technology, is an emerging treatment modality with special implications for underserved rural areas. This study found that a sample of rural residents seeking telepsychology services ($n = 94$) had low health-related quality of life (HRQOL), often due to cooccurring physical and mental health diagnoses including high rates of depression. However, a brief telepsychology treatment delivered to rural clients ($n = 40$) was associated with an improvement in mental health-related quality of life ($d = 0.70$, $P < .001$). These results indicate that despite the complex health needs of these underserved communities, telepsychology interventions may help offset the disparities in health service access in rural areas.

1. Introduction

Over 3.8 million of the 60 million rural United States residents live in Texas, which has more rural residents than any state in the country [1]. Approximately one in four rural residents has a mental illness or substance abuse problem [2]. However, the resources available to individuals living in rural areas are not equivalent to those available to their urban counterparts due to barriers such as lack of transportation, geographic isolation, low socioeconomic status, low educational attainment, and low rates of insurance coverage [3]. For instance, even though some mental health diagnoses occur at least as often in rural areas as in urban ones [4, 5], the negative impact of those diagnoses on health and quality of life may be greater in rural areas because of the barriers to availability, accessibility, and perceived stigma of mental health care services [6]. Rural-urban health disparities have been reported in groups ranging from clergy [7] to veterans [8].

Not only are rural residents confronted with unique barriers to service, but health care providers are less likely to deliver services in rural areas due to lower wages and compensation, increased ethical risk, and higher burn-out rates [9]. Given the range of rural health needs and the scarcity of specialty services, providers who do offer services in rural communities are often pressured to treat patients at the limits of their knowledge and expertise [10]. The unique features of the rural health care landscape require health policies, legislation, and interventions informed by these issues.

Telehealth, or the use of telecommunication technologies to provide health care services at a distance, is one way to offset the disparities in health care access found in rural areas. Telehealth describes a broad range of health-related services that may include use of internet, telephone, videoconferencing, email, chat, text messaging, and other technologies to improve access, affordability, and efficiency of service delivery. The American Psychological Association (APA) recently recognized the benefits of using *telepsychology* (i.e., psychological telehealth services) to increase access to underserved areas [11]. For the purposes of this paper, the term telepsychology is used to describe the delivery of individual psychotherapy via secure videoconferencing technology. In their guidelines for the use of this emerging treatment modality, APA suggested that health service providers should utilize telepsychology when research evidence supports its use for a particular client or population (p. 8). However, APA also pointed out that outcomes research for telepsychology may be lacking for many clients due to the developing nature of the field. The purpose of this paper is to (a) better understand the health needs of rural clients seeking mental health care services and (b) establish an evidence basis for telepsychology's effectiveness with rural clients. Meeting these two goals is an important step to increasing mental health care access for underserved rural areas.

A major challenge to providing health care services to rural communities—telehealth or otherwise—is the diversity of the rural communities themselves. As sociologist Daryl Hobbs said, "When you have seen *one* rural community, you have seen *one* rural community" (emphasis in original, p. 397) [12]. Rural health policies and interventions should be empirically and *locally* informed, based on the needs and resources of each unique community. Creating sustainable initiatives to meet health needs in rural areas often requires local collaboration among community stakeholders, including clinicians, researchers, students, community leaders, and other policy makers [13].

Understanding a rural community's available health resources is a vital first step in locally informed policy and intervention development. *Community capacity* describes a community's ability to mobilize its social, political, and organizational capital to meet unmet needs [14]. This begins with an assessment of needs and is followed by the development of deliberate, collaborative intervention strategies. The "build it and they will come" mentality will not lead to sustainability in rural areas. Universities may be powerful facilitators of community capacity, but they must collaborate with local stakeholders and maintain those relationships beyond their inception [15].

In 2006, the Center for Community Health Development (CCHD) at the Texas A&M Health Science Center (http://www.cchd.us/) conducted a survey in the Brazos Valley—a region of Texas comprised of seven counties, all of which are federally designated Health Professional Shortage Areas (HPSAs). Texas has the highest percentage of HPSAs in the country [16]. The 2006 survey found that mental health and public transportation were among the top needs of the region. Over half of respondents reported having at least one day of "poor mental health" in the last month, and 62% of respondents reported needing mental health services and being unable to get the needed services [17].

In response to the identified health needs of the area, a "town and gown" partnership was created between Leon County (one of the seven Brazos Valley counties) and Texas A&M University to provide telepsychology services to the area. A locally appointed health resource commission mobilized resources in Leon County to provide a physical location to conduct the telepsychology services, and in 2009 advanced doctoral level students in the Counseling Psychology program at Texas A&M University began providing long-distance services under the supervision of a licensed psychologist [18].

It was expected that many Leon County residents seeking telepsychology services would present with cooccurring physical and mental health conditions. Consequently, assessment of client needs, issues, and response to telepsychology treatment required an evaluation of client health-related quality of life (HRQOL). HRQOL is a multidimensional construct of well-being often encompassing physical, mental, emotional, and social functioning [19, 20]. The Centers for Disease Control and Prevention (CDC) suggest that measures such as the Medical Outcomes Study Short Form (SF-12) [21] can be used to identify needed services, inform policy and legislation, and evaluate outcomes of health interventions [22].

Three other studies of similar size have evaluated the impact of telepsychology and telemedicine for mental health treatment on HRQOL using the SF-12v2. In one Canadian study, telepsychiatry outperformed in-person psychiatry for mental health improvement [23]. In two European studies that included German-speaking clients in The Netherlands, Germany, Austria, and Switzerland, internet-based cognitive behavioral therapy (CBT) interventions for grief and post-traumatic stress disorder (PTSD) outperformed the waitlist control group for mental health improvement [24, 25]. While all three studies found moderate to large effects of telehealth interventions on mental health status, no effects on physical health status were detected.

The current study was developed with two goals. First, given the barriers to health experienced by many rural communities, we wish to better understand the physical and mental health status of rural residents receiving telepsychology services. We compare the physical and mental health scores for participants in the current study with established HRQOL norms for the overall US population and with a national sample of depressed individuals. We expect that participants presenting for telepsychology services will have a lower HRQOL than both the national standardization sample and the national sample of depressed individuals. We also briefly review the depressive symptoms reported by participants in order to better describe the clinical features of the sample.

Second, we examine the possible impact of telepsychology services on client HRQOL in this underserved area. We expect that participants who received four sessions of telepsychology services will demonstrate significant improvements in mental health status. However, we were uncertain of the degree to which telepsychology services would affect physical health functioning.

These two goals are independent but related: *What are the physical and mental health needs of this population? And given barriers to other health services, is telepsychology an effective treatment option for this group?* Answering these questions is essential for empirically and locally informed health policy development. We expect that a range of stakeholders in and outside of the Brazos Valley would benefit from a better understanding of (a) the HRQOL of this rural community and (b) the increased health service options made possible by emerging areas such as telepsychology.

2. Methods

2.1. Participants. Participants in the current study resided in Leon County, Texas, and received telepsychology services between 2009 and 2012. Leon County is a federally designated Health Professional Shortage Area (HPSA) for both medical and mental health services [16]. Participants were predominantly low-income and were treated for a variety of presenting concerns, including depression, anxiety, bipolar disorder, posttraumatic stress disorder (PTSD), and relationship concerns.

Two samples of participants were analyzed for this study. Participants in a larger sample ($n = 94$) completed self-report measures of physical and mental health (SF-12v2; the Patient Health Questionnaire, PHQ-9) [26] during their first telepsychology session, and those data were used in the first part of the study to make descriptive comparisons with nationally representative samples. Within those 94 participants, a smaller group ($n = 40$) was reassessed with the SF-12v2 at the fourth session. Those follow-up data were used in the second part of the current study to evaluate the effectiveness of telepsychology.

There were several reasons that 54 individuals in the larger sample did not participate in the follow-up portion of the study. In some cases, participants dropped out of treatment before the fourth session ($n = 37$). Clients dropped out of treatment for a variety of known and unknown reasons. Some clients discontinued services because their presenting concerns were met before the fourth session. Others dropped out because they lacked transportation, found other treatment providers, moved from the area, or were incarcerated. In some cases participants continued to receive treatment; however their assigned counselor did not participate in the follow-up study ($n = 17$) and SF-12 data were not collected at the fourth session. No inclusion or exclusion criteria were implemented in selecting clients for the follow-up study; rather the follow-up group counselors elected to readminister the SF-12. Supporting analyses not reported here found that the follow-up group ($n = 40$) and the non-follow-up group ($n = 54$) did not have statistically significant differences on their initial levels of physical health (PCS), mental health (MCS), or depression (PHQ-9), and the two groups were demographically similar. Based on these analyses, the 54 individuals not assessed for the follow-up group are not believed to represent a qualitatively different population of individuals, as their physical health, mental health, and demographic attributes were not different.

For the larger sample ($n = 94$), participants ranged in age from 14 to 73 years ($M = 41.3$, SD $= 13.6$). There were 71 women (75.5%) and 23 men (24.5%). The sample reflected the racial and ethnic composition of the county [27], with 71 white (75.5%), 5 black or African American (5.3%), 6 Hispanic or Latino (6.4%), 1 Asian (1.1%), and 1 biracial participants (1.1%), with 10 participants (10.6%) not reporting a race or ethnicity.

For the smaller sample ($n = 40$), participants ranged in age from 14 to 62 years ($M = 40.6$, SD $= 13.2$). There were 34 women (85.0%) and 6 men (15.0%). There were 34 white (85.0%), 2 black or African American (5.0%), 2 Hispanic or Latino (5.0%), 1 Asian (2.5%), and 1 biracial participants (2.5%).

2.2. Procedures. Clients were either self-referred or referred by a local physician to the telepsychology clinic. Initial phone screenings were conducted to screen out dangerous suicidal or homicidal ideation/intent and active psychosis. Clients were then seen in an intake interview to determine the presenting problem and to develop a treatment plan. All clients were verbally administered several assessments during the intake interview, including the SF-12v2. No clients were intentionally excluded from data collection, as the measures are part of normal clinic protocol. The SF-12v2 was verbally administered again during the fourth session to assess response to treatment.

Counseling sessions were approximately 50 minutes long and conducted via videoconferencing technology. Both the client and counselor sit in front of a 42-inch high definition television screen with at secure T1 connection meeting HIPAA guidelines for encryption and confidentiality. Counselors were doctoral level students in the Counseling Psychology program at Texas A&M University. Students were trained in a scientist-practitioner model and encouraged to use evidence-based treatments with clients. Common therapeutic approaches used by counselors include cognitive behavioral therapy, cognitive processing therapy, acceptance and commitment therapy, and other humanistic approaches to address the presenting and emerging problems identified by clients during the course of therapy.

2.3. Measures

2.3.1. SF-12v2. The SF-12 [28] is a 12-item, self-report measure selected to measure health-related quality of life. A valid shorter version of the SF-36, the second edition of the SF-12 reproduces the total and composite scores with at least 90% accuracy. It is one of the most widely used health surveys in the world due to its proven practicality, utility, and psychometric stability [21]. The SF-12v2 yields two composite scores, the Physical Component Summary score (PCS) and the Mental Component Summary score (MCS), which reflect the overall level of physical and mental health status, respectively. Higher PCS scores indicate a higher level of physical functioning, and higher MCS scores indicate a higher level of mental and emotional functioning. PCS scores have an internal reliability coefficient of $\alpha = .89$, and MCS scores have an internal reliability coefficient of $\alpha = .86$. The two composite scores have strong statistical power, or the ability to detect true differences in health status when they occur [21].

The SF-12 includes norms so that individual and group scores can be compared to other relevant groups. The norming data was collected in 1998 from 7,069 individuals. Households were selected to match US census data on geographical region, market size, age, income, and household size. Scores are reported as standard T-scores with a mean of 50 and standard deviation of 10. However, other means and

Table 1: SF-12v2 norm comparisons.

	Current study		National depressed sample [21]		National standardization sample [21]	
	PCS	MCS	PCS	MCS	PCS	MCS
Mean	44.46	30.72	45.77	36.85	49.70	49.48
SD	15.30	12.46	12.10	10.82	9.93	9.87
25th percentile	31.13	21.87	36.76	28.45	44.39	43.79
50th percentile	46.45	27.99	47.06	36.79	53.28	52.01
75th percentile	56.48	37.74	56.08	44.92	56.61	56.70
Minimum	16.16	−0.54	10.62	5.73	6.59	5.73
Maximum	70.78	63.19	71.82	65.53	71.82	71.01
N	94	94	1,000	1,002	7,690	7,697

standard deviations have been calculated for specific groups. Some of the norms include a sample representative of the noninstitutionalized US population and subgroups based on gender, age, and common chronic health conditions such as diabetes, hypertension, depression, and arthritis [21].

2.3.2. PHQ-9. The brief Patient Health Questionnaire [26] was administered at intake to assess depressive symptomology. Each item on the assessment corresponds to a single criterion from the *Diagnostic and Statistical Manual of Mental Disorders, Fourth Edition.* The items are scored on a Likert scale with the following options: 0 = not at all, 1 = several days, 2 = more than half the days, and 3 = nearly every day. Total scores range from 0 to 27. A total score of 10 or greater is a widely used cut-off score used to indicate a probable major depressive disorder diagnosis [29]. Scores can be interpreted based on the total score as well to classify severity: 0–4 indicates no depression; 5–9 mild depression; 10–14 moderate depression, 15–19 moderately severe depression, and greater than or equal to 20 severe depression. PHQ-9 scores have demonstrated stable psychometric properties with a test-retest coefficient of .84 and internal consistency estimates of $\alpha = .86$ and .89 [26].

2.4. Analyses. To assess the relative health status of the present study's clinical sample (as measured by the SF-12v2), physical (PCS) and mental (MCS) health status data for participants in the current study are compared with a national standardization sample and with a national sample of depressed individuals using one-way ANOVA with Bonferroni post hoc comparisons. Data are also presented indicating the proportion of participants who met criteria for depressive symptomology (as measured by cut-off scores on the PHQ-9).

Analytic methods consistent with similar outcomes research [23–25] were used to determine the efficacy of telepsychology for participants in the current study. Paired t-tests were used to examine the statistical significance of physical and mental health status improvement after four sessions of telepsychology services. The effect size of treatment was calculated with Cohen's d for repeated measures [30].

3. Results

3.1. Sample Description and Normative Comparisons

Health Status. SF-12v2 data for clients are presented in Table 1 along with norms for a nationally representative sample of depressed individuals and norms for the general US population. A one-way ANOVA indicated that the samples in Table 1 had statistically significant differences for physical health status; $F(2, 8781) = 69.44$, $P < .001$. Bonferroni post hoc comparisons using Welch's t-tests indicated that the PCS scores for the rural telepsychology sample were not significantly different than the national depressed sample; $t(104) = -0.81$, ns. However, the telepsychology sample had lower PCS scores than the national standardization sample; $t(93) = -3.31$, $P = .001$. Thus, the rural telepsychology sample had a lower physical health status than the nationally representative sample of the overall US population, whereas their physical health status was similar to a national sample of depressed individuals.

A second one-way ANOVA indicated that the samples in Table 1 had statistically significant differences for mental health status; $F(2, 8790) = 844.12$, $P < .001$. Bonferroni post hoc comparisons using Welch's t-tests indicated that the rural telepsychology sample had lower MCS scores than both the national standardization sample, $t(94) = -14.54$, $P < .001$, and the national depressed sample, $t(106) = -4.61$, $P < .001$.

Not only do the participants in the current study have poorer mental health status on average than a national sample of depressed individuals, but they occupy the extreme low end of the distribution of mental health status for the overall population. The average participant in the Leon County sample (MCS = 30.72) falls about two standard deviations below the mean of mental health status for the US population, well below the average individual.

Depression. Seventy-nine participants in the current study (84.0%) scored a 10 or greater on the PHQ-9, which is the most commonly used cut-off score for diagnosing major depressive disorder [29]. Thirty-eight participants (40.4%) scored at or above 20 on the PHQ-9, indicating a severe level of depression. Forty participants (42.6%) reported suicidal thoughts or thoughts of self-harm occurring for at least

TABLE 2: HRQOL outcomes at fourth telepsychology session.

	Initial session	Fourth session	P	Effect size
PCS	44.12 (16.86)	40.80 (14.64)	ns	—
MCS	31.50 (12.81)	40.23 (14.83)	<.001	0.70

Note: $n = 40$.

several days in the two weeks previous to their initial telepsychology session.

3.2. Effect of Telepsychology on HRQOL. Receiving four sessions of telepsychology services was associated with a statistically significant improvement in MCS scores between intake ($M = 31.50$, SD = 12.81) and session-four follow-up ($M = 40.23$, SD = 14.83), $t(39) = 4.43$, $P < .001$. An effect size for the improvement in mental health status was calculated using Cohen's d for repeated measures, $d = 0.70$, a moderate sized effect [30]. There was not a statistically significant change in PCS scores between intake ($M = 44.12$, SD = 16.86) and follow-up ($M = 40.80$, SD = 14.64), $t(39) = -1.94$, $P = .060$. These results are summarized in Table 2.

Due to the small number of participants in the study and the small number of men ($n = 6$) and participants of color ($n = 6$), analyses to detect differential treatment response for gender and race/ethnicity lacked sufficient statistical power for any meaningful interpretation.

As expected, age was associated with lower physical health status. A post hoc analysis found that the age of participants in the follow-up group had a statistically significant correlation with the PCS score of clients at intake ($r = -.395$, $P = .012$), and a similar correlation was found between age and PCS score for the larger sample of 94 participants ($r = -.375$, $P < .01$). No statistically significant correlations between age and mental health status were found.

4. Discussion

This study found that the health-related quality of life (HRQOL) of rural Texas residents presenting for telepsychology services is indeed poor. While participants in this study reported physical health problems, their mental health status was exceptionally low, with the average participant's mental health status score falling about two standard deviations below the average for the US population. Individuals seeking telepsychology services had even lower mental health scores than a national sample of individuals diagnosed with major depressive disorder. This finding is consistent with other studies of rural and urban HRQOL differences [7, 8].

Providing psychological services to clients in a Health Professional Shortage Area (HPSA) poses several challenges. Individuals seeking treatment are expected to present with cooccurring physical and mental health diagnoses, as was the case in the current study's sample. Many clients in this study's sample reported a range of chronic health and disability issues in addition to psychological concerns such as depression, trauma, substance abuse, and anxiety. Even with access to telepsychology services, many clients (and their counselors) may be undertreated for their physical health concerns. The ongoing lack of care experienced in rural HPSAs has clear implications for the provision of telepsychology services.

Despite the complexity of their presenting physical and mental health concerns, we found that telepsychology was effective at improving the mental health status of clients who were assessed after four sessions of therapy. These results add to the growing evidence base for telepsychology, and they show that this emerging treatment modality may be effective specifically for rural residents living in an underserved area. Our findings may be of special importance to health care providers in rural areas who have been encouraged to utilize telepsychology when outcomes research supports its use for that particular population [11].

While working in rural areas has its challenges, it is not without opportunities. As was seen in this study, utilizing academic-community partnerships provides opportunities to train future professionals in innovative service delivery models. There is also the potential for more collaborative care for health care consumers. In urban areas, it is virtually impossible for all the health providers to be familiar with the dozens or even hundreds of other providers in the area. But due to the small number of providers in rural areas, providers have the ability to know the names and faces of all other providers in the community. If interorganizational communication is encouraged and expected, community capacity can be built and consumers can expect more integrated care [31].

Sixty-two percent of individuals surveyed in the rural Brazos Valley region of Texas report being unable to access needed mental health services [4]. Given the numerous barriers to health experienced by many rural communities, it is possible that millions of rural US residents desire mental health care but are unable to access it. This study demonstrates that telepsychology services developed through an academic-community partnership are a viable option for rural residents in need of effective mental health care. Telepsychology is an emerging area of telehealth and telemedicine with rapidly growing evidence for its effectiveness, and its high accessibility has special implications for rural communities.

Limitations of the current study include the relatively small sample size, although this is a necessary aspect of studying groups living in sparsely populated areas. Due to the small number of participants, subsequent analyses lacked the statistical power to measure possible effects of gender or race/ethnicity on treatment outcome. While the focus of this study was on the response to a brief treatment (four sessions), future studies should also investigate the impact of long term treatment, especially given the chronic nature of many rural clients' presenting concerns. Counselors in the current study did not conduct a comprehensive assessment of all physical and mental health needs of clients; while global measures of HRQOL were used for this analysis, future studies may wish to investigate the prevalence and impact of specific diagnoses on response to telepsychology treatment. No clients were excluded from the study as long as they did not meet clinical exclusion criteria (e.g., high suicidal or homicidal risk, active psychosis); however several individuals seeking telepsychology treatment were unable to receive services because of mobility restrictions. All sessions were conducted at the community health center in Leon County, and individuals without cars were unable to attend weekly sessions. While this is a limitation of this study's design, many telehealth and telemedicine interventions use technology to deliver services directly to patients' homes [32–34]. Telepsychology researchers may wish to study in-home services as well; however special considerations should be made to ensure client confidentiality and safety [11].

Acknowledgments

This research was supported by Grant no. D06RH07934 from the Office of Rural Health Policy, Health Resources and Services Commission. The findings and conclusions presented here are the authors' and do not necessarily represent the official position of the Office of Rural Health Policy.

References

[1] U.S. Census Bureau, PctUrbanRural_State, 2010, http://www.census.gov/geo/reference/ua/ualists_layout.html.

[2] L. W. Roberts, J. Battaglia, and R. S. Epstein, "Frontier ethics: mental health care needs and ethical dilemmas in rural communities," *Psychiatric Services*, vol. 50, no. 4, pp. 497–503, 1999.

[3] C. M. Galambos, "Health care disparities among rural populations: a neglected frontier," *Health and Social Work*, vol. 30, no. 3, pp. 179–181, 2005.

[4] D. F. Brossart, M. L. Wendel, T. R. Elliott, H. E. Cook, L. G. Castillo, and J. N. Burdine, "Assessing depression in rural communities," *Journal of Clinical Psychology*, vol. 69, no. 3, pp. 252–263, 2013.

[5] T. Cellucci and P. Vik, "Training for substance abuse treatment among psychologists in a rural state," *Professional Psychology: Research and Practice*, vol. 32, no. 3, pp. 248–252, 2001.

[6] K. B. Smalley, C. T. Yancey, J. C. Warren, K. Naufel, R. Ryan, and J. L. Pugh, "Rural mental health and psychological treatment: a review for practitioners," *Journal of Clinical Psychology*, vol. 66, no. 5, pp. 479–489, 2010.

[7] A. Miles, R. J. Proescholdbell, and E. Puffer, "Explaining rural/non-rural disparities in physical health-related quality of life: a study of United Methodist clergy in North Carolina," *Quality of Life Research*, vol. 20, no. 6, pp. 807–815, 2011.

[8] W. B. Weeks, L. E. Kazis, Y. Shen et al., "Differences in health-related quality of life in rural and urban veterans," *American Journal of Public Health*, vol. 94, no. 10, pp. 1762–1767, 2004.

[9] S. L. Hastings and T. J. Cohn, "Challenges and opportunities associated with rural mental health practice," *Journal of Rural Mental Health*, vol. 37, pp. 37–49, 2013.

[10] L. G. Gamm, S. Stone, and S. Pittman, *Rural Healthy People 2010: A Companion Document to Healthy People 2010*, Texas A&M University System Health Science Center, Southwest Rural Health Research Center, College Station, Tex, USA, 2010.

[11] American Psychological Association, "Guidelines for the practice of telepsychology," *The American Psychologist*, vol. 68, pp. 791–800, 2013.

[12] D. L. Brown and L. E. Swanson, *Challenges for Rural American in the Twenty-First Century*, Pennsylvania State University Press, Pennsylvania, Pa, USA, 2003.

[13] C. E. McCord, T. R. Elliott, D. F. Brossart, and L. G. Castillo, "Mental health issues in rural areas," in *Rural Populations and Health: Determinants, Disparities, and Solutions*, R. Crosby, R. Vanderpool, M. Wendel, and B. Casey, Eds., pp. 323–339, Jossey-Bass, San Francisco, Calif, USA, 2012.

[14] E. J. Trickett, "Community psychology: individuals and interventions in community context," *Annual Review of Psychology*, vol. 60, pp. 395–419, 2009.

[15] C. E. McCord, T. R. Elliott, M. L. Wendel et al., "Community capacity and teleconference counseling in rural texas," *Professional Psychology: Research and Practice*, vol. 42, no. 6, pp. 521–527, 2011.

[16] Health Resources and Services Administration, "HPSA by state and county," 2008, http://hpsafind.hrsa.gov/HPSASearch.aspx.

[17] Center for Community Health Development, *Brazos Valley Health Status Assessment: Executive Report*, School of Public Health, College Station, Tex, USA, 2006.

[18] M. L. Wendel, D. F. Brossart, T. R. Elliott, C. McCord, and M. A. Diaz, "Use of technology to increase access to mental health services in a rural Texas community," *Family and Community Health*, vol. 34, no. 2, pp. 134–140, 2011.

[19] C. E. Ferrans, "Definitions and conceptual models of quality of life," in *Outcomes Assessment in Cancer*, J. Lipscomb, C. C. Gotay, and C. Snyder, Eds., pp. 14–30, Cambridge University Press, Cambridge, UK, 2005.

[20] World Health Organization, "The World Health Organization Quality of Life assessment (WHOQOL): position paper from the World Health Organization," *Social Science and Medicine*, vol. 41, pp. 1403–1409, 2005.

[21] J. E. Ware, M. Kosinski, D. M. Turner-Bowker, and B. Gandek, *User's Manual for the SF-12v2 Health Survey*, Quality Metric Incorporated, Lincoln, RI, USA, 2002.

[22] Centers for Disease Control and Prevention, "Health related quality of life," 2011, http://www.cdc.gov/hrqol/concept.htm.

[23] D. Urness, M. Wass, A. Gordon, E. Tian, and T. Bulger, "Client acceptability and quality of life - telepsychiatry compared to in-person consultation," *Journal of Telemedicine and Telecare*, vol. 12, no. 5, pp. 251–254, 2006.

[24] C. Knaevelsrud and A. Maercker, "Internet-based treatment for PTSD reduces distress and facilitates the development of a strong therapeutic alliance: a randomized controlled clinical trial," *BMC Psychiatry*, vol. 7, article 13, 2007.

[25] B. Wagner, C. Knaevelsrud, and A. Maercker, "Internet-based cognitive-behavioral therapy for complicated grief: a randomized controlled trial," *Death Studies*, vol. 30, no. 5, pp. 429–453, 2006.

[26] K. Kroenke, R. L. Spitzer, and J. B. Williams, "The PHQ-9: validity of a brief depression severity measure," *Journal of General Internal Medicine*, vol. 16, no. 9, pp. 606–613, 2001.

[27] U.S. Census Bureau, "State and county QuickFacts," 2010, http://quickfacts.census.gov.

[28] J. E. Ware Jr., M. Kosinski, and S. D. Keller, "A 12-item short-form health survey: construction of scales and preliminary tests of reliability and validity," *Medical Care*, vol. 34, no. 3, pp. 220–233, 1996.

[29] L. Manea, S. Gilbody, and D. McMillan, "Optimal cut-off score for diagnosing depression with the Patient Health Questionnaire (PHQ-9): a meta-analysis," *Canadian Medical Association Journal*, vol. 184, no. 3, pp. 191–196, 2012.

[30] J. Cohen, *Statistical Power Analysis for the Behavioral Sciences*, revised, Academic Press, New York, NY, USA, 1988.

[31] H. R. Clark, A. Ramirez, K. N. Drake et al., "Utilization of an interorganizational network analysis to evaluate the development of community capacity among a community-academic partnership," *Progress in Community Health Partnerships: Research, Education, and Action*, vol. 8, no. 1, pp. 41–51, 2014.

[32] S. Abbate, M. Avvenuti, and J. Light, "Usability study of a wireless monitoring system among Alzheimer's disease elderly population," *International Journal of Telemedicine and Applications*, vol. 2014, Article ID 617495, 8 pages, 2014.

[33] B. Lindberg, C. Nilsson, D. Zotterman, S. Söderberg, and L. Skär, "Using information and communication technology in home care for communication between patients, family members, and healthcare professionals: a systematic review," *International Journal of Telemedicine and Applications*, vol. 2013, Article ID 461829, 31 pages, 2013.

[34] A. Williams, R. LaRocca, T. Chang et al., "Web-based depression screening and psychiatric consultation for college students: a feasibility and acceptability study," *International Journal of Telemedicine and Applications*, vol. 2014, Article ID 580786, 9 pages, 2014.

15

Adapting a Database of Text Messages to a Mobile-Based Weight Loss Program

Selma Limam Mansar, Shashank Jariwala, Nawal Behih, Maahd Shahzad, and Aysha Anggraini

Information Systems Program, Carnegie Mellon University, Doha, Qatar

Correspondence should be addressed to Selma Limam Mansar; selmal@qatar.cmu.edu

Academic Editor: Miriam Vollenbroek-Hutten

Obesity has become a worldwide epidemic. Qatar, a rapidly developing country in the Middle East, has seen a sharp increase in the prevalence of obesity. The increase can be attributed to several reasons, including sedentary lifestyles imposed by a harsh climate and the introduction of Western fast food. Mobile technologies have been used and studied as a technology to support individuals' weight loss. The authors have developed a mobile application that implements three strategies drawn from proven theories of behavioral change. The application is localized to the cultural context of its proposed users. The objective of this paper is to present a method through which we adapted the messaging content of a weight loss application to the context of its users while retaining an effective degree of automation. The adaptation addressed body image, eating and physical exercise habits, and regional/cultural needs. The paper discusses how surveying potential users can be used to build a profile of a target population, find common patterns, and then develop a database of text messages. The text messages are automated and sent to the users at specific times of day, as suggested by the survey results.

1. Introduction

Tackling the weight issue is a significant undertaking. Worldwide, the number of obese people has doubled in the past 20 years [1]. We explored ways in which mobile technologies can be adapted to meet environmental and cultural norms and thereby support individuals in their effort to lose weight. In this paper, we examine the case of the Middle East through the example of Qatar.

According to the International Association for the Study of Obesity, the numbers for obesity for the Qatari population are alarming. The association ranks the country sixth on its list of the most obese countries worldwide. The numbers presented in [2] (cited by [3]) were overwhelming: for the 25–65 age group, 34.6% of the men were obese and 34.3% were overweight. For females in the same age group, 45.3% were obese and 33% were overweight. The figures are also alarming for children: [4] (cited by [3]) found that in the 12–17 age group, 28.7% of boys were overweight and 7.6% were obese. Additionally, 20.3% of the girls in the same age group were overweight and 4.5% were obese. A more recent study in Qatar [5] suggests slightly lower figures among children of 2–19 years old, but still a much higher percentage than the current 16.9% for American children in this age group as reported by the National Health and Nutrition Examination Survey (NHANES) [6]. Despite this disparity, the media regularly links the nation's weight problem to wealth and also to exposure to Western-style restaurants that allegedly are instilling foreign food habits [7, 8].

The implications of an overweight citizenry for a nation's healthcare system have been widely publicized. A major challenge in addressing the problem has been to find ways to communicate the health implications of overweight and to motivate the population to adopt a healthier lifestyle. The ubiquity of cellphones has attracted the attention of some researchers as both a communication and motivational tool. In Qatar, the mobile phones subscription rate was 142% in February 2012 [9]. Although the Supreme Council of Information and Communication Technology in Qatar (ICTQatar) did not give a specific number, smartphones are said to constitute a significant percentage among the mobile phones in use. The high rate of market penetration of smartphones suggests that users are accustomed to accepting and using mobile applications. Moreover, the results of a study by [10] support the use of mobile applications for weight loss. In their paper, the authors investigated the effects of a mobile phone weight loss program on healthy but overweight adults. The research involved a control group and an experimental group and tested both groups on the use of the mobile phone application. The application instructed participants on how to reduce food intake and take dietary precautions, relayed feedback about goals, and reported daily weight numbers. The outcome of the experiment relied on several variables, all of which indicated at the end of the experiment that the experimental group had lost a significant amount of weight, but the control group had lost only a small amount. The researchers concluded that the mobile phone weight loss program was effective because it helped in propelling and sustaining short-term and long-term weight loss in participants.

Few localized mobile applications on weight loss are available. Brunstein et al. (2012a) [11] conducted a study in the summer of 2012 in which they downloaded the smartphone applications (apps) available through application stores in the "Health and Fitness" category and other health-related categories. Hardly any content in either Arabic or English was found for the residents of the Middle East. The efficacy of customized applications is nevertheless no longer debatable. Many studies over the past decade support localization, at least for websites [12, 13].

An important feature of our application is the messaging between a nutritionist and the users of the mobile application. Using messaging for mobile applications is not new and has been proven to be effective. The messaging (SMS exchange messages) function is usually used to send reminders and motivational or educational messages. Research has proved various degrees of efficacy. For example, shoppers who received advice on food substitution via SMS continued buying healthier alternatives after the program ended [14]. Another study [15] showed that text messages sent to adolescents as part of a diet plan were well accepted, and still another study [16] demonstrated a positive impact from sending weekly e-mails on exercise and food diaries. Authors in [17] reported a similar result from sending biweekly SMSs.

One of the advantages of automated SMSs is the ability to reach many users instantly and deliver information and motivational messages. However, the messages must be well designed to meet the dietary and physical exercise needs of individual users. Indeed, highly personalized support could be achieved by sending differentiated messages to each user, but that would be too time consuming for a nutritionist assisting them. The objective of this paper is to present a method through which we adapted the messaging content of a weight loss application to the context of its users while retaining an effective degree of automation. The adaptation addressed body image, eating and physical exercise habits, and regional/cultural needs.

In this paper, we briefly describe our application, which can be used by any user who can read English or Arabic. Our mobile application uses three features: automated motivational messages and reminders or messaging with a nutritionist, social group support, and self-monitoring of preestablished small and attainable goals. We present the application in Section 2. In Section 3, we discuss our method for creating a well-tailored application for users in a specific region or culture. To prepare the bank of SMS messages, we derived a method that invited input from potential users of the application, then designed the messages, and determined the frequency and timing of their transmission. This method differs from those in other studies in which the acceptance of messages was tested after the experiment [18]. Section 4 presents the results of our method with a group of Arab female students, aged 18–25. Section 5 concludes with a critical discussion of the results and the method.

2. Mobile Application Design

The authors of this paper worked with physicians to understand the nutritional aspect of healthy living in Qatar. In [19], physicians at a large hospital in the country were interviewed. The interviews delivered three consistent messages as follows: (1) most adults and the elderly will prefer communication and technologies presented in Arabic. Young adults and teenagers may be more comfortable with English than their elders, but may still prefer Arabic; (2) most adults and the elderly will need support and guidance in the use of sophisticated technologies; the use of applications has to be straightforward; (3) there is an urgent need for prevention and for raising awareness concerning diets and physical exercise habits.

We also worked with nutritionists and psychologists to understand what may motivate individuals to start a healthful lifestyle or to continue one. Traditional weight loss programs may not trigger long-term change. Multiple simultaneous interventions achieve better results than single-intervention programs; the latter programs typically achieve only modest weight loss. Our analysis led to a description of how theories of behavioral change can be mapped into a mobile application to trigger change [20]. Psychologists advised using Stroebe's theory on behavioral change [21, 22] to address dieters' challenges over short-term intervals. The theory covers three dimensions of dieting.

(1) *Cognitive*: it is important to increase dieters' awareness of the goals they set up for themselves. Dieters often have many goals (such as to improve their body image, tone up, lose weight, and cut out fat). Frequent reminders of their goals help maintain dieters' motivation to stay on their program.

(2) *Motivational*: the results of neither diets nor physical exercise are immediately noticeable. this delay of gratification may lead to premature abandonment of a program. However, fostering motivation and self-efficacy through the design of more modest goals that can be attained faster helps keep dieters on track. For example, someone can specify a given week or

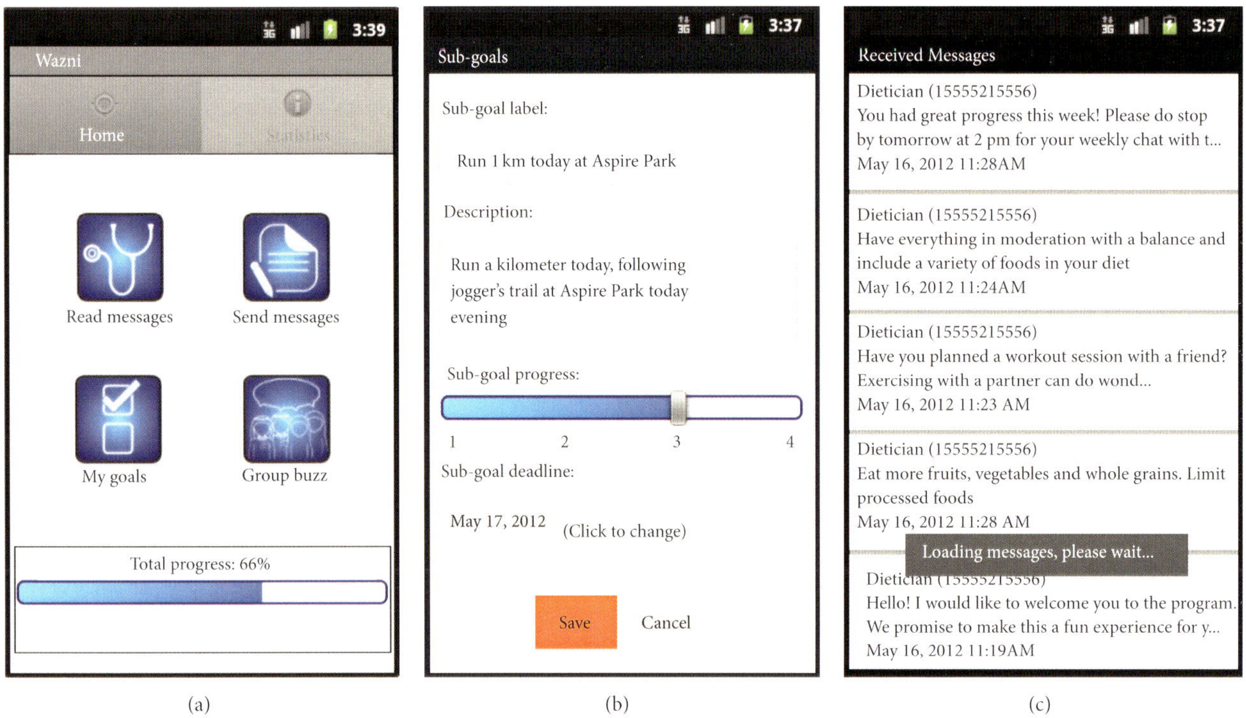

FIGURE 1: Screenshot of the mobile application (English version).

period of time to increase water intake or reduce the consumption of soft drinks.

(3) *Social*: dieters live in social environments in which temptations may be too strong. Eating and exercise habits need to be integrated into a social context, possibly one in which friends or relatives support the dieter in achieving his or her goals.

In [20], we proposed a mobile application that supports these three dimensions of behavioral change. To address the *cognitive* aspect, locally designed and tailored SMS messages can be sent daily to remind users of their goals. The *motivational* aspect can be addressed by a design feature in which participants enter incremental, achievable goals weekly. Participants can be asked to indicate daily whether they were successful in reaching each of their goals. In the *social* aspect of the application, social media can be leveraged. Participants can be invited to work toward a collective group goal.

The application was developed in both English and Arabic, using the Android platform. The usability of the application was tested and fully described in [23]. Figure 1 provides a snapshot of the application's interface and features.

In the following section, we describe the method we used to construct relevant messages.

3. A Method for Building Mobile Application Content

The effectiveness of automated messages will be increased if they are tailored to the targeted population group (the individuals pursuing weight loss). By tailoring we mean not only creating meaningful content but also the best times for transmitting this content and the frequency of transmissions as well. Hence, understanding the profile of participants is essential for the optimal customization of the content of these messages. We adopted the following methods.

3.1. Survey Design. Our first step was to design a survey to ascertain the most common eating and exercise habits of a targeted population. In the results section, we show the example of targeting a group of female Qatari college students. The survey consisted of questions pertaining to the following

(1) Demographics.

(2) Body mass index (BMI).

(3) A contour drawing rating scale (CDRS): it asks respondents to select the outline of a body that they perceive as most closely representing their own as well as one that represents their ideal figure. The CDRS was adapted from [24], Figure 2.

(4) Eating patterns and attitudes: this survey section was adapted from a questionnaire by [25]. It serves as a quick guide to identifying dietary habits as well as areas of indulgence or other unhealthful diet or eating patterns (diet type, daily frequency of meals, frequency of eating out, types of restaurants and cuisine, portion size, food pyramid, and beverage intake and type of beverage). An Eating Attitudes Test (EAT) [26] was included to evaluate patterns for behaviors found in anorexia nervosa patients.

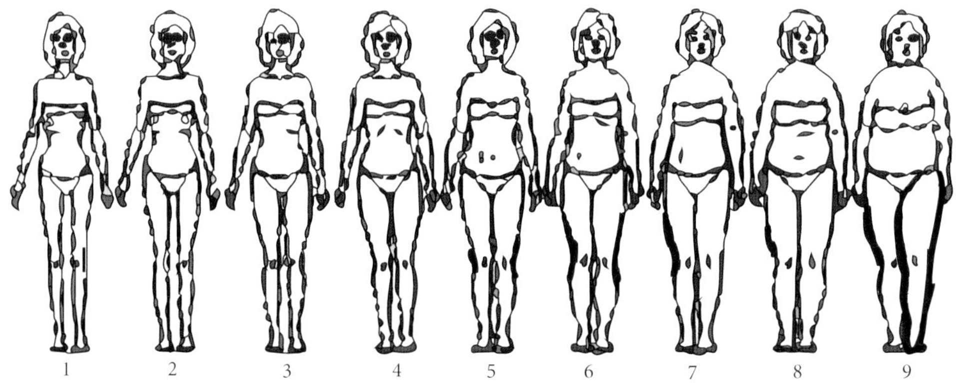

FIGURE 2: Body contour images used by participants.

The test consists of 40 questions reflecting factors such as food habits, perceived body image, vomiting, dieting, and perceived social pressure. Responses were recorded on a 6-point Likert scale: "always," "very often," "often," "sometimes," "rarely," or "never." Reponses were given a score of 3 in the extreme anorexic direction, with adjacent choices given scores of 2 and 1, respectively. All other responses were given a score of zero. A score of more than 30 points indicated symptoms of anorexia nervosa. Participants with the latter score were excluded from the results.

(5) Physical activity: this survey section asked respondents if they were physically active and about the amount of time they devoted to physical activity. The section seeks to determine whether respondents fall within the recommended activity levels of the World Health Organization (WHO). WHO defines physical activity in adults (18–64) as including "leisure time physical activity (e.g., walking, dancing, gardening, hiking, and swimming), transportation (e.g., walking or cycling), occupational (i.e., work), household chores, play, games, sports or planned exercise in the context of daily, family, and community activities" [27]. As per [27], we categorized degrees of physical activity as "inactive," "moderate intensity," and "vigorous intensity." The recommendations for healthy adults are a minimum of 30 minutes a day of activity of moderate intensity for five days a week or 20 minutes of vigorously intense activity for three days a week.

(6) Typical participant's profile: we used the survey to profile a typical participant's eating and physical exercise behaviors and patterns. The typical profile was used to later design appropriate messages as well as determine the timing and frequency for sending messages.

3.2. Database of Text Messages Design

(1) We used authoritative references on healthful lifestyles to build a database of messages. We then reduced the messages to short, concise text.

(2) We divided the messages into categories. The appropriate categories can be devised after analyzing the survey results and determining the typical eating and physical exercise patterns of a targeted population.

(3) We had the selected messages reviewed by a nutritionist to validate the health information.

(4) We had the messages reviewed by a psychologist to ensure they were motivational and appealing. Most of the comments from the psychologist related to rephrasing the messages to address small and achievable goals and to convey positive and supportive information.

(5) A database of messages was then created. The database arranged the messages according to the frequency and time of day a message from a given category would be sent (daily, weekly, etc.).

3.3. System's Architectural Design. See Figure 3.

4. Results: Profiling Potential Users in Context

The survey described in Section 3.1 was prepared and distributed by e-mail on September 18, 2012, to students of our university in Qatar. The survey was limited to females currently enrolled as students at the university. Filtering was achieved via the first two questions, which asked whether the responder was enrolled at the university and a female. A response of "No" to either question redirected the responder to the end of the survey. Sixty-eight respondents started the survey; eight of them were male and hence were redirected to the end of the survey. Forty-five of about 174 female students (52% of a total of 335 degree-seeking students) completed the survey, which was closed on September 29, 2012. This yields a response rate of 26%; all respondents are considered female students at the university. However, the total number of female native Arabic speakers at the university is not available.

4.1. Identifying Demographics, BMI Figures, and Body Image. Survey responses were further filtered, by selecting those who were native speakers of Arabic. These 26 responses were

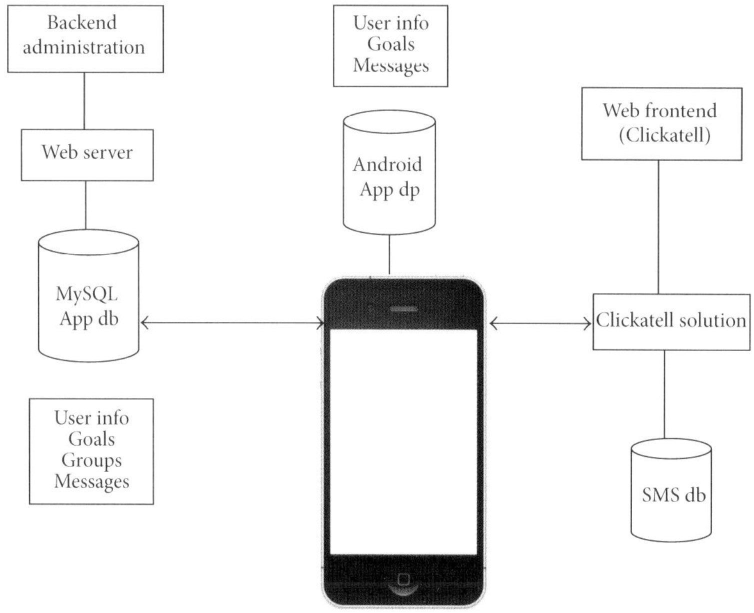

FIGURE 3: Application architecture.

TABLE 1: BMI profiles.

BMI range	Average	Median	Mode	Standard deviation	Perceived CDRS mode	Desirable CDRS mode
17–41.5	24.65	25.4	27.1	5.62	4	3

analyzed. About 65% of the native Arabic-speaking female students were 18–20 years old. The mean BMI of this group was 24.65 (which is in the normal range, overweight starting at 25 or above), in the range of 17 (underweight)–41.5 (obese class III); median and mode were 25.4 (overweight) and 27.1 (overweight), respectively, with a standard deviation of 5.62 (see Table 1). A strong correlation (0.87) was observed between the respondents' BMI and the CDRS figure they considered most like themselves. This suggests that most respondents were aware of their current weight and body figure: a BMI in a normal range translated to a normal range on the CDRS. However, one out of three obese participants and four of 11 who were overweight underestimated their body image. A similar lack of self-awareness was evident in one of the studies assessing the relationship between BMI and body image self-perception [28]. Another finding that corroborates with self-perception studies is that even females with BMI in the normal range (18.5–24.9 kg/m^2) would ideally like to lose weight [29]. Of the nine respondents with BMIs in the normal range, seven wanted to lose weight to ideally move further down the CDRS. Furthermore, none of the respondents marked the middle image on the CDRS as their ideal goal image. The highest selection was 4 on the 9-point scale, a selection still regarded as anorexic [24].

4.2. Identifying Eating Patterns and Attitudes. The most common diet was "halal" food, comparable to a kosher diet in the West. This is a religious and cultural norm, and almost all the respondents followed this particular diet. Of the 26 respondents, only two followed a low-fat diet, and two followed a vegetarian diet. These respondents with special diets, such as low fat, restricted their eating to at least two hours before sleeping or received specially planned meals from a diet shop. These persons were slightly above the normal BMI threshold and perceived their body images as normal (4-5, on a 9-point scale).

In terms of meals consumed, respondents on average consumed about two meals a day, with lunch—out of breakfast, brunch, lunch, and dinner—being the most frequent meal consumed. A large proportion of the group snacked in the afternoon (12) or throughout the day (12). The most common snacks included chocolate, chips, crackers and biscuits, cookies, cereals, and fruits.

An indicator of cultural eating habits may be the frequency with which young adults eat out or order "takeout" meals in [30]. We found that 23 of the 26 respondents ate out or had food delivered; 13 of them did so at least once a week. The most common dining facilities frequented were fast food restaurants (14), followed by eating at home and in the university cafeteria. The fast food option is not good news. As indicated in [31], regular fast food consumption leads to a steady increase in calories intake and hence to weight gain. The most popular cuisines were Italian, American, and Lebanese, followed by Chinese, Mexican, Indian, and traditional Qatari cuisines. However, there was no clear correlation between BMI and eating facilities or cuisine. The two most common food preparation techniques were frying (20) and boiling (20), followed by baking (19) and steaming (14).

TABLE 2: Eating patterns: food items.

Item	Freq.					
	Never	1-2	3–5	6–8	9–11	Total
Starch (bread, rice, pasta, and potato)	0	15	8	3	0	26
Fruits	0	20	6	0	0	26
Vegetables	0	16	10	0	0	26
Dairy	2	19	3	2	0	26
Meat, fish, poultry, and eggs	0	15	8	2	1	26
Fat	2	16	5	3	0	26
Sweets	1	18	5	2	0	26

TABLE 3: Beverages.

Item	Freq.			
	1–5	6–10	Not consuming	Total
Water (glasses)	20	6	0	26
Coffee	10	0	16	16
Tea	13	0	13	26
Soda	7	0	19	26
Alcohol	0	0	26	26
Others (juice, etc.)	6	0	26	26

Respondents were asked how frequently they ate various types of food, such as starch, dairy, meat, poultry, and fat. Table 2 shows the responses. The results are inconclusive. Indeed, the sizes of food portions were not captured and could play a larger role than just that of the frequency of intake [32]. Furthermore, the frequency of starch intake does not disclose the type of starch consumed, which could be either beneficial slow-digesting starch or undesirable starch sugars high in fructose, such as high fructose corn syrup, or even both [33].

Respondents were asked about their intake of beverages. We compared the consumption of water with the suggested adequate intake (AI) of water. Adequate intake is the average total water intake, including direct and indirect water consumption, by a group of healthy people [34]. The AI for young adult females is 2.7 L [35], a little over 11 glasses (8 fl. oz. each). Another category in which frequency may not translate to consumption is tea and coffee intake. Eighteen of 26 respondents have either tea or coffee 1–5 times a day, with five having both. The question does not capture how much sugar is added to these beverages, and high sugar content in beverages is detrimental even at 1–5 cups a day. Tea in this region, especially the local "karak" tea, which contains high amounts of sweetened condensed milk, typically contains a large amount of sugar.

The respondents were asked if they would like to change their eating habits, and 23 of 26 responded "Yes." The most common changes the respondents wanted to bring about were replacing unhealthful snacks with more healthful options, cutting down on junk food, reducing sugar intake, and making breakfast a regular daily meal, along with balanced meals in general (see Table 3).

The final segment of the survey included the Eating Attitudes Test (EAT) (see Section 3.1). From a total of 26 eligible respondents, four scored more than 30 on the EAT; of these, only one was underweight (BMI 17.2, EAT 41) and one of the participants had a BMI within the normal range (BMI 23.8, EAT 36). It is noteworthy that two participants were overweight, yet nevertheless scored high on the EAT (BMI 27.1, EAT 61 and BMI 28, EAT 41). We then consulted their responses on the 9-point CDRS to what they would ideally like to resemble [24]. Each of the participants had entered a selection corresponding to the lower range of the scale (2, 3, and 4) in which a selection of up to 4 correlated with symptoms of anorexia. Hence, we see that even healthy, or slightly overweight, females are expressing signs of anorexia. Healthy females scoring over 30 might be undergoing significant concerns regarding their body image and weight.

We believe that these behaviors—attitudes toward eating and concerns about body image in healthy or overweight females—may be attributable to the local social stigma pertaining to weight and body image. In the region, having a thin figure is part of what is deemed attractive. This puts social and peer pressure on females to "fit" the image of an attractive young woman. Young females are constantly concerned about their body image, and we find that even healthy females are dissatisfied with their perceived body images and want to lose weight (see the section on BMI-image dissatisfaction). These social and peer pressures, along with the social definition of attractive, may be the factors behind body image dissatisfaction and anorexic health behaviors and attitudes toward food (see Table 4).

4.3. Identifying Physical Exercise Patterns and Habits. The third section of the survey asked respondents if they were physically active (see Section 3.1). Ten of the 26 respondents were inactive; among those who were active, a majority (10) engaged in only 21–40 minutes of vigorous intensity per week (Table 5). Four respondents engaged in less than 30 minutes, 31–60 minutes, and 61–90 minutes of physical activity of moderate intensity (Table 6). Twenty-two respondents felt that they must change their physical activity habits and would like to do so by exercising more, engaging in some sorts of sports, enrolling in a gymnasium, or introducing fast walking into their daily routine.

Most of the respondents fell far short of the recommended amount of physical activity (see Table 5).

4.4. Deriving a Typical Respondent (Native Arabic Speaker) Profile. We targeted female respondents enrolled in our

Table 4: EATs values.

Range	Average	Median	Mode	Standard deviation	Cut-off score	Score greater than 30
5–61	21.85	21.5	14	12.93	30	4

Table 5: Vigorous-intensity physical activity.

Estimated engagement in vigorous-intensity physical activity (minutes per week)					
<20	21–40	41–60	61–75	>75	Physically inactive
3	7	4	1	1	10

Table 6: Moderate-intensity physical activity.

Estimated engagement in moderate-intensity physical activity (minutes per week)						
<30	31–60	61–90	91–120	121–150	>150	Physically inactive
4	4	4	3	0	1	10

university who are native speakers of Arabic. We had a total of 26 respondents from the target group after filtering out male respondents, those who were not currently enrolled, or those who were not native Arabic speakers.

The typical respondent, based on the survey, is a female native speaker of Arabic who is a student in our university and between the ages of 18 and 20. She has a normal range BMI of 24.65 (her self-perceived body image is 4.23, and her desirable body image is 2.92 on a 9-point scale).

In terms of eating patterns, she follows a halal diet. Her most regular meal of the day is lunch, with breakfast being the meal most often skipped. She also snacks throughout the day; her typical snacks are chocolate, chips, crackers, or biscuits. She eats out or orders takeout meals at least once a week, and fast food is typically her first choice. American or Italian is her usual cuisine of choice. She balances various types of food preparation, such as frying, boiling, and baking, but does not typically broil. In terms of food items, her diet is balanced between starch, vegetables, dairy, meat, fat, and sweets. She should, however, increase her daily fruit intake. In terms of fluid consumption, she does not consume alcohol, but she would benefit from reducing her intake of soda and juice and also by drinking 3 to 7 more glasses of water a day. She would like to change her eating habits, starting by replacing unhealthful snacks with healthier options, cutting down on fast food, reducing her sugar intake, and having balanced meals, a goal that includes making breakfast a regular part of her day.

This typical respondent is also moderately active physically. She does not engage in enough physical activity and would benefit from significantly increasing it. She would also like to change her exercise habits by engaging in activities with more vigorous intensity, increasing the weekly frequency of her workouts, enrolling in a gymnasium, and introducing fast walking into her physical activity. Finally, in terms of her eating attitudes, she does not exhibit symptoms of anorexia nervosa.

4.5. Building a Database of Text Messages. We used the survey results to compile a database of messages. The categories for the SMS database were discerned from the survey, based on the topics that needed to be addressed. The category of "eating habits" contained messages targeting a change in eating habits, such as having balanced meals, eating at a comfortable pace and within limits, fighting urges, and replacing sugary beverages with water. A majority of the survey respondents wanted to overcome unhealthful habits, to cut down on sugar, and to eat healthful and balanced meals. A category of junk food was introduced as well. It aimed at educating the participants on the detrimental effects of junk food and at suggesting healthier alternatives, reducing the frequency of eating junk food, and suggesting alternative food preparation techniques, such as grilling or broiling instead of frying. As we have seen in the eating patterns discerned from the survey, more than half of the respondents go to fast food restaurants and would like to switch to healthier options. Consequently, we included a category on restaurants to induce healthful eating behavior when eating out on weekends with friends or family. Typical messages suggested replacing side dishes with healthier options, such as replacing fried or mashed potatoes with a salad, replacing soda with water, sharing a dessert, and starting meals with soup and salad. Thirteen of the 23 respondents who ate out or ordered takeout meals did so at least once a week, and this is another instance of behavior that we can change for the better. We introduced a category on snacks to help participants make better choices instead of trying to stop snacking entirely. The messages promote a healthier approach to snacking, such as fighting the urge to snack all the time, avoiding snacks before bedtime, keeping healthier alternatives such as fruits in sight, and doing diet-conscious grocery shopping, such as picking up water-filled grapes because they occupy more stomach volume. Finally, a category on physical activity was included because, as mentioned earlier, almost all the respondents were far short of the recommended amount of physical activity. Moreover, most of the respondents, as is the case with a majority of the population in the region, lead sedentary lifestyles with insufficient outdoor physical activity because of the unfavorable climate. Most of the respondents, as is the case with a significant number of students here, are dropped off or picked up close to the doors of the university. Hence, our messages include such suggestions as parking farther away than usual at the university and also at shopping malls and taking stairs instead of elevators. Other messages encourage working out, visiting a gymnasium regularly (with friends, to keep up motivation), as well as general messages calculated to raise awareness of the benefits of exercise (see Table 7).

Table 7: SMS categories and frequency.

Category	Number of messages	Frequency	Typical timings	Sample message
Eating habits: driving change	23	Daily	Breakfast (7:15 am) Lunch (11:30 am) Dinner (8:00 pm)	A calorie is a calorie regardless of its source. Whether you're eating carbohydrates, fats, sugars, or proteins, all of them contain calories [36]
Junk food: alternatives and awareness	22	At least four times a week	Lunch (12:00 pm) on Friday Evening (6:00 pm) on Saturday Alternating lunch and evening on weekdays	Fast foods have no nutritional value. "They are very low in vegetables. Most of it is refined products and processed foods" [37]
Restaurants: alternatives and awareness	6	Weekends (Thursday, Friday)	Evening (6:00 pm)	Start your meal with a soup and salad and order vegetables as your side dish [38]
Snacks: good choices	30	Daily	Morning (10:30 am) Afternoon (3:00 pm) Evening (5:30 pm) Night (9:00 pm)	Having snacks in a convenient place to reach is helpful. Try putting fruit in a bowl on the counter, so you can grab an apple or orange when you're hungry [39]
Physical activity:	26	Daily	Morning (9:00 am) Afternoon (4:00 pm)	Hunt for the farthest parking space. If you drive to run errands, purposefully park your car a little farther from your store entrance [40]

5. Conclusions: Lessons Learned and Future Guidelines

This paper presented a method for designing text messages for use in a contextual mobile application. The application is designed to support achieving sustainable weight loss. With our method, text messages are not guesses aimed at targeting potential future users but are derived after creation of a profile of typical users. This profile was constructed through the use of a survey that adapted previous research into an overall design to elicit respondents eating and exercise habits as well as gain insights into their relationships to food and their perceptions of their bodies. After the typical user profile was constructed and the database of messages was developed, the messages were reviewed by a nutritionist and a by psychologist to validate their health information and to ensure they were motivational.

To illustrate our method, we ran the survey with the targeted background of young native Arabic-speaking females at our university. We analyzed their eating patterns and typical health behavior. Some of the important findings showed that the typical representative of the target population does not eat healthfully, skips meals while still maintaining a balanced diet, does not consume enough water, and does not engage in recommended amounts of physical activity. These findings allowed us to develop a customized database of text messages that can be used in a mobile application. The mobile application can be used to transmit timely text messages aimed at the nutrition and exercise habits of a typical respondent profile.

The results presented are localized to young Arab females attending universities. The derived profiles can be of interest to universities in the region as well as nutritionists concerned about healthful habits in the Middle East. However, our method does not depend on the context of the study and may be used to assess respondents' eating and physical activity profiles. Even if used on a nonhomogeneous group (say patients attending a weight loss clinic of mixed genders, ages, and ethnicities), it is possible, through statistical analysis of the surveys, to derive profiles and adapt sets of text messages. The survey would identify not just one but as many profiles as the studied group would suggest it encompasses.

The next step in our research will be to test the application as well as its culturally adapted content through a five-week pilot study. The study will test the effectiveness of each of the three components—the SMS exchange, goal setting and progress monitoring, and social support network—of the mobile application against traditional intervention methods. The usability questionnaires, distributed exclusively to the experiment group that uses smartphones, will help assess the adaptability of the mobile application to the local context and culture. On the other hand, the health behavior questionnaires, given to both the experiment and the control groups, will help track participants' changes in health behavior and attitudes; they also will yield qualitative information, such as temptations encountered and how participants overcame them.

A future study lasting 15 weeks would permit firmer conclusions about the application's effectiveness because it will enable measurement of behavioral changes and weight loss over a longer duration. This will help assess any sustainable weight loss and behavioral change. It will also enable researchers to evaluate each aspect of the mobile application and hence the underlying theories of behavioral change.

Acknowledgments

The authors would like to acknowledge that the work for this paper was partly funded by the Qatar Foundation for Education, Science and Community Development. The statements made herein are solely the responsibility of the authors and do not reflect any official position by the Qatar Foundation or Carnegie Mellon University.

References

[1] WHO, *Global Status Report on Noncommunicable Diseases*, World Health Organization, Geneva, Switzerland, 2010.

[2] A. Bener, J. Al-Suwaidi, K. Al-Jaber, S. Al-Marri, M. H. Dagash, and I. Elbagi, "The prevalence of hypertension and its associated risk factors in a newly developed country," *Saudi Medical Journal*, vol. 25, no. 7, pp. 918–922, 2004.

[3] IASO, *International Association for the Study of Obesity*, 2012, http://www.iaso.org/resources/world-map-obesity/.

[4] A. Bener, "Prevalence of obesity, overweight, and underweight in Qatari adolescents," *Food and Nutrition Bulletin*, vol. 27, no. 1, pp. 39–45, 2006.

[5] L. Davallow, A. H. Ayash, I. El Assad, and A. Khidir, "The prevalence of obesity amongst school children and adolescents in Qatar," in *Proceedings of the Qatar Foundation Annual Research Forum*, 2011.

[6] C. L. Ogden, M. D. Carroll, B. K. Kit, and K. M. Flegal, *Prelevance of Obesity in the United States*, National Center for Health Statistics, Hyattsville, Md, USA, 2012.

[7] M. Slackman, *Privilege Pulls Qatar Toward Unhealthy Choices*, 2010, http://www.nytimes.com/2010/04/27/world/middleeast/27qatar.html?_r=2&.

[8] C. Bell, *Obesity: A Big Problem for Fast Growing Qatar*, 2012, http://www.aljazeera.com/indepth/features/2012/07/2012722917422894.html.

[9] IctQatar, *Supreme council of information and communication technology*, 2012, http://www.ictqatar.qa/en/news-events/news/ictqatar-explores-everything-mobile.

[10] I. Haapala, N. C. Barengo, S. Biggs, L. Surakka, and P. Manninen, "Weight loss by mobile phone: a 1-year effectiveness study," *Public Health Nutrition*, vol. 12, no. 12, pp. 2382–2391, 2009.

[11] A. Brunstein, J. Brunstein, and S. L. Mansar, "Integrating health theories in health and fitness applications for sustained behavior change: current state of the art," *Creative Education*, vol. 3, pp. 1–5, 2012.

[12] S. T. Shen, M. Woolley, and S. Prior, "Towards culture-centred design," *Interacting with Computers*, vol. 18, no. 4, pp. 820–852, 2006.

[13] P. Sandrini, "Website localization and translation," in *Proceedings of the EU-High-Level Scientific Conference on Challenges of Multidimensional Translation (MuTra '05)*, 2005.

[14] A. Huang, F. Barzi, R. Huxley et al., "The effects on saturated fat purchases of providing Internet shoppers with purchase-specific dietary advice: a randomised trial," *PLoS Clinical Trials*, vol. 1, no. 5, article e22, 2006.

[15] S. J. Woolford, S. J. Clark, V. J. Strecher, and K. Resnicow, "Tailored mobile phone text messages as an adjunct to obesity treatment for adolescents," *Journal of Telemedicine and Telecare*, vol. 16, no. 8, pp. 458–461, 2010.

[16] E. Mattila, R. Lappalainen, J. Pärkkä, J. Salminen, and I. Korhonen, "Use of a mobile phone diary for observing weight management and related behaviours," *Journal of Telemedicine and Telecare*, vol. 16, no. 5, pp. 260–264, 2010.

[17] E. L. Donaldson and S. Fallows, "A text message-based weight management intervention for overweight adults," *Journal of Human Nutrition and Dietetics*, vol. 24, no. 4, pp. 385–386, 2011.

[18] J. Redfern, A. Thiagalingam, S. Jan et al., "Development of a set of mobile phone text messages designed for prevention of recurrent cardiovascular events," *European Journal of Preventive Cardiology*, 2012.

[19] S. L. Mansar and S. Kekre, "A founding framework for addressing obesity in Qatar using mobile technologies," *Communications in Computer and Information Science*, vol. 221, part 3, pp. 402–412, 2011.

[20] S. L. Mansar, A. Brunstein, S. Jariwala, and J. Brunstein, "Addressing obesity using a mobile application: an experiment design," in *Proceedings of the E-Health 2012, IADIS Multi Conference on Computer Science and Information Systems (MCCSIS '12)*, 2012.

[21] W. Stroebe, *Dieting, Overweight, and Obesity: Self-Regulation in Food-Rich Environment*, American Psychological Association Press, Washington, DC, 2008.

[22] W. Stroebe, W. Mensink, H. Aarts, H. Schut, and A. W. Kruglanski, "Why dieters fail: testing the goal conflict model of eating," *Journal of Experimental Social Psychology*, vol. 44, no. 1, pp. 26–36, 2008.

[23] S. L. Mansar, S. Jariwala, M. Shahzad, A. Anggraini, and N. Behih, "Localizing a weight loss mobile application," in *Information Systems and Technologies for Enhancing Health and Social Care*, R. Martinho, R. Rijo, M. M. Cruz-Cunha, and J. Varajão, Eds., pp. 1–348, 2013.

[24] M. A. Thompson and J. J. Gray, "Development and validation of a new body-image assessment scale," *Journal of Personality Assessment*, vol. 64, no. 2, pp. 258–269, 1995.

[25] R. F. Kushner, *Roadmaps for Clinical Practice: Case Studies in Disease Prevention and Health Promotion—Assessment and Management of Adult Obesity: A Primer for Physicians*, American Medical Association, Chicago, Ill, USA, 2003.

[26] D. M. Garner and P. E. Garfinkel, "The eating attitudes test: an index of the symptoms of anorexia nervosa," *Psychological Medicine*, vol. 9, no. 2, pp. 273–279, 1979.

[27] WHO (World Health Organization), *Physical Activity and Adults*, 2011, http://www.who.int/dietphysicalactivity/factsheet_adults/en/index.html.

[28] I. S. Kakeshita and S. D. S. Almeida, "Relationship between body mass index and self-perception among university students," *Revista de Saúde Pública*, vol. 40, no. 3, pp. 497–504, 2006.

[29] A. B. de Gonzalez, P. Hartge, J. R. Cerhan et al., "Body-mass index and mortality among 1.46 million white adults," *The New England Journal of Medicine*, vol. 363, no. 23, pp. 2211–2219, 2010.

[30] M. Badran and I. Laher, "Obesity in Arabic-speaking countries," *Journal of Obesity*, vol. 2011, Article ID 686430, 9 pages, 2011.

[31] R. Rosenheck, "Fast food consumption and increased caloric intake: a systematic review of a trajectory towards weight gain and obesity risk," *Obesity Reviews*, vol. 9, no. 6, pp. 535–547, 2008.

[32] J. H. Ledikwe, J. A. Ello-Martin, and B. J. Rolls, "Portion sizes and the obesity epidemic," *Journal of Nutrition*, vol. 135, no. 4, pp. 905–909, 2005.

[33] E. E. J. G. Aller, I. Abete, A. Astrup, M. Alfredo, and M. A. van Baak, "Starches, sugars and obesity," *Nutrients*, vol. 3, no. 3, pp. 341–369, 2011.

[34] Panel on Dietary Reference Intakes for Electrolytes and Water, *Dietary Reference Intakes for Water, Potassium, Sodium, Chloride, and Sulfate*, National Academies Press, Washington, DC, USA, 2005.

[35] B. M. Popkin, K. E. D'Anci, and I. H. Rosenberg, "Water, hydration, and health," *Nutrition Reviews*, vol. 68, no. 8, pp. 439–458, 2010.

[36] CDC, *Healthy Weight—It's Not a Diet, It's a Lifestyle!*, 2011, http://www.cdc.gov/healthyweight/calories/index.html.

[37] M. Saberi, *Expert Advice: Eat Less Fast Food*, 2011, http://gulfnews.com/news/gulf/uae/general/expert-advice-eat-less-fast-food-1.858844.

[38] Zuckerbrot, *Foods to Avoid at Popular Chain Restaurants*, 2009, http://www.foxnews.com/health/2009/01/19/foods-avoid-popular-chain-restaurants/.

[39] Glamour, *21 Healthy Snacking Tips*, 2010, http://www.glamour.com/health-fitness/2010/08/21-healthy-snacking-tips#slide=21.

[40] HSPH, *20 Exercise Tips*, 2012, http://www.hsph.harvard.edu/nutritionsource/staying-active/tips-for-getting-exercise-into-your-life/index.html.

16

A Real-Time Health Monitoring System for Remote Cardiac Patients Using Smartphone and Wearable Sensors

Priyanka Kakria,[1] N. K. Tripathi,[1] and Peerapong Kitipawang[2]

[1]*School of Engineering and Technology, Asian Institute of Technology, Phaholyothin Highway, Klong Luang, Pathumthani 12120, Thailand*
[2]*International College of Medicine, Thammasat University, Rangsit Campus, Phaholyothin Highway, Klong Luang, Pathumthani 12120, Thailand*

Correspondence should be addressed to Priyanka Kakria; priyankakakria08@gmail.com

Academic Editor: Fei Hu

Online telemedicine systems are useful due to the possibility of timely and efficient healthcare services. These systems are based on advanced wireless and wearable sensor technologies. The rapid growth in technology has remarkably enhanced the scope of remote health monitoring systems. In this paper, a real-time heart monitoring system is developed considering the cost, ease of application, accuracy, and data security. The system is conceptualized to provide an interface between the doctor and the patients for two-way communication. The main purpose of this study is to facilitate the remote cardiac patients in getting latest healthcare services which might not be possible otherwise due to low doctor-to-patient ratio. The developed monitoring system is then evaluated for 40 individuals (aged between 18 and 66 years) using wearable sensors while holding an Android device (i.e., smartphone under supervision of the experts). The performance analysis shows that the proposed system is reliable and helpful due to high speed. The analyses showed that the proposed system is convenient and reliable and ensures data security at low cost. In addition, the developed system is equipped to generate warning messages to the doctor and patient under critical circumstances.

1. Introduction

During the recent decade, rapid advancements in healthcare services and low cost wireless communication have greatly assisted in coping with the problem of fewer medical facilities. The integration of mobile communications with wearable sensors has facilitated the shift of healthcare services from clinic-centric to patient-centric and is termed as "Telemedicine" in the literature [1]. In the larger perspective, telemedicine can be of two types: (1) live communication type, where the presence of the doctor and patient is necessary with additional requirements of high bandwidth and good data speed, and (2) store and forward type, which requires acquisition of medical parameters such as vital signs, images, videos, and transmission of patients data to concerned specialist in hospital [2, 3].

According to existing medical surveys, telemedicine has been adopted to take care of the patients with cardiac diseases, diabetes, hypotension, hypertension, hyperthermia, and hypothermia [4–8]. The most promising application is in real-time monitoring of chronic illnesses such as cardiopulmonary disease, asthma, and heart failure in patients located far from the medical care facilities through wireless monitoring systems [9]. Heart diseases have become one of the leading causes of human fatalities around the world; for instance, approximately 2.8 million people die each year as a result of being overweight or obese as obesity can lead to adverse metabolic effects on blood pressure and cholesterol which ultimately increases the risks of coronary heart disease, ischemic stroke, diabetes mellitus, and a number of common cancers [10]. According to WHO, it has been estimated that heart disease rate might increase to 23.3% worldwide by the year 2030 [11]. The treatment of such chronic diseases requires continuous and long term monitoring to control threat.

The ubiquitous social connectivity can be used in telemedicine for remote monitoring and offsite diagnoses. It should be noted that over 94% of the world population, that is, 6.8 billion people, are the subscribers of cell phone and about

2.7 billion subscribers are using Internet [12]. Cell phone subscription is increasing rapidly and might reach the level of 8.5 billion by the end of 2016 with 70% of smartphone users from developing countries. In addition, smartphones technology comprises various services such as location tracking, short message service, and access of WLAN/GPRS/3G which provides ubiquitous connectivity. There are extensive studies on use of mobile phones in healthcare and clinical practices illustrating the use of inbuilt applications of smartphones like GPS and location enabled services which offer independent survival of old age patient with fragilities [13–16]. Existing studies have also highlighted the uses of inbuilt apps in continuous monitoring and maintaining individual records [17]; for instance, in [18] another study, the authors discussed the benefits of existing smartphone health apps considering their credibility for continuous data flow, feasibility, portability, and power consumption. Nevertheless, the discrepancies such as battery consumption, calibration, and generation of false alarms have challenged the capabilities of smartphone apps in the implementation of real-time health monitoring and diagnosis.

An alternative to inbuilt smartphone sensors is wearable sensors that have been used for continuous monitoring, storing, and sending medical data to healthcare givers over distance. Existing studies with wearable sensors offer monitoring in applications like physiological, biochemical, and motion sensing [19–21]. These sensors have been used in monitoring health indicators and body positions of the patients, as well as in keeping track of sports and other activities [22, 23]. These wearable sensors are becoming promising due to the fact that these sensors are low cost, easily available, user friendly, accurate, and reliable. Many studies explored the clinical applications of wearable sensors in cardiovascular, neurological, asthma, and hypertension diseases [24, 25]. For instance, [26] developed a system to monitor congestive heart failure in patients, comprising a biosensor in the form of a ring that monitors heart data. Similarly, systems have been designed to monitor respiratory diseases which record acoustic signals by placing a microphone on the neck of the patient while breathing [26]. The framework consisted of a band-pass filter to reduce noise and other distortions in signals which helped to achieve approximately 90% of measurement accuracy. The research work was then extended for detecting apneas using algorithms [27]. Wearable technology is also useful in solving the issues of monitoring in motion artifacts by using multiple sensors integrated on a single chip. Integration of different sensors on same platform (tight fitting in garment) in order to monitor respiratory diseases is another kind of application. These systems are found to be better than spirometry but still require advancements to minimize motion artifacts [28].

Further, although wearable technology has contributed heavily in the advancement of healthcare monitoring systems, concerns are there that may affect performance of the healthcare monitoring systems. These concerns include (1) failing to use real-time data in the monitoring systems during testing of application, (2) battery issues, (3) security and privacy of the data collected from patients, (4) requirement of medical professional's recommendations at each step of the development, (5) clinical validation or experts' acceptability, and (6) user friendliness for the patients and for healthcare professionals. The integration of wearable technologies with mobile networks can offer new potentials of rapid, reliable, and secure information transfer from patients to the doctors [21, 29, 30].

The current study addresses the issue of integrating a wearable sensor with mobile technology by developing a remote monitoring system for heart patients. In this study, we propose a location based real-time monitoring system comprising a wearable sensor, mobile application, and a web interface to overcome some of the issues, as mentioned in the literature. The wearable sensor has been used to generate patient's diagnostic information which is then transferred to a smartphone wirelessly via Bluetooth low energy technology. Further, the collected information on the smartphone is transferred to a web interface via Wi-Fi/3G. The proposed system has the ability to generate emergency alerts on the basis of predefined values by comparing patient's data to inform the doctor if there is a requirement of checkup or investigation. Furthermore, various types of sensors have been used and results are compared to identify the most promising sensor providing most accurate results close to the conventional systems. The developed system has been evaluated under the supervision of the experts.

2. Materials and Methods

This study develops a remote monitoring diagnostic framework to detect underlying heart conditions in real-time which helps avoiding potential heart diseases and rehabilitation of the patients recovering from cardiac diseases. The proposed real-time monitoring system is compatible to use various wearable sensors to extract medical information which helps finding out multiple parameters such as heart rate, blood pressure, and body and skin temperature at the same time. These cardiac parameters help early detection of diseases such as arrhythmia, hypotension, hypertension, and hyperthermia through alarming system based on upper and lower threshold values. Similar to the existing monitoring systems, the developed system has two interfaces, one for patients and other for the doctor. The patient interface is comprised of wearable sensors which extract medical information of the patients and transmit to an Android based listening port via Bluetooth low energy. The listening port transfers this information to web server which processes data to show reports on doctor interface. The details of the system architecture, components, data processing, and alarming system are explained as follows.

2.1. System Architecture. The system architect is three-tier comprising (1) a patient interface, that is, wearable biosensors' tier, (2) Android handheld device, that is, a smartphone, and (3) a web portal as shown in Figure 1.

The first tier of the system is patient's interface which consists of multiple wearable sensors used to collect medical information of the patient. This tier transmits real-time data

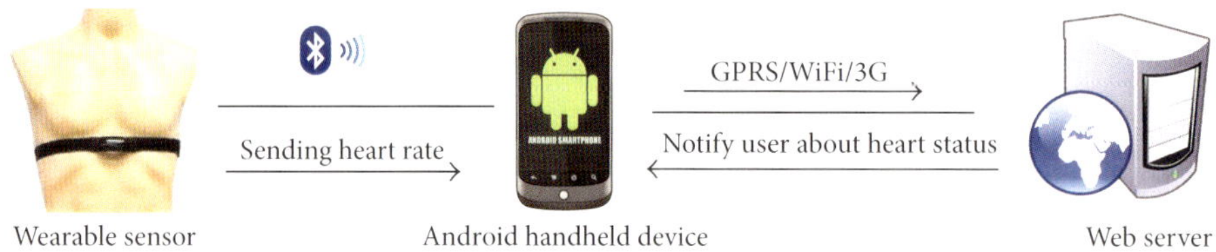

Figure 1: System architecture for remote patient monitoring system.

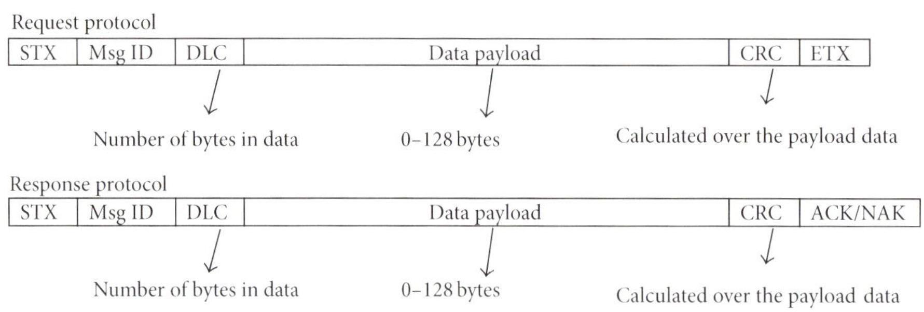

Figure 2: Message format for communication.

wirelessly from wearable devices worn by the patient to second tier of the system via Bluetooth low energy. The second tier consists of an Android smartphone used to extract patient's information from wearable sensors. Android smartphone with inbuilt wireless networking has the ability to communicate with web portal via GPRS, 3G, or other Wi-Fi networks. In addition, the inbuilt GPS application of the smartphone helps to find out the location of the individuals under observation. In third tier, web portal extracts data from SQLite internal data base and transfers data to online MySQL via GPRS/3G or Wi-Fi. Web portal is a platform that acquires the data of multiple patients wearing wearable sensors and displays them on web interface, also known as doctor's interface, along with location and personal information for identification. In this study, three types of wearable sensors are used to extract heart rate, blood pressure, and body temperature information of the patients.

The proposed system has the ability to use multiple sensors which enables simultaneous monitoring of several heart parameters from multiple patients. The facility of using multiple sensors at same time to obtain required data increases applicability of the developed system and assists in comparing the accuracy of various sensors. The focus of this study is to develop a real-time diagnostic system for remotely located heart prone patients by measuring heart rate, blood pressure, and body temperature using wearable sensors.

Heart rate or heart pulse is a palpable rhythmic expansion of an artery produced by electric flow of blood and recorded as number of pulses in one minute [31]. The change in pulse rate can be due to either body activity or any medical disorder. The effect of age on pulse rate considered as normal range is different for different age groups. The importance of measuring the accurate heart rate is understood and should not be ignored. The measuring accuracy of the sensor has direct impact on accuracy of the heart rate measurement in real-time monitoring systems. Therefore, the selection of an accurate heart rate monitoring device is of prime importance in early detection of underlying heart diseases.

Zephyr BT is a wearable sensor which has been used to extract heart rate information of the patients requiring continuous monitoring. The selection of Zephyr BT sensor is made on the basis of accuracy, reliability, cost, availability, and comfort. Bluetooth low energy technology makes this sensor feasible to use for longer time, which ultimately helps in increasing the system's durability and minimizes the risk of false alarms. Furthermore, Zephyr BT is compatible with Android version 4.4 and above.

The second measuring parameter of our monitoring system is blood pressure (BP). Blood pressure refers to the force exerted by the flow of blood against the atrial wall during heart contraction (systole) and heart expansion (diastole). An acute trend in BP (blood pressure) is considered as early indication which often helps medical experts diagnosing serious patients. Omron Wireless Upper Arm blood pressure monitor is used for extraction and wireless transmission of blood pressure information to the server. The Omron Wireless Upper Arm blood pressure monitor has been chosen due to its easy handling, light weight, and long term battery operating features. Furthermore, it has the ability to record 200 previous values of BP along with transmission to handheld listening port.

Body temperature of the patient is the third parameter under the scope of this study which is required to be measured for early detection and diagnosis purposes. G plus, Bluetooth based temperature sensor is used to monitor body temperature. The temperature information is then transmitted to handheld listening port using wireless communication.

2.2. Data Transmission from Wearable Sensors to Android Listening Port. The data transmission process from sensor to Android listening port via Bluetooth is shown in Figure 2. STX denotes the start of text in ASCII character by delimiting

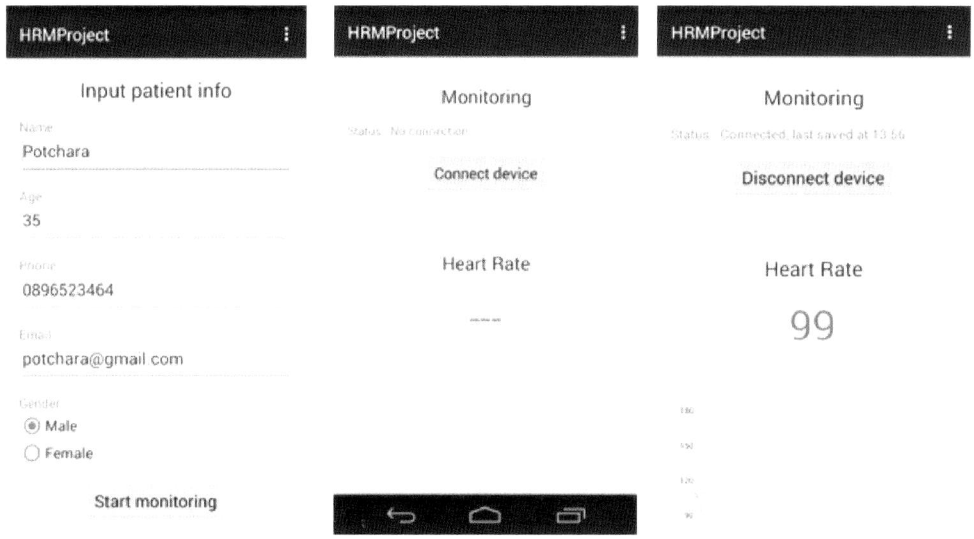

FIGURE 3: Application interface of listening port: patient basic information, connection notification, and real-time monitoring.

the message. Message ID is in binary format which is used to identify the type of message. The standard message ID of Zephyr BT for heart monitoring is 0 × 26. Number of bytes within the data payload has been specified by data length code (DLC). Data payload contains the actual data transferred from Zephyr BT to listening port of the smartphone comprising data ranges from 0 to 128 bytes. CRC is an 8-bit CRC polynomial of 0 × 8C (CRC-8). The accumulator is being initialized to zero before starting the CRC calculation. ETX is a standard ASCII control character that ends message. Bluetooth technology is a short wavelength radio transmission in ISM band from 2400 to 2480 MHz used for standard data transmission in short ranges. In current study, this technology is used as a serial port transmission having sufficient baud rate of 115200 bps.

2.3. Creating Interphase for Android Listening Port. The listening port application has been developed in Android studio interface. The developed listening port is installed in an Acer E3 smartphone which acts as an Android handheld listening port of the system to receive information from first tier of the system via BLE (Bluetooth low energy). Once the connection is established, the listening port of the system starts scanning process via *startLeScan()* to detect BLE sensor and it stops immediately as soon as the detection process is complete (connection is created using *connectGatt()* approach). Heart rate data collected on listening port of the system using GATT attributes is in hexadecimal code which is then converted to integer value to determine average heart rate. Once data is collected from the sensor, *close()* function closes the listening port application. Heart data from smartphone is then transferred to data processing server using extensive messaging and presence of protocol (XMPP) networks. For data security, the smartphone keeps history of the records in SD card memory. The data preprocessing server processes data to compute average heart rate with respect to time. Furthermore, data preprocessing server generates alarms in abnormal conditions to notify the doctor. In addition, inbuilt GPS in smartphone helps locating the geographic location of the patient.

The snapshots of listening port interface are shown in Figure 3. First interface of the listening port is a registration form which is designed to collect personal information of the patient such as name, age, gender, and contact details. Second interface shows the connectivity status between the sensor and listening port. In third interface, real-time heart rate data stream appears with respect to time.

2.4. Web Interface. Web interface enables several physicians, doctors, and medical centers to view and diagnose patients' medical status simultaneously. However, to ensure data visibility only to authorized doctor/physician, web portal requires user ID and password. Web interface is implemented using Larval PHP framework. The data from the listening port is presented to the doctor on web portal in order to check medical status of the patient. Web portal is an interface between doctor and patient as shown in Figure 4.

2.4.1. Modules of Web Interface

Patient Data. This module consists of the patient's personal and medical records. Real-time data acquired by wearable sensors has been shown with respect to time. It contains the medical history of individual patient after getting registered at Android listening port device.

Alarming Messages. This module contains alarming messages generated at Android handheld listening port. Extracted physiological parameters give the alarming signals after comparison with assigned threshold values. These alarming signals indicate abnormalities like arrhythmia, hypotension,

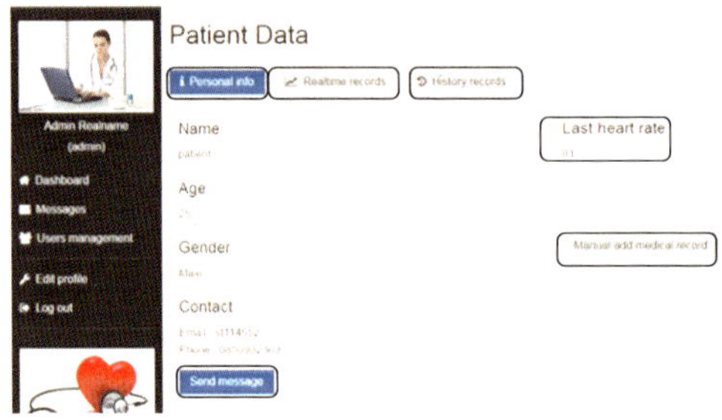

FIGURE 4: Patient data interface in web application.

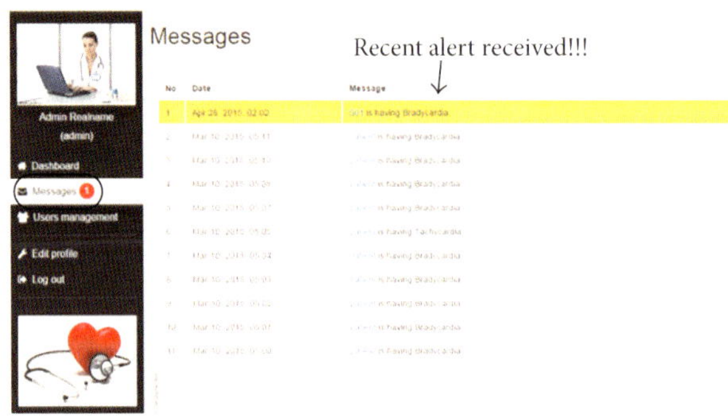

FIGURE 5: Alarming interface of remote patient monitoring system.

hypertension, fever, and hypothermia. Some real-time alarms from patients are shown in Figure 5.

User Management. User management allows the involvement of multiple doctors in the web application for diagnosing patients. In case of large data from multiple patients, several doctors can get involved in monitoring and diagnosing processes. User management module can contain 100 users including doctors, patients, and nursing staffs for keeping record of patients.

Location Records. The location records of patients are shown in Figure 6. After knowing about the abnormalities, the doctor can immediately track the current location of the patientwhich helps in both (1) reaching the patient and/or (2) sending ambulance to transfer the patient to hospital in case of serious emergency.

Figure 7 depicts data communication extracted by Zephyr BT (heart rate sensor) from patient to the doctor. For monitoring heart rate, patient needs to wear the sensors and once the connection is established, the sensors will start transmitting heart information of the patient to the listening port of the smartphone every 1.008 seconds at frequency of 1 Hz without requiring acknowledgements. A passkey has also been assigned for secured data acquisition from sensors to the listening port of the smartphone. From the Android listening port, the heart rate data is transferred to the web application.

2.5. Adaptive Alarming System. The proposed system contains adaptive alarming system which generates alarms to notify the concerned doctor in case of emergency. The alarming system is based on threshold algorithm as shown in Figure 8. The threshold values have been taken from the report of American Heart Association (AHA) [32] and European Society of Hypertension [33] and also after discussing with cardiologists, as shown in Table 1. The predefined handler task generates alarm if average heart data deviates from the threshold value. The alarming system also generates a message to notify the user about the abnormality.

Alarming mechanism basically consists of data visualization, statistical preprocessing, and notifications. These three components come under JAVA classes providing scalability application using polymorphism. Decisions in alarming mechanism are based on mathematical model [34], which describes the cardiovascular system during various activities.

The proposed alarming system is a generalized monitoring model that works on the principle of upper and lower threshold values. The threshold values on the basis of different age groups are presented in Table 2. The proposed alarming mechanism can be customized for individual monitoring due to the fact that the proposed alarming system accepts various threshold values, and values of the threshold levels can be defined on the basis of cardiac vital parameters of the individuals. The customized monitoring helps in setting adaptive boundary limits which keep on changing throughout the monitoring phase. The proposed system compares heart rate after every ten minutes with previous values to find out if any change occurred.

Robust scoring mechanism has been applied in alarming module. In this module, the information of heart rate, blood pressure, and body temperature is collected through sensors

Table 1: Threshold values for alarming mechanism.

Sinus rhythm type	Threshold value of heart rate, blood pressure, and temperature
Normal	$60 \leq$ HR ≤ 100 (beats/minute), BP = 100–140/60–80 mmHg, and temperature = 36.5–37.5°C
Bradycardia	HR ≤ 60 (beats/minute)
Tachycardia	HR ≥ 100 (beats/minute)
Hypertension (Stage 1)	Blood pressure = Sys/Dys $\geq$ 140/90 mmHg
Hypertension (Stage 2)	Blood pressure = Sys/Dys $\geq$ 150/95 mmHg
Hypotension	Blood pressure = Sys/Dys $\leq$ 90/60 mmHg
Fever	Temperature $\geq$ 37.8°C
Hypothermia	Temperature $\leq$ 35.0°C

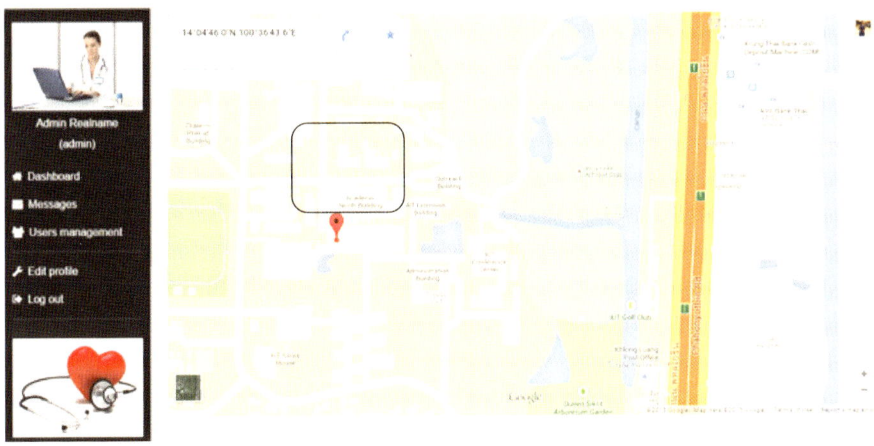

Figure 6: Location record of remote patient monitoring system.

which is then transmitted and collected on a platform called handheld listening port. Fuzzy logic approach is used to interpret the preprocessed data in association with diagnosis concepts such as bradycardia, tachycardia, hypertension, hypotension, fever, and hypothermia. Different threshold values have been derived using normal and abnormal vital sign ranges annotated by a physician as well as from the literature [35]. The alarming system works as shown in Box 1.

3. Result and Discussions

In this study, a real-time heart monitoring system is developed for chronic disease management. Various cardiac parameters such as heart rate, blood pressure, and temperature are being acquired using wearable sensors. Android listening port has been created to receive and store medical information of the patient which is then transmitted to the web interface using wireless communication. Web interface has been designed to be on the doctors' side so as to inform them of the medical status along with location of the patient in real-time. The accumulated data is stored in data server which pushes the information to doctor's web interface and ultimately, data of the patient located in remote area is made visible to the doctor sitting in super specialty hospital.

In this section, the practical implementation of the proposed real-time monitoring system is examined to determine the ability, accuracy, and performance of the system. The practical implementation process is comprised of real-time implementation of the system to heart prone patients in hospitals.

Prior to the integration of wearable sensors into the system, calibration of the wearable sensors has been done with respective conventional measuring devices, used in hospitals. In detail, Bluetooth based blood pressure sensor is evaluated with manual mercury column meter which shows that blood pressure sensor is more accurate on left-hand side. Heart rate sensors are tested with conventional machine and also with one-minute manual reading and results obtained are found to be accurate. Similarly, temperature sensor is calibrated with mercury thermometer and found to be accurate.

The practical implementation process of the system involves the participation of forty heart patients. Each patient was fitted with various wearable sensors to obtain medical information. Each subject was tested with respective conventional machines for evaluation. The testing protocol directed for each subject continued for a 10-minute acclimation period. Two data sets (wearable sensor and conventional devices) were assumed to have normal distribution and the resulting P value was 0.0003 (paired t-test). Statistical information of patients has been given in Tables 3 and 4.

The proposed system is designed to send alarm message immediately after getting arrhythmia. The system has the ability to notify the conditions of tachycardia and bradycardia. The experimental validation process has been done for

Table 2: Age-wise threshold values for adaptive alarming mechanism.

Parameters/age	18–35	36–64	Above 64
Normal heart rate	72–75 (BPM)	76–79 (BPM)	70–73 (BPM)
Bradycardia	HR ≤ 55	HR ≤ 60	HR ≤ 65
Tachycardia	HR ≥ 110	HR ≥ 120	HR ≥ 100
Hypertension	BP ≥ 150/100	BP ≥ 145/95	BP ≥ 140/90
Hypotension	Systolic BP < 85 mmHg	Systolic BP < 96 mmHg	Systolic BP < 117 mmHg
Fever	Temperature ≥ 37.2°C	Temperature ≥ 37.5°C	Temperature ≥ 36.9°C
Hypothermia	Temperature < 35.5°C	Temperature < 35.1°C	Temperature < 35.0°C

BPM represents beats per minute.

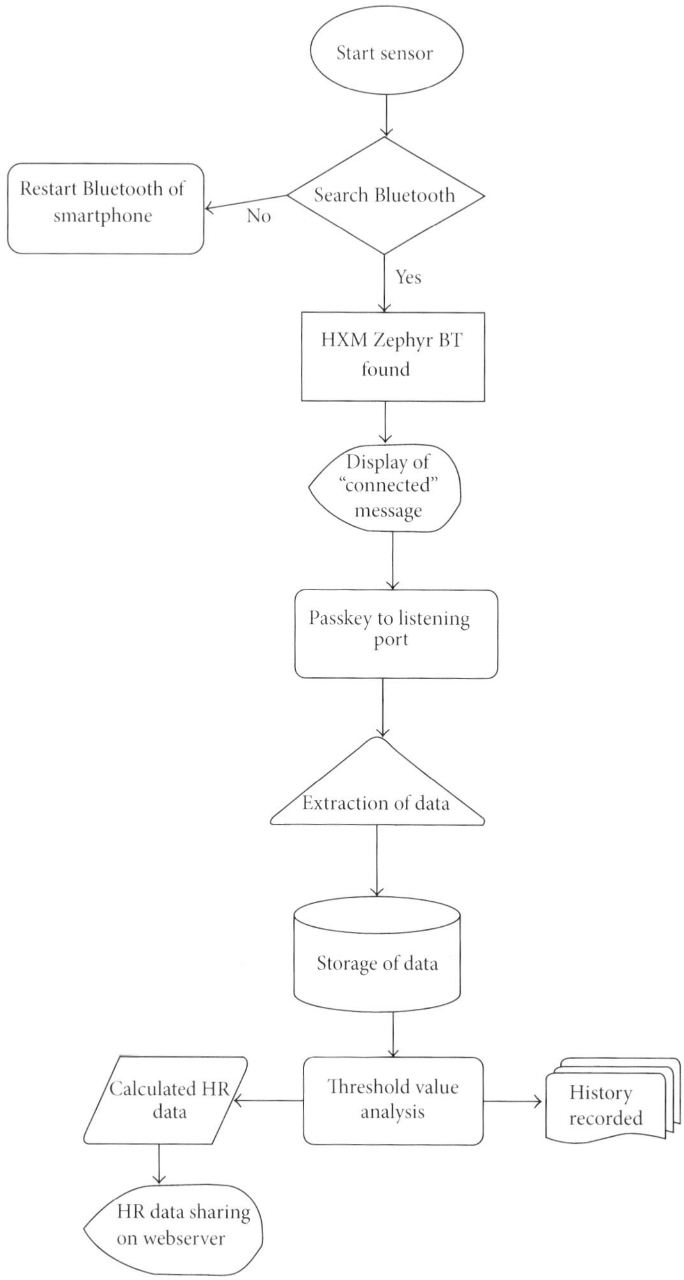

Figure 7: Flowchart of the remote patient monitoring system.

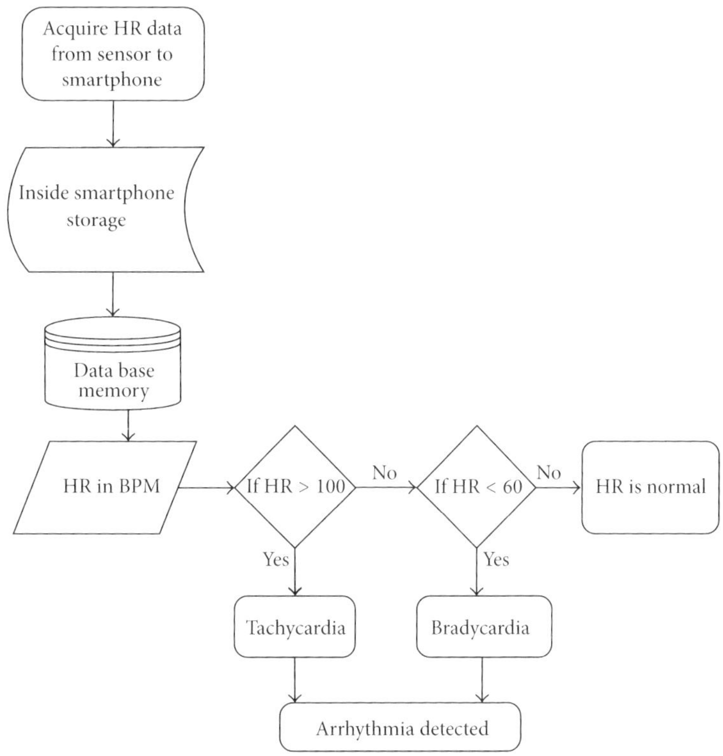

FIGURE 8: Flowchart of alarming mechanism.

IF (HR is L) and (BP is L/H) then "*Warning for Bradycardia*"
ELSE IF (HR is L) and (BP is L/L) and (Temp is L) then "*Warning for Hypothermia*"
  ELSE IF (HR is L) and (BP is L/L) then "*Warning for Hypotension*"
ELSE IF (HR is H) and (BP is L/H) then "*Warning for Tachycardia*"
ELSE IF (HR is H) and (BP is L/H) and (Temp is H) then "*Warning for Fever*"
  ELSE IF (HR is H) and (BP is HH/HH) then "*Warning for Hypertension*"
ELSE IF (HR is VL) and (BP is VL/VH) then "*Alarm for Bradycardia*"
ELSE IF (HR is VL) and (BP is VL/VL) and (Temp is VL) then "*Alarm for Hypothermia*"
  ELSE IF (HR is VL) and (BP is VL/VL) then "*Alarming for Hypotension*"
ELSE IF (HR is VH) and (BP is VL/VH) then "*Alarm for Tachycardia*"
ELSE IF (HR is VH) and (BP is VL/VH) and (Temp is VH) then "*Alarm for Fever*"
  ELSE IF (HR is VH) and (BP is VH/VH) then "*Alarming for Hypertension*"
ELSE Patient is normal (no signs of above mentioned diseases detected)
END IF
HR = Heart rate; BP = Blood pressure; Temp = Temperature; VL = Very low; L = Low; H = High; VH = Very high.

BOX 1

TABLE 3: Mean value of patient data.

S. number	Parameter	Mean values
1	Number of patients	40
2	Age	41
3	Gender (M/F)%	36/64
4	Heart rate	79 BPM
5	Blood pressure	123/71
6	Temperature	36.5°C

remote patients residing 10–100 km away from the hospital (server).

3.1. Alarming Response Time. The alarming system compares medical information of the patient with given threshold values and generates an alarming message if the measured value crosses upper or lower threshold limits. Typical 3G DTAC network has been used on Acer E3 (Liquid Model). Moreover, the performance of the system has been checked

TABLE 4: Statistical data of patients.

S. number	Parameter	Age	Heart rate	Blood pressure	Temperature
1	Minimum	25	62	67/45	32.5
2	Maximum	66	120	190/106	36.6
3	Range	41	93	123/61	4.1
4	Standard deviation	13.5	16.5	21.5/13/5	0.3
5	Median	37	96.5	126/68	36.5
6	Mode	49	84	124/68	36.6

TABLE 5: Average data transmission time using Wi-Fi and 3G.

Alarm for	Average time b/w sending and receiving alarm in Wi-Fi (H:M:S)	Average time b/w sending and receiving alarm in 3G network (H:M:S)
Tachycardia	00:00:29	00:00:58
Bradycardia	00:00:30	00:00:59
Hypertension	00:00:31	00:00:51
Hypotension	00:00:33	00:00:57

Note: the value for each type of alarm is the average value of 20 alarms.

for both Wi-Fi and 3G communication protocols. It is found that the time taken for sending an alarm message from patient to doctor is 30 seconds with Wi-Fi networks, while in case of 3G networks, the time taken by an alarm message from patient's interface to the doctor is 56 seconds. The average transmission time of an alarming message for Wi-Fi and 3G network is shown in Table 5.

According to American Heart Association (AHA), 90% of the patients cannot recognize themselves as being at high risk before cardiac attack. Hence, the risk can be minimized by giving them medically calibrated wearable sensors with alarms in case of abnormality [36]. AHA recommended that ideal time in between sudden fall or rise in cardiac vital signs and sending an alarm message to cardiologist is in between 4 to 6 minutes which is called the golden period of saving a heart patient. The time required for an alarm message in proposed monitoring system under both wireless protocols is less than the golden period. Even in outskirt areas with poor network, the data transmission rates are quite acceptable as per medical standards. Present study demonstrates the applicability of remote care monitoring and it assures 24/7 continuous screening of patients residing at a considerable distance from super specialty hospitals.

Some existing studies about Smart Vest [37] and LOBIN [38] share a similar approach to monitor remote patients using wearable textiles. Smart Vest uses wireless transmission from textile to a remote web server whereas LOBIN uses wireless transmission boards and distribution points in remote areas. Despite advantages of the systems, there are some concerns, like patient's comfort; they may find garments with wired sensors uncomfortable. By overcoming the concern, current system uses wearable sensors that are physically comfortable for wearing. Another important feature of the developed system is the use of 3G network which provides wide coverage area as compared to existing system. This wide area coverage allows free mobility of the patient which helps the patient to perform daily without disturbance while being monitored. In contrast, the systems proposed in the literature provided limited coverage area. For instance, in [39] authors designed a multihoping network for multipatient remote monitoring system that offered only 10-meter coverage area.

From the experiments, it has been found that one physician can monitor 15–25 patients if solely appointed on proposed system; however, this number reduces to 5–12 patients if a physician is requested to monitor patients through proposed system along with regular work in hospital. Furthermore, it is important to mention here that the number of patients depends on the condition of the patients in hospital as well as patients monitored by the proposed system.

4. Conclusion

Increasing rate of chronic diseases in aging population is becoming a serious concern due to lack of sufficient facilities and extremely high cost. The situation is even worse for the people residing in remote areas far from medical facilities as delay in diagnosis and treatment may lead to death. Timely diagnosis and treatment can solve these issues to a great extent. The advancements in wireless communications and wearable sensor technology open up the opportunity of real-time healthcare monitoring systems. In this study a real-time heart monitoring system for heart patients located in remote areas has been proposed. The developed system is comprised of wearable sensors, Android handheld device, and web interface. The system is adaptable and has the ability to extract several cardiac parameters such as heart rate, blood pressure, and temperature of multiple patients simultaneously. The extracted data is being transmitted to Android handheld device using Bluetooth low energy which is then transmitted to web application for further processing. Web application processes received data to show medical status of the patient along with personal information such as age, gender, address, and location on web interface. An alarming system based on threshold values has also been designed which sends alert message to the doctor in case of abnormalities such as arrhythmia, hypotension, hypertension, fever, and hypothermia.

In order to evaluate and show the practical implementation, the developed system has been used to monitor forty (40) cardiac patients located far away from the designed web application. The data obtained through the developed system is found to be significantly acceptable. Furthermore, for remote monitoring validation the system is tested under Wi-Fi and 3G wireless protocols to find out about time delay, that is, the time taken to send data from patient's interface to doctor's interface, and found that the message sending time for both wireless protocols is under acceptable range of medical standards (4 to 6 minutes as per American Heart Association).

The scope of this study is the development and implementation of real-time monitoring system for remote patients using wireless technology. The developed system would inform the doctor in case of emergency through alarms; however, delay in alarms might occur due to weak signals of 3G networks in some remote areas. Though the delayed alarming time is still within the golden period of time it should be considered in future research. As wireless technology is emerging day by day, the use of latest wireless technology may overcome these issues which ultimately increases the applicability and usefulness of the proposed remote monitoring system. Furthermore, false alarms can be generated due to the battery issues of sensors and smartphone. The research can be extended to overcome these battery and false alarm limitations.

References

[1] W. Ping, W. Jin-Gang, S. Xiao-Bo, and H. Wei, "The research of telemedicine system based on embedded computer," in *Proceedings of the 27th Annual International Conference of the Engineering in Medicine and Biology Society (IEEE-EMBS '05)*, pp. 114–117, IEEE, Shanghai, China, January 2006.

[2] H. S. Ng, M. L. Sim, C. M. Tan, and C. C. Wong, "Wireless technologies for telemedicine," *BT Technology Journal*, vol. 24, no. 2, pp. 130–137, 2006.

[3] A. M. Johansson, I. Lindberg, and S. Söderberg, "Patients' experiences with specialist care via video consultation in primary healthcare in rural areas," *International Journal of Telemedicine and Applications*, vol. 2014, Article ID 143824, 7 pages, 2014.

[4] A. Gani, A. V. Gribok, Y. Lu, W. K. Ward, R. A. Vigersky, and J. Reifman, "Universal glucose models for predicting subcutaneous glucose concentration in humans," *IEEE Transactions on Information Technology in Biomedicine*, vol. 14, no. 1, pp. 157–165, 2010.

[5] C. Takenga, R. Berndt, O. Musongya et al., "An ICT-based diabetes management system tested for health care delivery in the african context," *International Journal of Telemedicine and Applications*, vol. 2014, Article ID 437307, 10 pages, 2014.

[6] G. Bobrie, N. Postel-Vinay, J. Delonca, and P. Corvol, "Self-measurement and self-titration in hypertension: a pilot telemedicine study," *American Journal of Hypertension*, vol. 20, no. 12, pp. 1314–1320, 2007.

[7] M. A. Pervez, G. Silva, S. Masrur et al., "Remote supervision of IV-tPA for acute ischemic stroke by telemedicine or telephone before transfer to a regional stroke center is feasible and safe," *Stroke*, vol. 41, no. 1, pp. e18–e24, 2010.

[8] N. Petr, "Smartphones for in-home diagnostics in telemedicine," *International Journal of Medical and Biological Sciences*, vol. 6, pp. 36–40, 2012.

[9] S. Meystre, "The current state of telemonitoring: a comment on the literature," *Telemedicine Journal & e-Health*, vol. 11, no. 1, pp. 63–69, 2005.

[10] World Health Organization, *Health Statistics and Health Information Systems*, World Health Organization, 2012.

[11] W. H. Organization, *Global Status Report on Noncommunicable Diseases 2010*, World Health Organization, Geneva, Switzerland, 2011.

[12] M. N. K. Boulos, S. Wheeler, C. Tavares, and R. Jones, "How smartphones are changing the face of mobile and participatory healthcare: an overview, with example from eCAALYX," *BioMedical Engineering Online*, vol. 10, article 24, 2011.

[13] J. Coughlan and R. Manduchi, "A mobile phone wayfinding system for visually impaired users," *Assistive Technology Research Series*, vol. 25, no. 2009, p. 849, 2009.

[14] S. J. Lane, N. M. Heddle, E. Arnold, and I. Walker, "A review of randomized controlled trials comparing the effectiveness of hand held computers with paper methods for data collection," *BMC Medical Informatics and Decision Making*, vol. 6, article 23, 2006.

[15] M. N. K. Boulos, A. Anastasiou, E. Bekiaris, and M. Panou, "Geo-enabled technologies for independent living: examples from four European projects," *Technology and Disability*, vol. 23, no. 1, pp. 7–17, 2011.

[16] C. Free, G. Phillips, L. Felix, L. Galli, V. Patel, and P. Edwards, "The effectiveness of M-health technologies for improving health and health services: a systematic review protocol," *BMC Research Notes*, vol. 3, no. 1, article 250, 2010.

[17] S. Patel, H. Park, P. Bonato, L. Chan, and M. Rodgers, "A review of wearable sensors and systems with application in rehabilitation," *Journal of NeuroEngineering and Rehabilitation*, vol. 9, no. 12, pp. 1–17, 2012.

[18] A. Kailas, C.-C. Chong, and F. Watanabe, "From mobile phones to personal wellness dashboards," *IEEE Pulse*, vol. 1, no. 1, pp. 57–63, 2010.

[19] P. Pierleoni, L. Pernini, A. Belli, and L. Palma, "An android-based heart monitoring system for the elderly and for patients with heart disease," *International Journal of Telemedicine and Applications*, vol. 2014, Article ID 625156, 10 pages, 2014.

[20] M. Singh, A. Agarwal, V. Sinha et al., "Application of handheld Tele-ECG for health care delivery in rural India," *International Journal of Telemedicine and Applications*, vol. 2014, Article ID 981806, 12 pages, 2014.

[21] F. Wu, H. Zhao, Y. Zhao, and H. Zhong, "Development of a wearable-sensor-based fall detection system," *International Journal of Telemedicine and Applications*, vol. 2015, Article ID 576364, 11 pages, 2015.

[22] K. J. Fraser, V. F. Curto, S. Coyle et al., "Wearable electrochemical sensors for monitoring performance athletes," in *Organic Semiconductors in Sensors and Bioelectronics IV*, vol.

8118 of *Proceedings of SPIE*, International Society for Optics and Photonics, San Diego, Calif, USA, September 2011.

[23] D. Morris, B. Schazmann, Y. Wu et al., "Wearable sensors for monitoring sports performance and training," in *Proceedings of the 5th International Summer School and Symposium on Medical Devices and Biosensors (ISSS-MDBS '08)*, pp. 121–124, IEEE, June 2008.

[24] S. Patel, H. Park, P. Bonato, L. Chan, and M. Rodgers, "A review of wearable sensors and systems with application in rehabilitation," *Journal of NeuroEngineering and Rehabilitation*, vol. 9, no. 1, article 21, 2012.

[25] F. Palumbo, J. Ullberg, A. Štimec, F. Furfari, L. Karlsson, and S. Coradeschi, "Sensor network infrastructure for a home care monitoring system," *Sensors*, vol. 14, no. 3, pp. 3833–3860, 2014.

[26] S. A. Taplidou and L. J. Hadjileontiadis, "Wheeze detection based on time-frequency analysis of breath sounds," *Computers in Biology and Medicine*, vol. 37, no. 8, pp. 1073–1083, 2007.

[27] P. Corbishley and E. Rodríguez-Villegas, "Breathing detection: towards a miniaturized, wearable, battery-operated monitoring system," *IEEE Transactions on Biomedical Engineering*, vol. 55, no. 1, pp. 196–204, 2008.

[28] A. Lanata, E. P. Scilingo, E. Nardini, G. Loriga, R. Paradiso, and D. De-Rossi, "Comparative evaluation of susceptibility to motion artifact in different wearable systems for monitoring respiratory rate," *IEEE Transactions on Information Technology in Biomedicine*, vol. 14, no. 2, pp. 378–386, 2010.

[29] J. A. Fraile, J. Bajo, J. M. Corchado, and A. Abraham, "Applying wearable solutions in dependent environments," *IEEE Transactions on Information Technology in Biomedicine*, vol. 14, no. 6, pp. 1459–1467, 2010.

[30] K. Ernest, C. Lamei, S. Mohamed, M. Shakshuk, I. Badreldin, and I. ElBabli, "A ZigBee-based telecardiology system for remote healthcare service delivery," in *Proceedings of the 1st Middle East Conference on Biomedical Engineering (MECBME '11)*, pp. 442–445, IEEE, Sharjah, United Arab Emirates, February 2011.

[31] T. L. Stedman, *Stedman's Medical Dictionary for the Health Professions and Nursing*, Lippincott Williams & Wilkins, Baltimore, Md, USA, 2005.

[32] P. M. Rautaharju, B. Surawicz, and L. S. Gettes, "AHA/ACCF/HRS recommendations for the standardization and interpretation of the electrocardiogram: part IV: the ST segment, T and U waves, and the QT interval a scientific statement from the American Heart Association Electrocardiography and Arrhythmias Committee, Council on Clinical Cardiology; the American College of Cardiology Foundation; and the Heart Rhythm Society Endorsed by the International Society for Computerized Electrocardiology," *Journal of the American College of Cardiology*, vol. 53, no. 11, pp. 982–991, 2009.

[33] G. Committee, "2003 European Society of Hypertension European Society of Cardiology guidelines for the management of arterial hypertension," *Journal of Hypertension*, vol. 21, no. 6, pp. 1011–1053, 2003.

[34] T. M. Cheng, A. V. Savkin, B. G. Celler, S. W. Su, and L. Wang, "Nonlinear modeling and control of human heart rate response during exercise with various work load intensities," *IEEE Transactions on Biomedical Engineering*, vol. 55, no. 11, pp. 2499–2508, 2008.

[35] J. E. W. Beneken and J. J. van der Aa, "Alarms and their limits in monitoring," *Journal of Clinical Monitoring*, vol. 5, no. 3, pp. 205–210, 1989.

[36] H. J. J. Wellens, A. P. Gorgels, and H. de Munter, "Cardiac arrest outside of a hospital how can we improve results of resuscitation?" *Circulation*, vol. 107, no. 15, pp. 1948–1950, 2003.

[37] P. S. Pandian, K. Mohanavelu, K. P. Safeer et al., "Smart Vest: wearable multi-parameter remote physiological monitoring system," *Medical Engineering & Physics*, vol. 30, no. 4, pp. 466–477, 2008.

[38] G. López, V. Custodio, and J. I. Moreno, "LOBIN: E-textile and wireless-sensor-network-based platform for healthcare monitoring in future hospital environments," *IEEE Transactions on Information Technology in Biomedicine*, vol. 14, no. 6, pp. 1446–1458, 2010.

[39] M. R. Yuce, "Implementation of wireless body area networks for healthcare systems," *Sensors and Actuators A: Physical*, vol. 162, no. 1, pp. 116–129, 2010.

17

On Using a Mobile Application to Support Teledermatology

Juan Pablo Sáenz,[1] Mónica Paola Novoa,[2] Darío Correal,[3] and Bell Raj Eapen[4]

[1] *Dipartimento di Automatica e Informatica, Politecnico di Torino, Turin, Italy*
[2] *Fundación Universitaria de Ciencias de la Salud, Hospital de San José, Bogotá, Colombia*
[3] *Departamento de Ingeniería de Sistemas y Computación, Universidad de los Andes, Bogotá, Colombia*
[4] *McMaster University, Hamilton, ON, Canada*

Correspondence should be addressed to Juan Pablo Sáenz; juan.saenz@polito.it

Academic Editor: Andrés Martínez Fernández

Background. The use of mobile applications in dermatology to support remote diagnosis is gaining acceptance, particularly in rural areas, where dermatology services are commonly managed by healthcare personnel with no specialty training. Moreover, ontologies—sets of concepts that represent knowledge in a given domain—are increasingly being used to support medical diagnosis. A specific case is ONTODerm: an ontology to aid dermatological diagnosis. However, there is little information on the combined use of mobile applications and ontologies as support solutions in dermatology. *Objective.* Assessing the reliability of ONTODerm as a tool to support remote dermatological diagnosis when used together with a mobile dermatological application in underprivileged areas. *Methods.* A mobile application that allows characterization of skin lesions was developed, and the information about the lesions was sent to ONTODerm. An exploratory study was conducted in a remote area without access to a dermatologist. A total of 64 dermatological queries were recorded in the application and consulted with ONTODerm. Later, an experienced dermatologist evaluated the characterization and diagnosis of each query to determine the accuracy of the system. *Results.* The results showed that the probability of obtaining a correct diagnosis was between 64.4% and 85.6% with a confidence interval of 95%. A higher accuracy rate was obtained when the skin lesion occurred on the face or when its border was categorized as poorly demarcated. *Conclusions.* This study demonstrates the implementation of a teledermatology strategy based on mobile applications and domain ontology-driven knowledge base to provide timely assistance to healthcare professionals. This approach was found to be pertinent in the Colombian rural context, particularly in forest regions, where dermatology specialists are not available. The results of this article do not represent a final validation of the proposed approach; they suggest how the ontology can be improved to effectively support medical staff in marginalized regions.

1. Introduction

The use of mobile health applications (or mHealth) to support telemedicine is becoming widely adopted. The ease of use and the ubiquity of mobile phones make their use in remote diagnostic applications increasingly viable [1–3].

Mobile applications are also popular in teledermatology [4–8]: the use of telecommunication technologies to support the diagnosis and treatment of skin conditions. These applications are particularly relevant in remote locations, where the possibility of finding a dermatology practice is low. In Colombia, according to the Colombian Association of Dermatology, there were 1.25 dermatologists per 100,000 inhabitants in 2011, with a large number of them in larger and more densely populated cities (3 per 100,000 inhabitants), thus leaving rural areas without specialized dermatological care options [9].

In rural areas, dermatological services are commonly provided by medical staff without dermatology expertise. Consequently, complex queries are sent to specialists by email, and the answers may take several days to arrive. Under these circumstances, the use of mobile applications to enable real-time dermatological diagnosis (in a rural context) has a great potential in countries like Colombia [10].

1.1. Ontologies. An ontology is a model of a particular domain, built for a particular purpose [11]. Computational ontologies are a means to formally model the structure of a system through the relevant entities and relations that emerge from its observation [12]. When domain knowledge is formally declared, it is possible to make explicit inferences about the concerned domain and get a common understanding of the concepts that are modeled in the ontology. The relevance of ontology in the health sector is described by Kiong et al. [13]. The authors present the development of a health ontology system aimed at integrating relational data (stored in the form of databases) with a set of concepts and their associated semantics. This integration would enable the machines to make interpretations over that information through semantic agents for healthcare domain. Likewise, Maragoudakis et al. [14] describe an approach to the use of ontologies for reducing the ambiguity of dermatological terms. Through a domain ontology, authors attempt to standardize the protocols and terminology in the domain of skin lesions, facilitating a better understanding of the symptoms and development of early skin cancers.

ONTODerm [15] is an ontology for dermatology that was designed to be collaboratively developed by domain experts to analyze, modify, and visualize the data in a convenient and accurate manner, without the need for technical instructions. DKB is a Resource Description Framework (RDF) based knowledge base built using ONTODerm. DKB offers four main features: (I) describing the characteristics of a given disease, (II) identifying the differential diagnosis for a given set of features, (III) listing the differential diagnoses of a given disease, and (IV) enumerating the synonyms of a given disease.

Our study made use of the second feature. DKB receives a set of terms corresponding to the characterization of a skin lesion (i.e. "women, macule, multiple, confluent, poorly demarcated, and face") and, making use of its inference ability, determines a set of possible differential diagnoses and retrieve them in a list. For example, in the above query, the ontology returns the following result: "ChloasmaFaciei 46, Melasma 46, Ephelides 46, Freckles 46, Lichenoid Keratosis 46, Mask Of Pregnancy 46, Benign Lichenoid Keratosis 46, Lupus Panniculitis 36."

The associated number is an arbitrary scale for the degree of match and can be used by external applications to prioritize the arrangement.

1.2. Teledermatology. Several proposals concerning mobile devices in dermatology have already been developed [16]. In fact, mobile teledermatology is established as a technically feasible and diagnostically reliable method of increasing access to dermatologic expertise in poorer regions of the world, where access to computers with Internet is unreliable or insufficient. Azfar et al. [17] demonstrated that HIV-positive patients, in a resource-limited setting in Botswana, find mobile teledermatology acceptable for specialist consultations when face-to-face consultations may be difficult to obtain. Ebner et al. [18] and Schreier et al. [19] present two successful mobile teledermatology approaches that rely on sending mobile phone camera images to a dermatologist. However, to the best of our knowledge, studies reporting the use of ontologies and mobile applications for supporting teledermatology are scarce.

In this article, we present Skinhealth, a system that supports the diagnostic process of skin lesions by using an ontology and a knowledge base system integrated with a mobile application (1). This application was developed conjointly by the Systems and Computing Engineering Department at Universidad de los Andes (DISC) and Colombian dermatologists. Skinhealth is composed of a client application and a server application that runs on the DISC. Figure 1 presents a schematic view of the proposed solution.

To illustrate our proposal, let us consider the process presented in Figure 1. In step one, the healthcare professional in a remote area uses the Skinhealth mobile application to characterize a dermatologic lesion according to a fixed set of parameters. The mobile application then connects to an application server located in the DSIC in Bogotá and transfers the data. In step two, the application server transfers the query to ONTODerm using a web service hosted on an external server (http://gulfdoctor.net/dermbase). Once the external web service receives the request, it formulates a query to ONTODerm. In step three, the web service returns eight differentials to the application server in Bogotá. In step four, the application server stores the differentials obtained for the query and sends them to the mobile app in the rural area. This information is used by the healthcare professional during the diagnosis process. Figure 2 presents the mobile application used by the healthcare professional in the remote area.

1.3. Health Brigades. This paper reports the results of the first-time use of Skinhealth in a rural area in Colombia [20]. The use of the app was made within the context of a program called Health Brigades in Colombia. Health brigades have been carried out since 2003 and are organized by the foundation "Alas Para la Gente" (Wings for the People) [21]. These brigades have dozens of volunteering doctors and support of the Colombian Air Force and the Colombian military since they are usually conducted in remote areas with potential public order problems.

1.4. Objective. The objective of this study is to identify the pertinence and accuracy of ONTODerm and DermKnowledgeBASE when used as a tool to support remote dermatological diagnosis, in conjunction with a mobile dermatological application in a rural environment.

2. Methods

A health brigade conducted in a rural area in Colombia without immediate access to a dermatologist was selected as the scenario to analyze the ability of Skinhealth and ONTODerm in supporting remote diagnosis of dermatological lesions. The study population included all patients who attended the brigade without any exclusion criteria.

The study was conducted in two stages. The first stage involved a general physician in the health brigade (with no special training in dermatology) and an assistant in charge

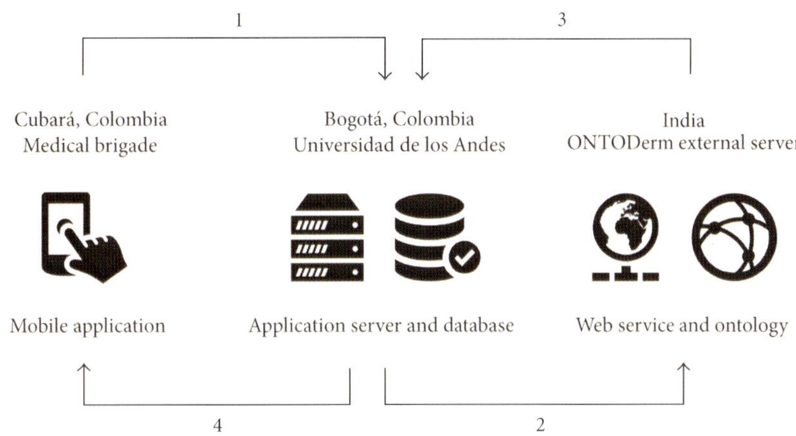

FIGURE 1: Skinhealth overall perspective view.

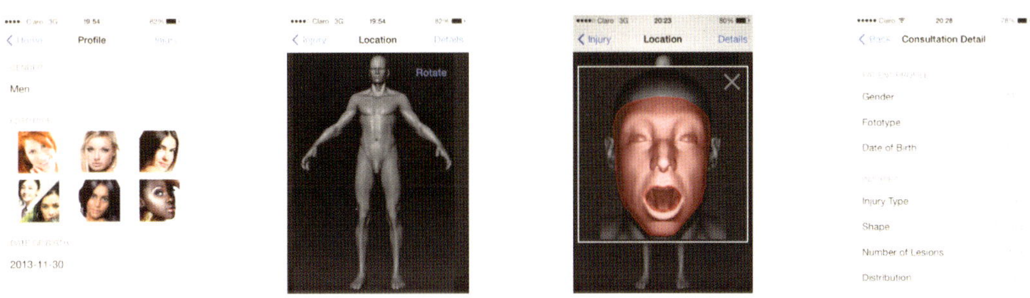

FIGURE 2: Screenshots of the mobile application.

of the Skinhealth mobile app. At every visit, the physician characterized the skin lesions according to a set of parameters. These parameters and the possible values that they could assume are presented in Table 1. The characterization of the skin lesion made by the physician, along with his suggested diagnosis, was registered by the assistant in the mobile application. Then, this characterization was submitted to the main server, in Bogotá, which invoked the DKB web service. The response from the web service was forwarded from the main server to the mobile application. Finally, the assistant verified that Skinhealth received and stored the result given by DKB, and the visit is completed. It is important to note that the general practitioner neither knows nor has access to the results sent by DKB to avoid being influenced by the ontology.

The second stage was performed once the health brigade concluded. A dermatologist with broad experience in skin diseases examined the characterization of each query and compared this information with the diagnosis made by the general practitioner, as well as with the results obtained from the web service. Based on this review, each diagnosis was classified as accurate or inaccurate, for both the diagnosis given by the general physician and the differentials obtained from the web service. The physician's diagnosis was marked as accurate if it matched with the dermatologist's diagnosis. In the case of the ontology, the set of eight differentials was marked as accurate if at least one of the differentials was consistent with the dermatologist's diagnosis.

2.1. Outcomes Measures. This study measured five characteristics that we considered important in determining the behavior of Skinhealth and ONTODerm. These measurements are presented below.

2.1.1. Demographics. The demographic information of the patients treated in the brigade is presented for the purpose of illustrating the general characteristics of the population addressed.

2.1.2. Percentage of Accuracy. The second measure is the percentage of correct diagnoses retrieved by the knowledge base; it indicates the proportion of queries in which the differentials were accurate given a certain lesion characterization. Confidence intervals were used to establish a more objective measure.

2.1.3. Evaluation of Results. The third measure accounts for the accuracy of the ontology by identifying those cases in which the ontology has better performance and those in which it fails to suggest accurate differentials. To calculate this indicator an inferential statistical analysis was performed recognizing the influence that the values of certain parameters have on the accuracy of a query. We believe that the observations arising from this measure will help understand the circumstances under which the ontology can be improved.

Table 1: The parameters that the application takes into account to describe dermatologic lesions.

Parameter	Possible values
Birth date	—
Sex	Female, male
Phototype (Fitzpatrick scale)	Phototype I, phototype II, phototype III, phototype IV, phototype V, phototype VI
Lesion type	Atrophic, cyst, macule, nodule, patch, plaque, pustule, ulcer, vesicle
Shape	Annular, circinate, dome-shaped, ragged, oval, pedunculated, rounded, umbilicated
Lesion number	Disseminated, multiple, recurrent, solitary
Lesion distribution	Asymmetrical, confluent, scattered, symmetrical
Affected areas	Abdomen, genital, arm, dorsal, buttocks, chest, foot, hand, ears, face, finger, hand, nail, finger, head, leg, neck, palmar, hair, plantar, finger, foot, nail
Border	Poorly demarcated, well demarcated
Appearance date	—
Symptoms	Alopecia, blanching, desquamation, pain, edema, eruption, excoriation, exfoliation, hemorrhage, pigmentation, pruritus, fever, facial paralysis, weight loss, systemic symptoms
Past	Anemia, arthritis, malnutrition, diabetes, epileptic, hypertension, hypotension, myocarditis, neuropathy

2.1.4. Filtering Based on Inferential Analysis. Based on the results of the inferential analysis, the values that negatively affected the accuracy of the differentials retrieved by DKB were excluded from the queries.

2.1.5. Specialist's Feedback. The fifth measure categorizes the reasons why certain queries, according to the expert, were classified as not accurate; thus, this measure provides some considerations to improve the precision of the ontology.

2.1.6. General Physician's Diagnostic Accuracy. Considering that the app is portrayed as a support tool for general practitioners, this measure describes the cases in which the lesion characterization made by the general practitioner was not consistent with his suggested diagnosis.

2.2. Statistical Analysis. A descriptive statistical analysis of the results was performed to identify the demographic characteristics of the population and the most frequent values in the characterization of the lesions. Subsequently, in order to draw conclusions regarding these characterizations, an inferential statistical analysis was conducted. The purpose of the inferential analysis was to determine which parameter values influence positively an accurate diagnosis and against which values the ontology is more likely to yield inaccurate results. In this inferential analysis, confidence intervals were applied to the parameters in which the sample size was big enough. Therefore, the results of the inferential analysis help to identify the expected behavior from the specific population where the brigade was carried out.

3. Results

Phase 1 of this study was conducted on the 26, 27, and 28 July 2013 in Colombian municipality Cubará, which has a population of 3,118 inhabitants: 1,551 women and 1,567 men, most of them belonging to the U'wa indigenous tribe. The nearest medical center with a dermatologist available is 166 kilometers away in Cúcuta city, at an eight-hour overland journey through a jungle area.

During the three-day brigade, 895 medical consultations were performed, distributed as follows: optometry, 18.43% ($n = 165$), general medicine, 14.18% ($n = 127$), pediatrics, 14.07% ($n = 126$), internal medicine, 9.72% ($n = 87$), alternative medicine, 8.04% ($n = 72$), gynecology, 7.26% ($n = 65$), dermatology, 7.26% ($n = 65$), orthopedics, 6.25% ($n = 56$), dentistry, 5.92% ($n = 53$), veterinary, 4.69% ($n = 42$), vaginal cytologies, 3.46% ($n = 31$), and outpatient surgeries, 0.67% ($n = 6$). Medical services were provided in the health center and in classrooms of the village school. A general physician attended dermatological visits between 8 am and 5 pm. Skinhealth was installed on a tablet with version 4.2 of the Android OS.

3.1. Demographic Information. The number of men who attended the dermatological consultation ($n = 20$) was less than half the number of women ($n = 44$), and the standard deviation of the averages ($n = 17$) and ranges of ages accounted for the demographic diversity of patients evaluated during the brigade. The most common skin phototypes were III ($n = 24$) and IV ($n = 23$). There were no people with skin phototypes I or VI.

Most women were between 15 and 38 years old, whereas most males were between 15 and 50 years old. The number of patients below the age of 12 or older than 60 years was small, comprising only eighth of the total number of patients (Table 2).

3.2. Ontology's Percentage of Accuracy. Phase 2 of the study took place in Bogotá two weeks after the brigade. In this phase, the dermatologist followed the established validation protocol; namely, she analyzed the values given by the general practitioner for each parameter of Table 1 during phase 1. The characterizations of the lesions were validated along with

Table 2: Demographic information.

Sex	n	%
Male	20	31
Female	44	69
Total	64	100
Age	Average (years)	SD
Male	38	16
Female	31	19
Total	33	17
Age range	Minimum age	Maximum age
Male	15	83
Female	2	74
Total	2	83
Phototype (Fitzpatrick scale)	n	%
Phototype I	0	0
Phototype II	16	25
Phototype III	24	37
Phototype IV	23	36
Phototype V	1	2
Phototype VI	0	0
Total	64	100

Table 3: Percentage of accurate results.

	Total	Male	Female
Sample size (n)	64	20	44
Point estimate	0.75	0.75	0.75
95% CI	[0.644; 0.856]	[0.560; 0.940]	[0.622; 0.878]

the diagnosis given by both the general physician and the ontology, and each query was assessed by the dermatologist as accurate or inaccurate.

In 75% ($n = 48$) of the cases, the ontology provided accurate results. Table 3 presents the point estimate and three confidence intervals for the entire sample segmented by gender.

Coincidentally, the point estimate of the proportion of correct diagnoses in men and women was the same. It should be noted that the sample size for men is not large enough; thus, confidence intervals are very broad and do not provide accurate information. In contrast, confidence intervals for women are smaller and allow the formulation of more precise observations. Table 3 shows that there is no difference between the proportions of correct diagnoses in men and women. Figure 3 presents the diagnoses of the consultations rated as accurate, while Figure 4 presents diagnoses of the consultations rated as not accurate.

3.3. Evaluation of Results. We noticed some interesting observations regarding "affected areas," "border," and "type of lesion" as detailed below.

3.3.1. Affected Areas. As can be seen in Table 4, most skin lesions were identified in the face and hair, comprising 60% of total observations. Since the volume of pooled data was high,

Table 4: Most frequent values for each parameter class.

	n	%	Accurate (%)	Not accurate (%)
Lesion type				
Patch	21	32.8	14 (66.6)	7 (33.3)
Macule	12	18.7	9 (75.0)	3 (25.0)
Total	33	51.5		
Number				
Solitary	26	40.6	17 (65.4)	9 (34.6)
Multiple	23	25.9	19 (82.6)	4 (17.4)
Total	49	76.5		
Shape				
Annular	18	28.2	10 (55.5)	8 (44.5)
Ragged	14	21.8	11 (78.6)	3 (21.4)
Total	32	50		
Distribution				
Asymmetrical	23	35.9	12 (52.2)	11 (47.8)
Confluent	13	20.3	11 (84.6)	2 (15.4)
Total	36	56.2		
Border				
Poorly demarcated	43	67.1	35 (81.4)	8 (18.6)
Total	43	67.1		
Affected areas				
Face	25	39.0	24 (96.0)	1 (4.0)
Hair	13	20.3	7 (53.8)	6 (46.2)
Total	38	59.3		

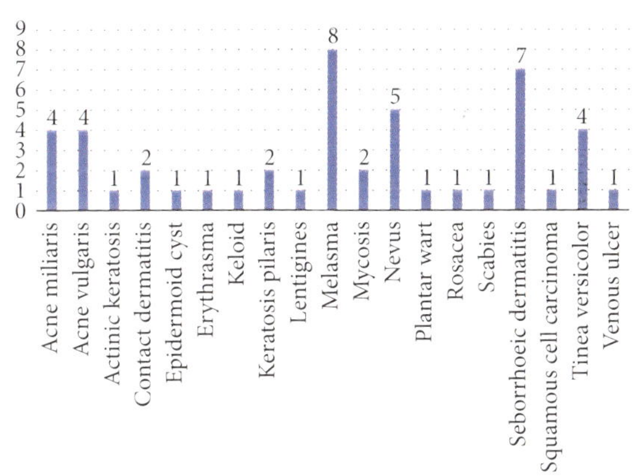

Figure 3: Diagnoses of the consultations rated as accurate.

it was possible to separately analyze the queries of lesions on the face and the queries of lesions on the hair in order to determine the degree of accuracy in each case.

The percentage of accurate queries in which the face was identified as the affected area was 96%. It was noted that, for "face," the values of other parameters were not recurrent. The above shows that, regardless of the value of the other parameters, the predictive power of web service is favorable when the lesion occurs on the face.

In contrast, when the affected area is the hair, the inaccuracy of the results cannot be explained not only due to the affected area but also due to other parameters that

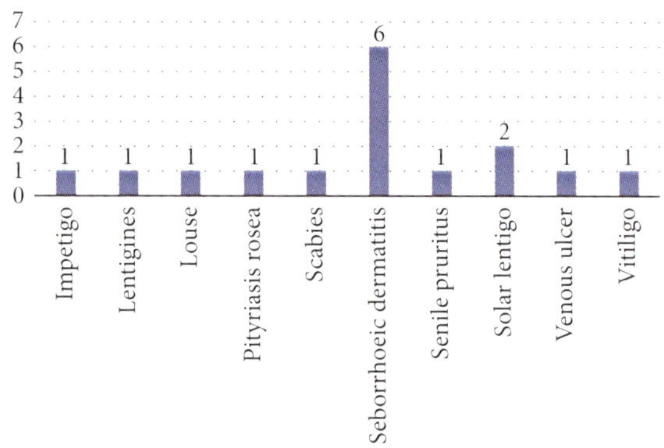

Figure 4: Diagnoses of the consultations rated as not accurate.

were recurrent among these queries involving dermatologic lesions in the hair area. A special case is one in which the affected area is the hair; the lesion is patch-type, the number is solitary, the distribution is asymmetrical, and the shape is annular.

3.3.2. Border. The ontology showed greater accuracy for those lesions with an indistinct border. An individual analysis of the behavior of queries by type of demarcation showed that 81.40% of poorly demarcated lesions were correctly identified by the ontology, while the percentage of those well demarcated was 61.90%.

When excluding queries in which the affected area was the hair or face, 85.71% of ill-demarcated lesions were accurate, while in well-demarcated lesions this percentage was 58%. Similarly, we analyzed the queries with strong demarcation and inaccurate validation and determined that there is no second feature repeated in these consultations. This allows us to infer that the system is less accurate when the lesion is well demarcated.

In contrast, we found that when lesions with ill-demarcated border were inaccurate, it also occurred that most of them corresponded to the case that was identified by analyzing the affected areas; that is, in the case in which the affected area was the hair, the lesion was patch-type, the number was solitary, the distribution was asymmetric, and the shape was annular. Thus, the failure in accuracy could not be attributed to the fact that the lesion was poorly demarcated.

This observation leads to the conclusion that the ontology performs better in cases in which the demarcation is indistinct, except for the case mentioned above.

3.3.3. Distribution of the Lesion. When the distribution of the lesion was asymmetric, differentials provided by the ontology were deemed accurate in approximately 50% of cases. However, when the distribution was not asymmetric, this percentage increased to 85% of cases. Hence, the system performs better for asymmetrically distributed lesions.

3.3.4. Special Case. From inferential analysis of parameters such as the affected area, border, and distribution of the lesion, we identified a particular case in which a precise combination of values generated a set of differentials categorized as inaccurate. In this specific case, the affected area was the hair, the lesion was patch-type, the number was solitary, the distribution was asymmetric, and the shape was annular. It occurred 11 times and accounted for 37.50% of queries catalogued as inaccurate. These incidences correspond to inquiries in which the general practitioner diagnosed seborrheic dermatitis. Just in two cases, the diagnosis of seborrheic dermatitis coincided with the differentials suggested by the ontology.

Table 5: Results obtained when the Special Case (SC), the Strong Demarcation and Special Case (SD and SC), and the Asymmetrical Distribution (AD) were excluded.

	SC	SC and SD	AD
Consultations (n)	53	32	41
Certitude (%)	81.0	94.0	88.0
95% CI	[0.706; 0.917]	[0.85; 1.0]	[0.788; 0.978]

3.3.5. Other Parameters. Other parameters were not analyzed individually because the ontology did not display performance problems in any case. Similarly, it was determined that inaccurate cases were mainly associated with a strong demarcation, an asymmetric distribution, or the particular case described above.

We performed an analysis of the sample excluding the queries with these values that seemingly had a negative impact on the accuracy. Table 5 presents the proportion of accurate queries and the probability of obtaining an accurate result with a 95% confidence interval.

Special Case (SC). When queries corresponding to the special case were subtracted from the sample ($n = 53$), the point estimate of the proportion of accurate queries increased from 75% to 81%, and the probability of obtaining an accurate result with the ontology fluctuated between 70.6% and 91.7%.

Strong Demarcation and Special Case (SD). If, furthermore, lesions with strong demarcation are excluded ($n = 32$), the proportion of accuracy in the point estimate rises to 94% with a probability greater than 85%.

Asymmetrical Distribution (AD). On the other hand, when lesions with asymmetric distribution are excluded, the point estimate of the proportion of accurate queries rises to 88%, with a probability between 77.85% and 97.8%.

3.4. Feedback from Specialist. The dermatologist provided feedback on the reasons why the differentials supplied by the ontology for certain queries were classified as inaccurate. The reasons for rejection of results were categorized as follows.

Age. The diagnoses suggested by the ontology represented diseases that do not occur in the age range of the patient.

Gender. The diagnoses suggested by the ontology represented diseases that do not occur in people of the patient's gender.

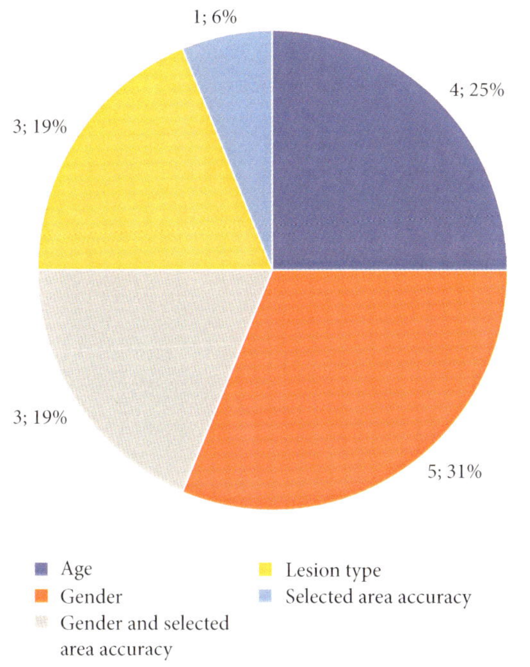

FIGURE 5: Frequency of referral to previously stated reasons for declaring a query inaccurate.

Accuracy in the Affected Area Selection. The degree of specificity of ontology in relation to areas of the body was not enough for the suggested diagnoses to be related to the patient's affected area.

Type of Lesion. The suggested diagnoses do not correspond to the type of lesion identified in the characterization.

Figure 5 summarizes the frequency of referral to previously stated reasons for declaring a query as inaccurate.

3.5. Level of Accuracy of the General Physician. An experienced dermatologist determined that, in eight queries, characterization of the lesion was not consistent with the diagnosis submitted by the general practitioner. Of these eight queries, the ontology tossed accurate results in six of them, despite incorrect characterization.

4. Discussion

At first, without classifying or segmenting results, the ontology provides favorable diagnoses with a probability between 64.4% and 85.6% (95% confidence interval), regardless of patient and lesion characteristics. Similarly, it was determined that there is no statistical difference concerning the effectiveness of the program when the patient is male or female; in both cases, the program gave positive results for 75% of queries.

Regardless of other parameters, ontology had great accuracy when the area of the lesion was the face. In contrast, results were more likely to be inaccurate when the lesion's borders were well demarcated and had asymmetric distribution.

We identified a particular case in which, irrespective of whether borders were weakly demarcated, the results were not favorable. When excluding queries with strong demarcation and those corresponding to the particular case previously stated, the effectiveness of the program increased significantly.

4.1. Limitations. All the statistical analysis was performed on a sample of 64 dermatologic consultations. It should be remarked that the conclusions drawn from this sample can be generalizable just to the population from which the sample was extracted, notwithstanding that a sample size greater than 30 was considered high enough for cases in which inferential statistics are carried out. During the development of this study, we were limited to the number of dermatology patients attending the brigade. We are aware that the size of the sample is small, and it is necessary to use Skinhealth in future medical brigades to validate our findings.

5. Conclusions

In the present study, we proposed the integration of a mobile app and its respective connectivity and portability features with the ability of inference and learning of a dermatological ontology. We tried to ascertain the potential of this solution in dermatological diagnostic work carried out by general practitioners in rural and geographically marginalized municipalities, where there are no specialists.

Overall, this study represents the first controlled evaluation of a teledermatology strategy that relies on mobile applications and domain ontology to immediately assist a general practitioner who answers dermatological consultations. This approach was found to be relevant in the Colombian context, particularly in geographically and economically marginalized regions. We believe that the results help to understand the circumstances under which the ontology can be improved to effectively support the general practitioners in the diagnosis of dermatologic lesions. However, since the sample size is small, more studies would be necessary to validate the findings. The conclusions drawn in this paper do not represent a final validation of Skinhealth but a preliminary evaluation to determine its potential as a tool that can support medical staff in regions where there are no dermatology specialists.

Abbreviations

DISC: Departamento de Ingeniería de Sistemas y Computación
DKB: DermKnowledgeBASE.

Acknowledgments

This study was made possible thanks to the support of the foundation Alas Para la Gente that organized and carried out several health brigades, such as the one in which this research was conducted.

References

[1] World Health Organization, *mHealth: New Horizons for Health through Mobile Technologies: Based on the Findings of the Second Global Survey on eHealth*, vol. 18 of *Global Observatory for eHealth*, 2011, http://www.who.int/goe/publications/goe_mhealth_web.pdf. Archived at: http://www.webcitation.org/6LkPFNqYx.

[2] Vital Wave Consulting., *mHealth for Development: The Opportunity of Mobile Technology for Healthcare in the Developing World*, 2009, http://www.unfoundation.org/news-and-media/publications-and-speeches/mhealth-for-development-1.html. Archived at: http://www.webcitation.org/6LomHPWJQ.

[3] D. Vatsalan, S. Arunatileka, K. Chapman et al., "Mobile technologies for enhancing eHealth solutions in developing countries," in *Proceedings of the 2nd International Conference on eHealth, Telemedicine, and Social Medicine (ETELEMED '10)*, pp. 84–89, IEEE, Philipsburg, Sint Maarten, February 2010.

[4] A. C. Brewer, D. C. Endly, J. Henley et al., "Mobile applications in dermatology," *JAMA Dermatology*, vol. 149, no. 11, pp. 1300–1304, 2013.

[5] G. R. Kanthraj, "Classification and design of teledermatology practice: What dermatoses? Which technology to apply?" *Journal of the European Academy of Dermatology and Venereology*, vol. 23, no. 8, pp. 865–875, 2009.

[6] E. T. Wurm and H. P. Soyer, "Mobile Teledermatology," in *Telemedicine in Dermatology*, M. Binder, A. C. Smith, and E. M. T. Wurm, Eds., pp. 79–85, Springer, Berlin, Heidelberg, 2012.

[7] F. Kaliyadan, T. T. Amin, J. Kuruvilla, and W. H. A. B. Ali, "Mobile teledermatology - patient satisfaction, diagnostic and management concordance, and factors affecting patient refusal to participate in Saudi Arabia," *Journal of Telemedicine and Telecare*, vol. 19, no. 6, pp. 315–319, 2013.

[8] "There's an app for that: The emergence of mobile applications in dermatology," *Journal of the American Academy of Dermatology*, vol. 68, no. 4, p. AB90, 2013.

[9] A. F. Ramírez, J. G. Chalela, and J. Ramírez, "Cuántos dermatólogos hay en Colombia? Análisis de los datos de la Asociación Colombiana de Dermatología y Cirugía Dermatológica," *Rev AsocColombDermatol*, vol. 20, no. 1, pp. 21–26, 2012, http://www.revistasocolderma.com/numeros/pdf/relacion%20de%20dermatologos.pdf. Archived at: http://www.webcitation.org/6LkPTA4ky.

[10] C. Rey-Moreno, J. S. Reigadas, E. E. Villalba, J. J. Vinagre, and A. M. Fernández, "A systematic review of telemedicine projects in Colombia," *Journal of Telemedicine and Telecare*, vol. 16, no. 3, pp. 114–119, 2010.

[11] G. Antoniou and F. vanHarmelen, *A Semantic Web Primer*, The MIT Press, Cambridge, MA, USA, 2nd edition, 2008.

[12] N. Guarino, D. Oberle, and S. Staab, "What Is an Ontology?" in *International Handbooks on Information Systems*, S. Staab and R. Studer, Eds., pp. 1–17, Springer, Berlin, Heidelberg.

[13] Y. C. Kiong, S. Palaniappan, and N. A. Yahaya, "Health ontology system," in *Proceedings of the 2011 7th International Conference on Information Technology in Asia: Emerging Convergences and Singularity of Forms, CITA'11*, Malaysia, July 2011.

[14] M. Maragoudakis, I. Maglogiannis, and D. Lymberopoulos, "A medical, description logic based, ontology for skin lesion images," in *Proceedings of the 8th IEEE International Conference on BioInformatics and BioEngineering, BIBE 2008*, Greece, October 2008.

[15] B. R. Eapen, "ONTODerm—A domain ontology for dermatology," *Dermatol Online J*, vol. 14, no. 6, Article ID 18713597, p. 16, 2008.

[16] K. Tran, M. Ayad, J. Weinberg et al., "Mobile teledermatology in the developing world: Implications of a feasibility study on 30 Egyptian patients with common skin diseases," *Journal of the American Academy of Dermatology*, vol. 64, no. 2, pp. 302–309, 2011.

[17] R. S. Azfar, J. L. Weinberg, G. Cavric et al., "HIV-positive patients in Botswana state that mobile teledermatology is an acceptable method for receiving dermatology care," *Journal of Telemedicine and Telecare*, vol. 17, no. 6, pp. 338–340, 2011.

[18] C. Ebner, E. M. T. Wurm, B. Binder et al., "Mobile teledermatology: A feasibility study of 58 subjects using mobile phones," *Journal of Telemedicine and Telecare*, vol. 14, no. 1, pp. 2–7, 2008.

[19] G. Schreier, D. Hayn, P. Kastner, S. Koller, W. Salmhofer, and R. Hofmann-Wellenhof, "A mobile-phone based teledermatology system to support self-management of patients suffering from psoriasis," in *Proceedings of the 30th Annual International Conference of the IEEE Engineering in Medicine and Biology Society (EMBS '08)*, pp. 5338–5341, Vancouver, BC, Canada, August 2008.

[20] J. P. Sáenz, M. P. Novoa, D. Correal, and B. R. Eapen, "Skinhealth, a mobile application for supporting teledermatology: A case study in a rural area in Colombia," *Lecture Notes of the Institute for Computer Sciences, Social-Informatics and Telecommunications Engineering, LNICST*, vol. 192, pp. 160–163, 2017.

[21] "Alas para la Gente," http://alasparalagente.com. Archived at: http://www.webcitation.org/6LkPWh7Oo.

18

Clinical Outcomes of Telemonitoring for Patients on Warfarin after Discharge from Hospital

Natthaporn Sudas Na Ayutthaya,[1,2]
Itsarawan Sakunrak,[2] **and Teerapon Dhippayom**[2]

[1]*Department of Pharmacy, Kamphaeng Phet Hospital, Mueang Kamphaeng Phet, Thailand*
[2]*Faculty of Pharmaceutical Sciences, Naresuan University, Phitsanulok, Thailand*

Correspondence should be addressed to Teerapon Dhippayom; teerapond@nu.ac.th

Academic Editor: Carlos De Las Cuevas

Objective. To evaluate the impact of telephone follow-up service on clinical outcomes in patients on warfarin when discharged from hospital. *Methods.* This randomized controlled trial was conducted at a general hospital in Thailand. Patients aged ≥20 years who were prescribed warfarin when discharged were eligible to participate in this study. They were randomly allocated, using a computer generated random number, to receive either telephone follow-up intervention or usual care. Participants in the intervention group received telephone follow-up by hospital pharmacists for three months. During each telephone call, pharmacists performed medicine use reviews and addressed any problems identified. *Key Findings.* A total of 50 patients participated in this study. The proportion of international normalized ratio (INR) values in the target range for the telephone follow-up group (36/79, 45.6%) was higher than that in the usual care group (19/79, 24.1%), p=0.005. The mean time in the therapeutic range (TTR) in the telephone follow-up group was also higher than that in the usual care group (49.8±34.3 versus 28.0±27.5, p=0.017). All patients in the usual care group experienced one or more out-of-range INR values (25/25, 100%) compared to 21 out of 25 (84%) in the telephone follow-up group, p=0.037. There was no difference between the two groups in the incidence of complications or adverse events associated with warfarin. *Conclusions.* The telephone follow-up service in recently discharged patients helps them achieve and maintain their INR target. This anticoagulant supportive service should be promoted to patients receiving warfarin therapy after discharge. This trial is registered with TCTR20180614006 (Thai Clinical Trials Registry).

1. Introduction

Warfarin is a well-established oral anticoagulant used for the prevention and treatment of thromboembolism and thromboembolic complications in patients with atrial fibrillation, heart valve replacement, or myocardial infraction [1]. Due to its narrow therapeutic index and dosage variability among patients, individuals receiving warfarin therapy require dose adjustment based on the international normalized ratio (INR) to reduce the risk of adverse reaction such as thrombotic and bleeding events that could lead to hospitalization or life-threatening conditions [2].

Several studies have demonstrated that pharmacist-managed anticoagulation clinics improve time in therapeutic range, lower the incidence of adverse events, and reduce the need for frequent office/anticoagulant clinic visits [3]. Anticoagulant management can be achieved through office visits or telephone visits, which proved to be comparable [4–6]. The advantages of telephone-based management of warfarin are that it provides time and cost savings, increases access to care, provides convenience, and reduces the risk of anticoagulation therapy related complications. Homebound patients have also reported a high degree of satisfaction with telephone-based anticoagulation management [7]. However, anticoagulant management via telephone calls might not be feasible everywhere as it requires INR measurements, and healthcare structures in some areas may not support the implementation of this service due to limited access to INR measurement facilities outside hospital settings. A previous study revealed that continuous warfarin follow-up counseling through phone calls and home visits helped improve INR control in patients discharged on warfarin [8].

However, the intensive intervention employed in this study, i.e., weekly telephone and fortnightly home visit for three months, may not be a practical approach for many settings. Also, telephone-based management of warfarin is deemed suitable for patients with stable INRs, while those with an unsteady INR may require alternative approaches.

Hospitalization is one of the potential causes of INR fluctuations in the postdischarge period, particularly among patients who newly initiated therapy [9]. Patients who are discharged on warfarin require close follow-up monitoring to ensure the safe and effective use of warfarin as their clinical conditions may not be as stable as ambulatory patients. Telephone follow-up adds another layer of service; currently, no evidence exists to justify that a telephone follow-up service could help patients achieve their INR target. The objective of this study is therefore to evaluate the impact of telemonitoring using a telephone follow-up service on clinical outcomes in patients on warfarin after discharge from a hospital.

2. Methods

This study is a randomized controlled trial with parallel group design and a 1:1 allocation ratio. It was conducted between May and September 2016 in Kamphaeng Phet Hospital, a 410 bed general hospital in the Lower Northern Region of Thailand. The study protocol was approved by Naresuan University Institutional Review Board (NU-IRB no. 119/59). Informed consent was obtained from all patients before their participation in this study.

2.1. Participants. Patients aged 20 years or older were eligible for inclusion if they (i) were prescribed warfarin upon discharge, (ii) had no scheduled surgery within three months after discharge, (iii) were able to manage their own medication, (iv) could communicate in Thai, and (v) possessed a telephone. Those who were prescribed warfarin prior to admission and had INR values in target ranges throughout the preceding three months were excluded.

As no similar study was found that could be used for sample size calculations, the number of participants in this study was based on a recommendation by Collins et al. for experimental research design [10]. Accordingly, a minimum of 21 participants per group was needed to detect statistically significant differences in one-tailed and/or two-tailed tests with 80% power and a 5% alpha level. Taking into account a predicted dropout rate of 20%, the number of participants per group in this study was 25.

2.2. Interventions. Participants in the telephone follow-up group and the usual care group received standard pharmacy services for patients discharged on warfarin, which included (i) assessing appropriateness of the warfarin dose, (ii) checking for warfarin drug interaction with other concomitant medicines, (iii) educating patients about the indication and the use of warfarin, (iv) assessing and identifying factors associated with warfarin adherence for those who had been using warfarin prior to admission, and (v) checking for patients' understanding of the given information.

Three clinical pharmacists who worked in medical wards were informed about the telephone follow-up procedures and were checked for their fidelity to the study protocol on a monthly basis. After discharge of the participants in the telephone group, pharmacists made one phone call before the next in-person follow-up based on the following schedules: day three for a one-week scheduled visit, day seven for a two-week scheduled visit, and day fourteen for a three- or four-week scheduled visit. For the second and subsequent visits within the three-month study period, pharmacists continued to make telephone calls on a regular interval as follows: day three for a 1-week scheduled visit; days three and seven for a two-week scheduled visit; days three, seven, and fourteen for a three-week scheduled visit; and days seven, fourteen, and twenty-one for a four-week scheduled visit.

During each 10–25-minute telephone call, pharmacists performed medicine use review by asking patients about problems/obstacles with managing warfarin including adverse events and complications, assessing medication adherence, and giving reminders for the next scheduled visits. Pharmacists promptly addressed any problems identified during the telephone call with patients.

2.3. Outcomes and Data Collection. The primary outcomes were the proportion of INR values in range, time in therapeutic range (TTR), proportion of INR out of range, and the number of patients with one or more out-of-range INR values. Safety outcomes were the frequency of complications or adverse events associated with warfarin, i.e., bleeding events, thromboembolic events, emergency room visits, and hospitalization. Bleeding in the following locations was classified as major bleeding: intracranial, intraspinal, intraocular, retroperitoneal, intra-articular, pericardial, and intramuscular [11]. Other complications included depletion of hemoglobin to 1.24 mmol/L or less and bleeding that required more than 2 units of blood transfusions.

All INR testing was performed with ACL TOP 300 CTS machine, which was calibrated by technicians from the instrument's company every month. The TTR was calculated with the Rosendaal method using INR measurements from all warfarin clinic visits for each patient. The medical technologists were not aware of the study groups when they performed and reported the participants' INRs.

Demographic characteristics, indication for warfarin therapy, and goal INR were extracted from medical records for each patient. Warfarin clinic records were the source of data on outcomes of interest. At each clinic visit, patients were asked to report complications/adverse events such as bleeding and thrombosis. Pharmacists at the warfarin clinic then checked for signs and symptoms of reported safety outcomes. Participants were also asked to report any emergency room visits or hospitalization, which was subsequently confirmed with hospital records.

2.4. Randomization. The study population was stratified by experience of using warfarin, i.e., individuals who had used warfarin before admission and naïve users who were first prescribed warfarin during the course of the current admission. A random allocation sequence was created using a computer

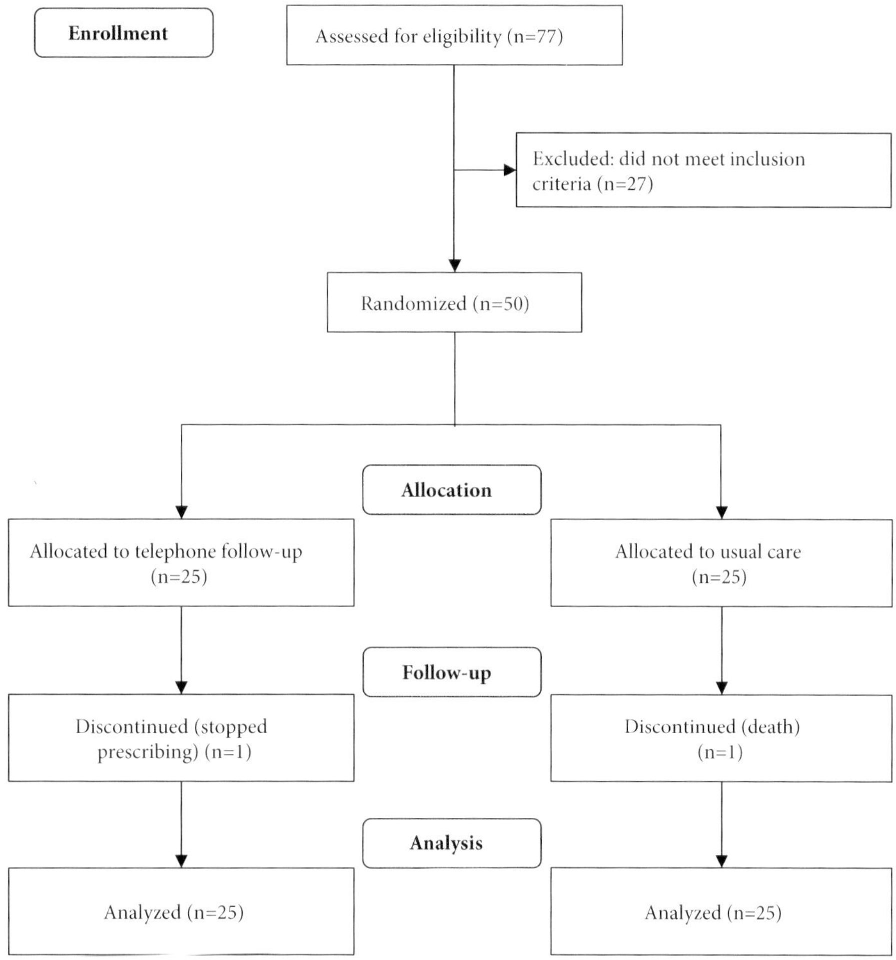

Figure 1: CONSORT flow diagram.

generated random number table. Random numbers were subsequently put into opaque envelope and sealed. Clinical pharmacists who worked on medical wards identified eligible patients and obtained signed informed consent before they were discharged. During the recruitment phase, information about newly enrolled participants was sent to the principal investigator to assign participants to an intervention.

2.5. Statistical Analysis. Participant demographic characteristics were compared using either the chi-squared test for nominal data or the *t*-test for continuous data. All INR measurements, except measures after readmission, in each group were used to calculate the percentage of INR values in therapeutic and out of therapeutic range (subtherapeutic and supratherapeutic). The chi-squared test was used to compare the difference in INR values in therapeutic range, INR values out of range, patients with one or more out-of-range INR values, and safety outcomes. TTR was calculated from INR value records for each patient during the study period. INR records after readmission were not used for TTR calculations. The overall mean TTR in both groups was compared using a *t*-test. All statistical analyses were performed using SPSS, version 17.0; SPSS Inc.; Chicago, IL). A p-value of <0.05 was used to determine statistical significance.

3. Results

The recruitment period took place between May and June 2016. Once enrolled, each participant was followed for three months with the last follow-up ending in September 2016. A total of two, out of fifty, participants did not complete the study. One participant from the telephone follow-up group no longer required warfarin due to an improvement in indicated condition (deep vein thrombosis), while one individual from usual care group died (Figure 1).

The majority of participants in the telephone follow-up group were female (18/25, 72%), which was different in the usual care group (12/25, 48%). Mean age of participants in both groups was not different, i.e., 56.6±11.9 years and 58.7±10.0 years in telephone follow-up and usual care group, respectively. Participants who were prescribed warfarin for the first time accounted for half of the participants in each group (13/25, 52%). The main indication for warfarin in

Table 1: Demographic characteristics.

Characteristics	Telephone (n=25)	Usual care (n=25)	p-value
Gender, female	18 (72%)	12 (48%)	0.083
Age, years	56.6±11.9	58.7±10.0	0.506
Experience of using warfarin			
Naïve	13 (52%)	13 (52%)	1.00
≤3 month experienced	5 (20%)	3 (12%)	0.440
>3 month experienced	7 (28%)	9 (36%)	0.544
Indication			
Valvular heart disease	6 (24%)	8 (32%)	0.529
Mechanical prosthetic valves	2 (8%)	1 (4%)	0.552
Atrial fibrillation	14 (56%)	17 (68%)	0.382
Deep vein thrombosis	8 (32%)	6 (24%)	0.529
Pulmonary embolism	0 (0%)	1 (4%)	0.312
Comorbidities			
Diabetes	4 (16%)	5 (20%)	0.713
Hypertension	9 (36%)	15 (60%)	0.089
Dyslipidemia	7 (28%)	8 (32%)	0.758
Ischemic heart disease	3 (12%)	1 (4%)	0.297
Heart failure	5 (20%)	6 (24%)	0.123
Chronic kidney disease	5 (20%)	6 (24%)	0.733
Others	3 (12%)	2 (8%)	0.637
Warfarin dosing on discharge (mean±SD)	18.2±6.7	18.1±4.6	0.922
Target INR			
2.0-3.0	23 (92%)	24 (96%)	0.552
2.5-3.5	2 (8%)	1 (4%)	0.552

INR: international normalized ratio.

both groups was atrial fibrillation, i.e., 56% in the telephone follow-up group and 68% in the usual care group. Other prescribed indications included valvular heart disease, mechanical prosthetic valves, deep vein thrombosis, and pulmonary embolism. Participants in both groups shared common comorbidities such as diabetes, hypertension, and dyslipidemia. Almost all participants had the same target INR of 2.0-3.0. Only two (8%) participants in the telephone follow-up group and one (4%) in the usual care group had their INR goal at 2.5-3.5 (Table 1).

Pharmacists made a total of 179 successful telephone calls to participants in the telephone follow-up group with an average of 7.16 calls for each participant (range 7–10 calls). During the three month study period, participants in both groups had their INR measured on average 3.4 times. Specifically, a total of 79 INRs were measured in each group. Thirty-six INRs (45.6%) were in range for the telephone follow-up group, whereas only 19 INRs (24.1%) in the usual care group had INR values in the target range, p=0.005 (Table 2). The mean (standard deviation) TTR in the telephone follow-up group was also higher than that in the usual care group, 49.8 (34.3) versus 28.0 (27.5), p=0.017. For out-of-range INR values, the proportion of supratherapeutic INR values in the telephone follow-up group (9/79, 11.4%) was significantly lower than those in the usual care group (19/79, 24.1%), p=0.037. However, this was not the case for subtherapeutic INR values as the proportions of subtherapeutic INRs in the telephone follow-up group and the usual care group were not different, 34/79 (43.0%) versus 41/79 (51.8%), p=0.265. When taking into account the number of patients experiencing one or more out-of-range INR values, it was found that all participants in the usual care group had at least one previous record of an INR value out of target range (25/25, 100%) compared to 21 out of 25 (84%) in the telephone follow-up group, p=0.037.

Complications reported in both groups were not different. A total of three major bleeding events occurred during the study period; two were from the telephone follow-up group, and the other from the usual care group. Although not statistically significant, thromboembolic events and warfarin-related hospital admissions in the telephone follow-up group seemed to be relatively lower than those in the usual care group, 3/25 (12%) versus 6/25 (24%), p=0.259, and 4/25 (16%) versus 7/25 (28%), p=0.306, respectively (Table 3).

4. Discussion

To the best of our knowledge, this is the first study in the field using a RCT design to evaluate the impact of a telephone follow-up service in patients on warfarin. Hospitalized patients who were discharged on warfarin and received the telephone follow-up service had a higher rate of INR in target range and a higher TTR percentage than those who received usual care. The telephone follow-up service also decreased the number of patients experiencing out-of-range INRs after hospital discharge. This study also proved that the service is safe for patients as both study groups experienced rare and similar rates of thromboembolic and bleeding complications.

Most previous studies [4–6] explored the effects of telephone interactions for anticoagulant management based

TABLE 2: Therapeutic outcome measures.

Outcomes	Telephone	Usual care	p-value
INR values in range†	45.6% (36/79)	24.1% (19/79)	0.005
TTR‡	49.8$\pm$34.3	28.0$\pm$27.5	0.017
Out of range INR values			
Subtherapeutic†	43.0% (34/79)	51.8% (41/79)	0.265
Supratherapeutic†	11.4% (9/79)	24.1 % (19/79)	0.037
Patients with $\geq$1 out of range INR value	84.0% (21/25)	100.0% (25/25)	0.037

†Percentage of INR values out of all INR measures. ‡Mean $\pm$ standard deviation. INR: international normalized ratio. TTR: time in therapeutic range.

TABLE 3: Complications.

Outcomes	Telephone (n=25)	Usual care (n=25)	p-value
Bleeding events			
Major bleeding	2 (8%)	1 (4%)	0.552
Minor bleeding	3 (12%)	4 (16%)	0.684
Thromboembolic events	3 (12%)	6 (24%)	0.259
Warfarin-related hospital admission	4 (16%)	7 (28%)	0.306

on INR readings, while the telephone follow-up in this study focused on medicine use review to evaluate issues in managing warfarin and to assess medication adherence. This may explain why this telephone intervention showed improvement in the proportion of INR values in range and TTR percentage while telephone-management services in previous studies were comparable to standard warfarin management [4–6]. Another explanation is that most patients in previous studies had consistently stable INR values; hence, it would be difficult to see any additional benefit in these patients.

The beneficial effects of a telephone follow-up service found in this study are well aligned with findings from Ibrahim et al. which showed that follow-up counseling through phone calls every week and home visit biweekly for three months improved INR control [8]. However, the present study demonstrated that telephone follow-up alone without home visits is sufficient to help patients achieve and maintain their INR target. This telephone follow-up approach might be more practical and cost effective than the combination of telephone and home visits in patients discharged on warfarin, although it requires a head-to-head comparative trial to explore which intervention is more effective.

Despite patients who received telephone follow-up service having a higher percentage of TTR compared with those in the usual care group, they were only at goal 44% of the time, which does not indicate a good response to warfarin management, i.e., 60% or more [12]. A number of potential factors have been shown to affect discharge INRs including new initiation of warfarin therapy on hospital admission, shorter hospital stay periods, and concurrent infection [13]. Current recommendations for the initiation of warfarin therapy are 3–5 mg per day although the initial dose could be lower in some patients such as elderly patients, patient with increased risk of bleeding, or patients with liver disease [14, 15]. In this study, warfarin initiation doses prescribed in both groups were lower than current recommendations due to participants' comorbidities and complications prior to admission. This could explain the relatively low TTR and high proportion of subtherapeutic INR values that were observed in this study. It was also suggested that the TTR measurement is not recommended for the first month after initiating warfarin [16]. Using INR measurements for the first month after discharge for patients whose clinical conditions were unstable may reduce the calculated TTR as found in this study.

There are some limitations in this study. First, the duration of the telephone follow-up period was only 3 months, which may not be sufficient to observe effects that require long-term follow-up such as death or rehospitalization related to warfarin therapy. The sample size in this study also appeared relatively low compared with other trials. Nonetheless, it was adequate to statistically identify the difference in INR values in range and TTR between the telephone follow-up and usual care groups. The limitation of this small sample size was that it restricted the ability to undertake further subgroup analysis. Another limitation is that patients were recruited from one hospital, which may not represent the general population. It should be noted, however, that several characteristics of these patients including age, comorbidities, warfarin indication, and target INR suggest that they are comparable with general patients who receive warfarin after discharge.

5. Conclusion

This randomized controlled trial demonstrated that a telephone follow-up service when combined with usual care in recently discharged patients on warfarin helps patients achieve and maintain their INR target. Further studies with more participants and longer study periods may be needed to explore the impact of this service on complications of warfarin therapy. This anticoagulant supportive service could be a feasible approach to improve clinical outcomes and should be promoted to patients receiving warfarin therapy after discharge.

Acknowledgments

This research work received financial support from Naresuan University Postgraduate Student Fund. The authors acknowledge all patients participating in the study for their time. The authors would also like to thank clinical pharmacists who helped perform the interventions and all related healthcare personnel for their support during the course of this study. Special thanks are due to Dr. Alicia Ritscher, Pharm.D., Clement J Zablocki Veterans Affairs Medical Center, for improving the English language of the manuscript.

References

[1] M. Pirmohamed, "Warfarin: almost 60 years old and still causing problems," *British Journal of Clinical Pharmacology*, vol. 62, no. 5, pp. 509–511, 2006.

[2] W. Ageno, A. S. Gallus, A. Wittkowsky, M. Crowther, E. M. Hylek, and G. Palareti, "Oral anticoagulant therapy: antithrombotic therapy and prevention of thrombosis, 9th ed: American College of Chest Physicians evidence-based clinical practice guidelines," *CHEST*, vol. 141, no. 2, supplement, pp. e44S–e88S, 2012.

[3] B. S. Manzoor, W.-H. Cheng, J. C. Lee, E. M. Uppuluri, and E. A. Nutescu, "Quality of Pharmacist-Managed Anticoagulation Therapy in Long-Term Ambulatory Settings: A Systematic Review," *Annals of Pharmacotherapy*, vol. 51, no. 12, pp. 1122–1137, 2017.

[4] A. G. Staresinic, C. A. Sorkness, B. M. Goodman, and D. W. Pigarelli, "Comparison of outcomes using 2 delivery models of anticoagulation care," *JAMA Internal Medicine*, vol. 166, no. 9, pp. 997–1006, 2006.

[5] K. T. Blissit, M. L. Mullenix, and K. G. Brittain, "Evaluation of Time in Therapeutic Range on Warfarin Therapy between Face-to-Face and Telephone Follow-Up in a VA Medical Center," *Journal of Pharmacy Technology*, vol. 31, no. 2, pp. 78–83, 2015.

[6] A. K. Wittkowsky, E. A. Nutescu, J. Blackburn et al., "Outcomes of oral anticoagulant therapy managed by telephone vs in-office visits in an anticoagulation clinic setting," *CHEST*, vol. 130, no. 5, pp. 1385–1389, 2006.

[7] S. Hassan, A. Naboush, J. Radbel et al., "Telephone-based anticoagulation management in the homebound setting: A retrospective observational study," *Journal of General Internal Medicine*, vol. 6, pp. 869–875, 2013.

[8] S. Ibrahim, J. Jespersen, and L. Poller, "The clinical evaluation of International Normalized Ratio variability and control in conventional oral anticoagulant administration by use of the variance growth rate," *Journal of Thrombosis and Haemostasis*, vol. 11, no. 8, pp. 1540–1546, 2013.

[9] C. Van Walraven, A. Jennings, N. Oake, D. Fergusson, and A. J. Forster, "Effect of study setting on anticoagulation control: A systematic review and metaregression," *CHEST*, vol. 129, no. 5, pp. 1155–1166, 2006.

[10] K. M. T. Collins, A. J. Onwuegbuzie, and Q. G. Jiao, "A mixed methods investigation of mixed methods sampling designs in social and health science research," *Journal of Mixed Methods Research*, vol. 1, no. 3, pp. 267–294, 2007.

[11] S. Schulman and C. Kearon, "Definition of major bleeding in clinical investigations of antihemostatic medicinal products in non-surgical patients," *Journal of Thrombosis and Haemostasis*, vol. 3, no. 4, pp. 692–694, 2005.

[12] J. S. Dlott, R. A. George, X. Huang et al., "National assessment of warfarin anticoagulation therapy for stroke prevention in atrial fibrillation," *Circulation*, vol. 129, no. 13, pp. 1407–1414, 2014.

[13] M. I. Abdel-Aziz, M. A. S. Ali, A. K. M. Hassan, and T. H. Elfaham, "Factors influencing warfarin response in hospitalized patients," *Saudi Pharmaceutical Journal*, vol. 23, no. 6, pp. 642–649, 2015.

[14] C. T. January, L. S. Wann, J. S. Alpert et al., "2014 AHA/ACC/HRS guideline for the management of patients with atrial fibrillation," *Circulation*, CIR. 0000000000000041, 2014.

[15] R. A. Nishimura, C. M. Otto, R. O. Bonow et al., "2014 AHA/ACC Guideline for the Management of Patients With Valvular Heart Disease: Executive Summary: A Report of the American College of Cardiology/American Heart Association Task Force on Practice Guidelines," *Circulation*, vol. 129, no. 23, pp. 2440–2492, 2014.

[16] K. W. Phillips and J. Ansell, "Outpatient management of oral vitamin K antagonist therapy: Defining and measuring high-quality management," *Expert Review of Cardiovascular Therapy*, vol. 6, no. 1, pp. 57–70, 2008.

19

Qualitative Assessment of the Feasibility, Usability, and Acceptability of a Mobile Client Data App for Community-Based Maternal, Neonatal, and Child Care in Rural Ghana

Jessica D. Rothstein,[1,2] Larissa Jennings,[1,2] Anitha Moorthy,[3] Fan Yang,[1] Lisa Gee,[1] Karen Romano,[3] David Hutchful,[3] Alain B. Labrique,[1,2] and Amnesty E. LeFevre[1,2]

[1]*Department of International Health, Johns Hopkins Bloomberg School of Public Health, 615 N. Wolfe Street, Room E5030, Baltimore, MD 21205, USA*
[2]*Johns Hopkins University Global mHealth Initiative, 615 N. Wolfe Street, Room 5635, Baltimore, MD 21205, USA*
[3]*Grameen Foundation, No. 25 Labone Crescent, Accra, Ghana*

Correspondence should be addressed to Jessica D. Rothstein; jrothstein@jhu.edu

Academic Editor: Malcolm Clarke

Mobile phone applications may enhance the delivery of critical health services and the accuracy of health service data. Yet, the opinions and experiences of frontline health workers on using mobile apps to track pregnant and recently delivered women are underreported. This evaluation qualitatively assessed the feasibility, usability, and acceptability of a mobile Client Data App for maternal, neonatal, and child client data management by community health nurses (CHNs) in rural Ghana. The mobile app enabled CHNs to enter, summarize, and query client data. It also sent visit reminders for clients and provided a mechanism to report level of care to district officers. Fourteen interviews and two focus groups with CHNs, midwives, and district health officers were conducted, coded, and thematically analyzed. Results indicated that the app was easily integrated into care, improved CHN productivity, and was acceptable due to its capacity to facilitate client follow-up, data reporting, and decision-making. However, the feasibility and usability of the app were hindered by high client volumes, staff shortages, and software and device challenges. Successful integration of mobile client data apps for frontline health workers in rural and resource-poor settings requires real-time monitoring, program investments, and targeted changes in human resources.

1. Introduction

An estimated 66% of maternal deaths and 50% of deaths in children under the age of 5 occurred in sub-Saharan Africa in 2015 [1, 2]. Although Ghana's health indicators largely surpass many African nations, the country has faced significant challenges in improving maternal and child survival. Despite nearly halving the number of maternal deaths since 1990, approximately 319 women die each year out of 100,000 live births from pregnancy- and birth-related complications—a figure nearly twice that of the Millennium Development Goal [1, 3]. Among children under five, while overall deaths have declined by 51% since 1990, neonatal deaths occurring within 28 days after birth have largely remained stagnant, changing only from 30 to 29 deaths per 1,000 live births [2, 4].

A vast majority of maternal, neonatal, and child deaths are preventable [1, 5–8]. However, limited access and utilization of skilled antenatal, delivery, and postpartum care services hinder the timely and safe delivery of life-saving interventions [6–9]. In addition, reliable and comprehensive data on the implementation of maternal, neonatal, and child health services are needed to monitor and ensure that life-saving services are provided across the care continuum [10–12]. However, the inability of traditional health information systems to track new mothers and babies once they leave health facilities as well as inadequate communication

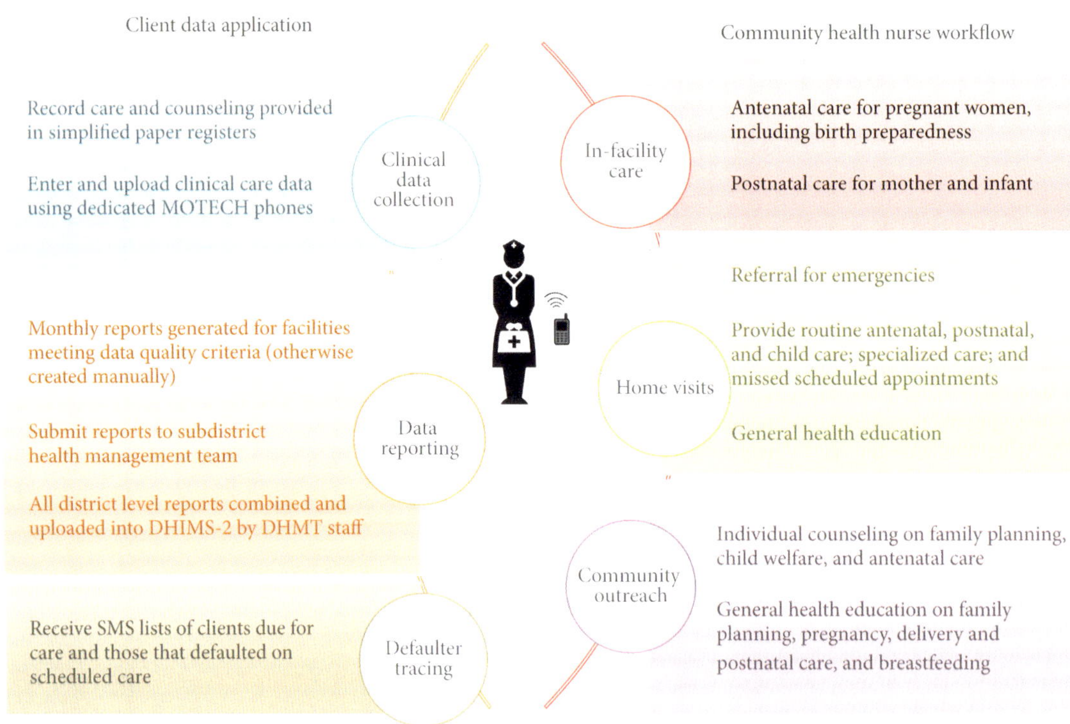

Figure 1: Functional summary of MOTECH's mobile Client Data App.

between health workers at different levels of the health system has led to slower progress towards maternal, neonatal, and child health goals [13–15].

Global penetration of mobile phones has the potential to optimize delivery of high quality maternal, neonatal, and child health information and access to services [16–21]. In particular, mobile apps, or software applications developed specifically for use on small, wireless computing devices such as smartphones or tablets, have been shown to improve the quality of care provided to pregnant and recently delivered women through electronic decision support [17, 18, 22], health worker planning [23, 24], and data collection and reporting [19, 25–27]. The reported ease of use and adaptability of mobile apps (or applications) for diverse populations also makes them an attractive, low-cost platform for developing health education and clinical care strategies [28–30]. Nonetheless, to increase efficacy and sustainability of mobile health applications, previous studies have underscored the importance of ensuring high user acceptance and usability of the technological innovation [31–33]. User-centered design and robust needs assessments are recognized as best practices for development technology [34]. Equipping frontline health workers with mobile phone applications may enhance the delivery of maternal, neonatal, and child health services as well as the accuracy of data capture and recording [16, 26, 35, 36]. Yet, little research exists on health worker perceptions of mobile applications intended to improve maternal, neonatal, and child data management, despite user views being critical to product uptake and implementation [37–39]. In addition, the opinions and experiences of frontline health workers in sub-Saharan Africa on using mobile applications to track pregnant women and mother-infant pairs are underreported. Such information is critical for improving the long-term impact and sustainability of mobile health (mHealth) strategies for clinical and community health settings.

Evaluation Objective. This evaluation aimed to qualitatively examine the feasibility, usability, and acceptability of the Client Data Application (or Client Data App) that was part of the Mobile Technology for Community Health (MOTECH) program to support frontline health workers in the delivery of maternal, neonatal, and child care in rural Ghana.

The MOTECH program was initiated in 2009 as a partnership between the Ghana Health Service, Grameen Foundation, and Columbia University Mailman School of Public Health to leverage mobile technology to increase quantity and quality of maternal and infant care in rural areas and ultimately improve health outcomes. The Client Data App enabled community health nurses (CHNs) to use mobile phones to digitize care provided to women and children and thereby track pregnant women and mother-infant pairs needing care (Figure 1). CHNs then received reminders and alerts about clients' upcoming and missed care. Parallel care reminders and alerts, in addition to other actionable health information, were sent to pregnant women and mothers with infants less than 12 months of age as part of a mutually supportive "Mobile Midwife" program within MOTECH [40]. A separate evaluation, not discussed in this manuscript, is planned to examine health workers' views on MOTECH's Mobile Midwife service.

2. Methods

2.1. Setting. Data were collected in 2014 in two districts: Awutu Senya and Gomoa West. MOTECH was implemented in Awutu Senya in 2011 and then replicated in Gomoa West and three other districts in 2013. Both districts are located in Ghana's Central Region and have among the highest rates of under-five and neonatal mortality in the country [4, 40]. This region additionally has significant human resource shortages. In the Central Region of Ghana, there are over 25,000 individuals to one doctor compared to the nationwide ratio of nearly 12,000 individuals to one doctor [41, 42]. The region also suffers from high vacancy rates of nurse-midwives trained to manage basic and emergency obstetric care [43–45]. Under these circumstances, mobile technologies that expand the reach of health workers are critical to overcoming barriers to care. Although telecommunication connectivity in the Central Region can be unreliable and mobile phones are not ubiquitous, phone ownership and access are high among health workers [46].

Maternal, neonatal, and child health services within Ghana's health system are primarily delivered via public health centers and community health posts. The health centers are staffed primarily by skilled health professionals (such as nurses and midwives) who offer comprehensive preventive and basic curative services, including minor surgeries and uncomplicated deliveries. In contrast, as part of Ghana's Community-based Health Planning and Services (CHPS) Initiative, community health posts are staffed by lower-skilled CHNs who provide health education, outreach and counseling, and basic curative services to clients via home visits and facility-based care [47]. Community health posts (referred to locally as CHPS facilities) are typically staffed by 2 to 3 CHNs who are required to have completed a two-year postsecondary certificate program in obstetrics as well as general and community health nursing. MOTECH Ghana was originally designed for use in community health posts and later extended to the health centers, hospitals, and other private health facilities. Within the two evaluation districts, MOTECH was implemented in a total of 46 facilities, including 35 community health posts and 11 health centers.

2.2. Description of the Client Data App. The mobile Client Data App used in this evaluation was delivered by low-cost GSM mobile Nokia 1680 and Nokia Asha 200 feature phones provided by Ghana Health Service, which helped CHNs and other users to digitize and track care delivered to mother-infant pairs in their area. The system's architecture was based on field-tested open-source software, including OpenXData for mobile data collection and OpenMRS for electronic medical records [48]. The client data system used a Java 2 Platform Micro Edition (J2ME) application to capture and store client data. All clients were assigned a unique MOTECH identification (ID) number upon registration to protect confidentiality and enable tracking across multiple facilities. During client encounters, CHNs first recorded care provided using five "simplified paper registers," which were developed by MOTECH to condense more than a dozen registers and streamline data collection. CHNs later entered data into digital forms on their mobile phones (Figure 2(a)). General packet radio service (GPRS) data channels were used to transfer these data from the phone to a central clinical data system that was stored on the MOTECH server (Figure 2(b)).

The data app system then crosschecked uploaded clinical information on timing and type of care given with national guidelines to estimate specific due dates for routine care. As a result, health workers received a weekly list via short message service (SMS) of pregnant clients and mother-infant pairs in their catchment area who were either due for or defaulted on care. CHNs were also able to query client data, enabling them to retrieve lists of defaulters or women due to deliver in the upcoming week, and to search for details about individual clients (Figure 2(c)). In addition, the Client Data App generated preselected monthly health reports that were required for national reporting, if client data were at least 85% complete and accurate three consecutive months. Previously, monthly health reports were numerous, redundant, and compiled by hand. Therefore, the Client Data App was intended to improve accuracy and processing speed.

The MOTECH developers designed the Client Data App for low-skilled health providers in rural and resource-poor settings. To account for anticipated power and mobile network breaks, the Java-enabled Nokia handsets allowed for mobile forms to be completed and stored offline for uploading at a later time. Phones had dual subscriber identity module (SIM) capacity and were equipped with SIM cards from two different mobile operators in case of network or congestion problems [46]. Field testing during the prototyping stage served to align the app's features with user needs, including the simplification of data entry using check boxes, radio buttons, lists, and number fields. CHNs received in-person training as well as a detailed training manual. They could also refer to a MOTECH call center for technical assistance. Monthly prepaid airtime units were provided to all users to upload information. The Client Data App's interface was available for use in English. Phones were password-protected, and user authentication schemes were built into Java forms to maintain confidentiality of client data [46].

2.3. Measurement. Qualitative in-depth interviews and focus groups were used to examine health worker perceptions on the Client Data App's feasibility, usability, and acceptability. For purposes of this evaluation, we defined the assessment areas as follows: *Feasibility* was defined as whether implementation of the Client Data App was easily and conveniently done, accounting for advantages and disadvantages to integrating the application into routine workflow. *Usability* was defined as whether the Client Data App could be used by CHNs to adequately record, track, and summarize data, including whether it functioned in a way that enhanced productivity or led to unproductive tasks due to errors. *Acceptability* was defined as whether CHNs and other stakeholders found the Client Data App likeable, including its interface and navigation features. These definitions were derived from similar prior research that qualitatively assessed user experiences for mHealth applications [28, 49–55].

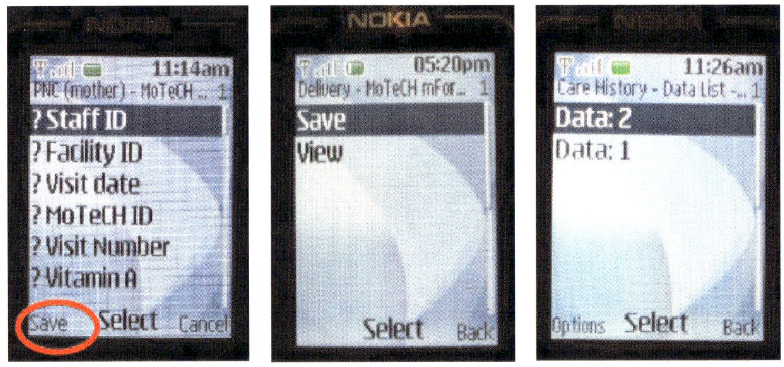

(a) CHNs used bottom left "Save" icon to save a mobile form. Forms were then listed under each form section

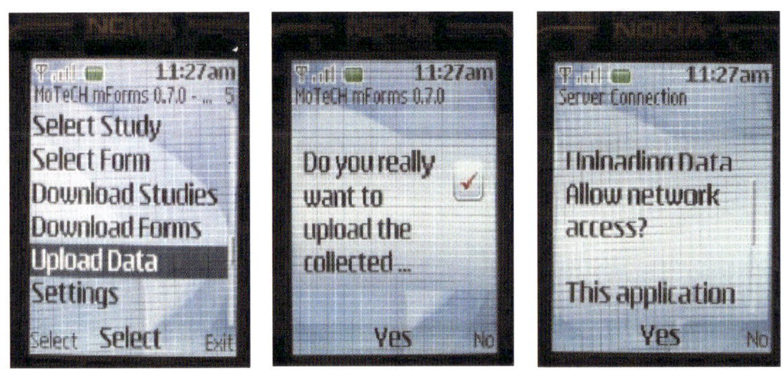

(b) To upload forms, CHNs selected "Upload Data" and answered a series of questions. CHNs received a message when the upload was completed

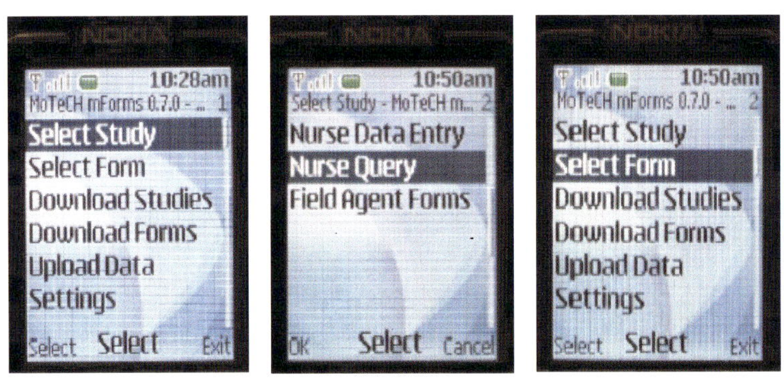

(c) CHNs queried the system by selecting "Nurse Query" and selecting the appropriate query form from a number of options

Figure 2: Screen shots of the MOTECH Client Data App's saving, uploading, and query forms.

2.4. Data Collection. Data were collected at three levels of the health system: community health posts (referred to locally as CHPS facilities), health centers, and district health directorates. Semistructured interview guides were used at all levels. In-depth interviews with CHNs and midwives asked them to describe perceived benefits and drawbacks of the Client Data App, as well as their experience using it during clinic and community outreach activities. CHNs and midwives were also asked to assess advantages and disadvantages of using the Client Data App for tasks such as recording care, tracking clients, and verifying data with automatic health reports. Skilled nurses working at the health centers did not use the Client Data App and therefore were not recruited for data collection. Interviews with district health directors and district health information officers explored how the Client Data App affected the quality of data provided by CHNs and their ability to use and supervise submission of monthly health reports. Questions also examined views regarding local and scaled-up implementation. Other district health directorate staff, including disease control officers and public health officers, who did not engage with the Client Data App were not interviewed. Focus groups with CHNs were included to further investigate findings from the individual interviews and to obtain CHNs' recommendations for modifying the MOTECH data management system. Focus groups with midwives are not conducted given the limited number of midwives available at participating sites.

All interviews and focus groups were conducted in English by a local Ghanaian and a US researcher, both with experience conducting qualitative research. The Ghanaian researcher occasionally translated local terminology in Akan used by participants. The interviews were conducted at community health posts and health centers and ranged from 40 to 120 minutes. Focus groups were conducted in a centrally located and neutral space. The discussions and lasted approximately 90 minutes. Each interview and focus group was digitally recorded and transcribed verbatim.

2.5. Sample Selection. One health center and three community health posts were randomly selected from each of the two participating districts. Purposive sampling was then used to identify CHNs, midwives, district health information officers, and district health directors with a minimum of six months experience using MOTECH's Client Data App. The target interview sample size was 14 individuals, representing one CHN and one midwife per health center, one CHN each from three community health posts in each district, and the district health director and district health information officer in each district. The target focus group sample size was two groups each with 7 to 8 CHNs. Given resources available, this sample size was expected to enable the evaluation to reach saturation in which no new findings emerged [56].

2.6. Analysis. A qualitative thematic analysis was conducted by two public health graduate students. Interview and focus group transcripts were manually coded using *a priori* topical codes according to the evaluation's three assessment areas: feasibility, usability, and acceptability. Emergent subcodes were then developed based on patterns within each concept and which were relevant to the literature. We then followed an iterative process of developing a codebook, identifying salient themes, and integrating core findings [57]. When new themes were identified throughout this process, transcripts were reanalyzed to find evidence that verified or modified those themes. Later-stage interviews and focus groups were used to validate responses among member participants [58]. We also confirmed findings based on feedback from MOTECH implementation partners during various stages of data collection and analysis [59].

2.7. Ethics Approval. The evaluation was approved by the institutional review board at the Johns Hopkins Bloomberg School of Public Health in Baltimore, Maryland, USA. As part of the MOTECH implementation plan, the Ghana Health Service in Accra, Ghana, also approved the evaluation's activities. All participants provided oral informed consent prior to data collection. This manuscript complies with the mHealth evidence reporting and assessment (mERA) checklist on reporting of health interventions using mobile technologies [60].

3. Results

Several findings emerged from our analyses, revealing both the achievements and challenges of MOTECH's implementation of the Client Data App. The emergent themes within each of the three assessment areas (feasibility, usability, and acceptability) are illustrated below with exemplary quotations. Key findings are summarized in Figure 3.

3.1. Participant Characteristics. A total of 14 individual interviews were conducted, representing eight CHNs and two midwives as first-line users of the Client Data App, as well as two district health information officers and two district health directors (Table 1). Two focus groups were additionally carried out, consisting of a total of 15 CHNs. The majority of participants were female and within the ages of 26 to 30 years.

3.2. Feasibility. We defined feasibility as whether implementation of the Client Data App was easily and conveniently achieved, accounting for advantages and disadvantages to integrating the application into routine care.

3.2.1. Easily Integrated into Routine Care. Participants generally reported that the Client Data App was easily integrated into their workflow and data capture. CHNs were able to incorporate registration of eligible individuals, including issuing their MOTECH IDs, into their client visits. CHNs also noted being able to readily incorporate information provided by MOTECH alerts into their weekly routines. Based on the ease of integration, users were able to envision the Client Data App becoming a permanent part of their work.

> *When a pregnant woman comes here, you start reviewing her records. When there is a new client, you give her an ANC booklet; you fill the form for her, taking the vitals of the client. Then you take their mobile phone number and register the woman into MOTECH .... (CHN, health center)*

> *... Every Monday morning, ... the MOTECH system sends us alert messages to remind us on those who are due for care. And those who are defaulters too ... So, every Monday morning I checked the phone and gets tracked on the data, and the details on those who are due for care and those who are defaulters and follow them and give the care to them. (CHN, community health post)*

> *We just hope that the MOTECH project comes to stay forever and incorporate it into Ghana Health Service, forever. (District health information officer)*

3.2.2. Hardware and Uploading Requirements Posed Some Inconveniences. However, limited mobile network connectivity in more rural areas of the district posed significant challenges to uploading client data. Consequently, CHNs had to preoccupy themselves with locating places with adequate connectivity in order to upload the mobile forms. This presented an added inconvenience, particularly for those CHNs

Table 1: Number and type of users enrolled in the evaluation by qualitative method and by total.

User characteristics	Individual interviews	Focus groups	Total
Total number of interviews or discussions	14	2	16
Number of interviews or discussions by health system level			
Health center	4	0	4
Community health post	6	2	8
District health directorate	4	0	4
Total number of enrolled users	14	15	29
Number of enrolled users by health worker type			
Community health nurse	8	15	23
Midwife	2	0	2
District health director	2	0	2
District health information officer	2	0	2
Number of enrolled users by age (in years)			
<26	0	2	2
26–29	7	13	20
≥30	7	0	7
Number of enrolled users by gender			
Female	11	13	24
Male	3	2	5

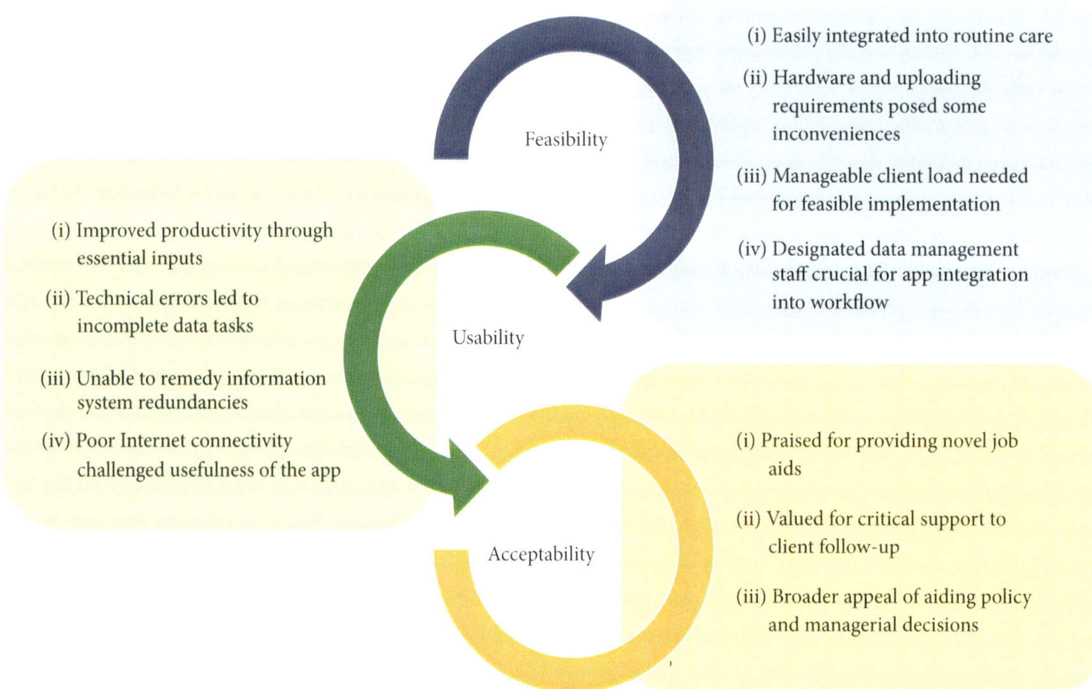

Figure 3: Summary of key qualitative findings by assessment area.

working in remote areas. For some CHNs, accommodating network connectivity challenges also required them to extend their workday.

> *We also have problems with network connectivity. For example, so the uploading may be a challenge. And sometimes they're typed, but it doesn't go through. Sometimes it doesn't go through at all. You have to go and climb a tree. (District health information officer)*

> *We try to find a place where the network is good. For example, when the network is good, you can upload everything. Let's say, my house, the*

network is good, I have to take the phone and upload there. (CHN, health center)

CHNs and other users additionally expressed concerns about the hardware used, as the small size and tedious typing functionality of the Nokia 1680 phones made data entry time-consuming. This rendered the Client Data App as a less feasible option in the long run, especially at high-volume health centers. Requests to be equipped with larger screen devices with keypads such as laptops or tablets were given by over half of interview participants, who stressed the challenges associated with their current handsets.

The numbers are quite huge numbers. If you are doing about 30 a day ... They have to enter them. Thirty people. It's tedious. So maybe they get a laptop or something bigger .... (District health information officer)

They also should give us laptop, or tablet, as we are typing, we can't speed it. I would prefer a smart phone because in smart phone, when you type something you don't have type everything, it will just [automatically] fill. (CHN, health center)

Another challenge involved the omitted generation of automated reports for some facilities because reporting completeness and accuracy had not reached 85% for the required three consecutive months. Limitations in meeting completion and accuracy thresholds and the corresponding failure to receive automated reports left many users frustrated.

Tomorrow I will be thinking I have to submit the report by Monday. Then I will be sitting here and do[ing] the uploads. If we are supposed to submit on Monday, there is a lot to do. But the reports are not coming, oh. We did three months and so automation ... will generate reports for you. I was so happy, but up to now I didn't see anything. (CHN, community health post)

3.2.3. Manageable Client Load Needed for Feasible Implementation. Feasible implementation was also hindered by a shortage of CHNs or other data entry staff, especially in health centers where client volume outweighed staff availability. High client caseloads interfered with CHNs' capacity to submit clinical data and receive timely alerts on clients who were due for or missed care. The significant clinical responsibilities of trained midwives at health centers and the unpredictability of their workdays also posed challenges to the consistent use of the Client Data App. The imbalance between client loads and health worker availability was compounded by high CHN attrition rates, which required retraining of staff on the Client Data App.

Because we are the health center, unlike the CHPS zone, concerning our volume, after the outreach, you have to do all the uploads. We cannot do the uploads rapidly because of our workload. Maybe they can take out the health centers or have something done to help because our workload is intense. (CHN, health center)

... By the end of the day, maybe you have a lady who haven't deliver[ed] yet, so after you close the antenatal phase, you have to go to the labor ward and be monitoring this labor case. Then by the end of the day, ... you are coming back to load the MOTECH ... In fact it's a headache. (Midwife, health center)

... In non-urban settings, like this place, staff attrition is very high. ... For the past about three years, we've been receiving an average of about 20 community health nurses every year. ... These are new people. So they don't know anything about MOTECH. They have to be trained. (District health director)

3.2.4. Designated Data Management Staff Crucial for App Integration into Workflow. Many participants commented that the feasibility of the Client Data App would be improved if staff were designated to data management rather than responsible for multiple care tasks, especially during community outreach activities. Others suggested that health worker shortages could be overcome by training health extension workers (who had previously been discontinued) for routine data entry. In addition, some participants proposed recruiting other MOTECH staff to assist with routine data entry during care provision.

I do have some problems with ... recording the care given. Sometimes ..., at the child welfare clinic, I have to take the height and the MUAC [mid-upper arm circumference] of the babies. ... I will be doing the weighing, the immunizing and the recording, and a whole lot of it. Sometimes I even forgot to take the MUAC or the height ... There is no help. We need some nurses to help us. (CHN, community health post)

If we can get other cadre of staff, who are not necessarily well trained, so that they can do this ....We did train some health extension workers, and then other staff ... [but]—they are not professionals. We did train them, but unfortunately they've all been exited out of the system, so that has compounded the problem. (District health director)

Would that be possible? To train personnel from MOTECH, and then they join us on the field? Or join us in our health facility? Because basically in Ghana, our work is very broad. Very huge. So, together with MOTECH help, it should end. (District health information officer)

3.3. Usability. We defined usability as whether the Client Data App could be used by CHNs to adequately record, track, and sum data, including whether it functioned in a way that enhanced productivity or led to unproductive tasks due to errors.

3.3.1. Improved Productivity through Essential Inputs. CHNs reported that MOTECH's simplified paper registers were a significant improvement over the previous data collection process. The mobile forms were perceived as straightforward and easily navigable. CHNs reported that they were generally able to transfer clinical information from the simplified registers to the mobile forms in approximately two minutes. In addition, by enabling CHNs to avoid redundant paper registers, the Client Data App saved time and allowed for more case entries per day and week.

> *I think MOTECH has made our work much easier. Before there is a lot of writing, then after MOTECH, maybe the important information will be portioned, so maybe when you write, it's easier. (CHN, health center)*

> *We don't rule lines anymore and the immunizations, we can write the actual number, everything else is there. (CHN, health center)*

3.3.2. Technical Errors Led to Incomplete Data Tasks. Nevertheless, the Client Data App's usability was hampered by technical errors which interfered with completing registration and data submission. The most commonly reported error involved identical MOTECH ID numbers designated to different clients. User delays resulting from these errors were also exacerbated by difficulties reaching the technical support team. In addition, data entry was often interrupted when the software froze unexpectedly.

> *They will say "the MOTECH ID is already in use." The MOTECH ID says it's new. So I stopped registering them. I have five clients who are not registered now. If I use those MOTECH ID numbers, they will just send me errors. (CHN, community health post)*

> *Sometimes there are errors. I uploaded, and I called the call center, but they don't respond. Like I have been contacting them but no answer. (CHN, community health post)*

> *It's sometimes ....an experience ... on the phone. I think sometimes it freeze, when you are working on some forms, you realize that it stops ... then you realize it's freeze. (CHN, health center)*

3.3.3. Unable to Remedy All of the Information System Redundancies. Usability challenges also arose because MOTECH was not interoperable with the national health information system. While the integration of MOTECH data with the District Health Information Management System 2 (DHIMS-2) was beyond the program's resources and scope, participants expressed frustration with this disconnect. The process of recording and summarizing client data was also delayed because it was not possible for MOTECH to automate all of the monthly reports for qualifying facilities.

> *Mind you, we have been advocating that if the MOTECH system and the DHIMS-2 would be on the same platform - so that this one will fit into this. So you don't have to print out, before you re-enter. That will save a lot of time. (District health information officer)*

> *We do the entry at the sub-district level, all the facilities in MOTECH. Change our phone and get us [a] tablet. Then we can do the DHIMS-2 ourselves at the sub-district level. (CHN, community health post)*

> *There is nothing about antenatal care. Even though they take [mobile] data on antenatal care, which they upload. There's nothing on family planning—they also take [mobile] data on family planning. So, the core areas which we think should be there because of MOTECH for the [mobile] reports are omitted. (District health information officer)*

Finally, some of the information needed to identify and track clients in their communities was not readily available through the Client Data App's alerts or queries. CHNs suggested including client addresses and travel instructions to ease follow-up in remote areas and the overall usability of the application.

> *The reminder is good, but the difficulty in tracing the defaulters is the address. To get the address, we still have to go back to the simplified registers to locate the defaulters. When the phone is in your pocket and you look at it, you see the person ... [but] it only comes with the name and the care. The addresses are not there. (CHN, health center)*

3.3.4. Poor Internet Connectivity Challenged the Usefulness of the App. The usefulness of the Client Data App was likewise affected by interruptions in network connectivity. Inconsistent connectivity led to difficulties in uploading clinical data and/or errors. This delayed receipt of timely alerts of clients requiring care. The discrepancy between data collection and submission also hindered the Client Data App's tracking functionality and the accuracy of the aggregate numbers in the automated monthly reports.

> *The internet connection is not that stable ... It is time-consuming when you are doing the uploads because you have to try it, try it, try it. When the network is good, we just do it once and it hits the system ... The network is not stable. The thing indicates it's connecting, for five minutes—it's still connecting. So you have to wait, waiting, waiting, waiting ··· (CHN, community health post)*

> *Because sometimes we upload the forms but it doesn't go through. ... It means it wouldn't be captured by the system. The report generated from the form will be different from what we have here. It is a challenge we have. ... Yesterday the phone I uploaded, it didn't go through. It is only today .... (CHN, community health post)*

In order to minimize delays due to connectivity interruptions, one CHN suggested that MOTECH incorporate additional feedback loops between users and the central database.

> *... Maybe on Mondays, if they can send us what we've uploaded for us to cross check. If it's not uploaded we will re-send it ... It will be easier and faster than just waiting for them. Otherwise we always complain about the automated generated report, because it's not tallying what's really happened. So given the reminders, they should also give us the reminders of the uploads. (CHN, health center)*

3.4. Acceptability. Acceptability was defined as whether CHNs and other stakeholders found the Client Data App likeable, including its interface and navigation features.

3.4.1. Praised for Providing Novel Job Aids. The Client Data App was acceptable to users given that it introduced new tools to assist health workers in performing their assigned tasks. In general, CHNs were satisfied with MOTECH's alert system. In particular, CHNs and those at community health posts found that the automated monthly reports eased their workload for data reporting and motivated them to capture and use data.

> *Sometimes, when you go to the outreach ... it's difficult for you to go to the register and find out which community you went to and which not. When you go to the reminders on MOTECH, it will just tell you because you uploaded the information after the outreach. So MOTECH has been really helpful to us, especially in the remote areas. (CHN, community health post)*

> *It is so rewarding when at the end of month, you receive your computer-generated reports. And then you don't have to go through the registers and do the targets. Even that, there's some incentive for those who receive the computer degrees and reports .... (District health information officer)*

Conversely, CHNs who worked at facilities that were not receiving the automated reports due to incomplete submitted data were less enthusiastic about the Client Data App. They expressed a desire to see these new job aids materialize.

> *I wish MOTECH system could generate all the reports for me. Then I will be motivated to upload everyday! I'd be more motivated if I see the reports. (CHN, community health post)*

3.4.2. Valued for Critical Support to Client Follow-Up. The Client Data App was also valued for improving the efficiency of client follow-up through weekly reminders, which eliminated the need for CHNs to conduct time-consuming searches through paper registers. In addition, CHNs noted that the weekly defaulter lists helped structure their community outreach and home visit schedules, maximizing the follow-up care provided.

> *Before MOTECH, sometimes we don't trace defaulters. It's better to trace. It's very helpful. Because if you don't trace, you don't know what's happening to your clients. Everything about the clients is on the phone. The vaccine [and] the routine. (CHN, community health post)*

> *Before the MOTECH, we don't have the reminders, I write it somewhere else, sometimes I remember it. Sometimes you remember. Sometimes it makes it easier to have the reminders, because you can't remember everything. The defaulters are about five to six, the reminders come on Monday morning. I can trace them by the end of day. (CHN, community health post)*

> *It helps trace our important clients and the message it gave, it tells them ... it saves mothers and pregnant women. (CHN, health center)*

3.4.3. Broader Appeal of Aiding Policy and Managerial Decisions. Administrators and data management staff working in the district health directorates were most satisfied with the Client Data App for its capacity to summarize data for timely decision-making. The automated monthly reports provided by MOTECH enabled a new level of scrutiny for data collection and aggregation in health centers and community health posts.

> *It's very good ..., For instance, the fact that the data, you can get everything at the facility level. But before that came into being, everything was allocated at the health center level or sub-district level. So we're not getting the details. It is all about the details. Now we can get more detailed data at the CHPS [health post] level than used to be. I think to me that is what I can put my finger on—more details. (District health director)*

District health directors felt the Client Data App brought about a better awareness of how data were collected and used and, therefore, a better appreciation for accuracy and completeness. District health directors also noted that, for staff with limited data analytical skills, the Client Data App assisted in synthesizing data rapidly and in a user-friendly format. Having more valid, aggregated data additionally enabled administrators to monitor trends and determine what needed to be improved.

> *To a large extent, because it is automated, I think I have to concede that the capacity of a good number of our staff at especially the lower levels are inadequate when you are talking about data analysis. So when it is ready-cooked like this, of course it's easy for them to—if it's [a] graphical presentation ... you can visualize everything that you want. And that is very handy. (District health director)*

> *As you know, these things are needed to help with decision-making ... at that level. You can clearly*

see the trends. You can clearly see where you are doing well [and] where you are not doing well. It is so good. (District health director)

4. Discussion

Our data indicate that MOTECH's Client Data App was a feasible, usable, and acceptable tool to aid health workers in collecting and tracking data to improve maternal, neonatal, and child health services. Health workers agreed that the Client Data App simplified individual client data collection, was easily integrated into their workflow, and enhanced their capacity to deliver follow-up services across the care continuum. These findings align with other studies that have demonstrated the benefits of equipping health workers with data management technologies to improve the continuity of care in rural populations [27, 61]. At the same time, our results highlight several challenges that would need to be addressed to optimize the utility of a client data management system using mobile devices in resource-poor settings.

First, our findings suggest that the successful integration of mobile applications into service delivery may necessitate targeted changes in human resources available at certain health facilities [62]. The greatest obstacle to implementation of the Client Data App was the combined effect of high client volumes, staff shortages, and poor network connectivity. CHNs tended to integrate mobile data entry into client care by waiting until the end of the day or week to upload data to the MOTECH server. Yet, the number of clients seen by health workers at the health centers and the long delays in uploading data precluded real-time submission. Thus, while data uploads were manageable for CHNs working at the community health posts, they were generally not manageable at health centers. Similar issues emerged within the context of a telemedicine program in Ghana's Amansi-West district, in which providers assumed a greater workload without a reduction in other tasks or increased personnel [63]. Our participants suggested training less skilled data staff or community health volunteers to assist with data entry, particularly for older providers who were sometimes less proficient with mobile apps [64]. In the context of future mHealth deployments, it will be important for implementing partners to work closely with the national health system and other government agencies to assess health workers' capacity to absorb additional mobile-based responsibilities and to explore possibilities for hiring and maintaining data staff.

Second, given the current cellular network in rural Ghana, it may have been possible to minimize network challenges through a more advanced monitoring system. Our results revealed that the lack of network reliability compromised the efficiency and usability of the Client Data App, notwithstanding the technological systems put in place to address these complications. Other studies have shown that poor network coverage and signal strength are often a major limitation to implementation of mobile technologies [23, 27, 31, 65, 66]. While the MOTECH team took careful measures to mitigate connectivity challenges, such as instituting a customer support call center and using high-storage devices with offline and multinetwork functionality, users still grew frustrated with the efforts required to upload data. The longs lags between data collection and submission, which CHNs reported as sometimes taking up to two weeks, limited the capacity of MOTECH to reliably track all client needs. A mechanism that allowed health workers to directly access clinical data to fix errors from incomplete uploads, rather than relying on a customer support center, may have enabled more immediate troubleshooting [40]. In addition, it is critical for implementers to carefully select what minimal clinical data are required for decision-making, rather than digitizing all paper registers or entry fields in order to maximize entry quality and speed.

Third, our findings shed light on the interconnectedness of the evaluation's assessment areas. Acceptance of the Client Data App was closely linked to its perceived usefulness to generate automated reports. When no problems were encountered during uploading, CHNs felt that the automated reports were a time saver. The MOTECH team had anticipated this would be the primary incentive for CHNs to engage with the Client Data App [46]. However, several health center-based CHNs were less motivated to enter data when the reports were not generated. These findings align with other research studies that have found technical issues such as screen freezes and delayed uploads impede efficient use and limit user uptake of mobile health applications [27, 55, 67]. A lower threshold of data completeness and accuracy for receiving automated reports may have improved usability. Similarly, engaging dedicated data staff to manage the Client Data App may have enhanced its usefulness and acceptance by increasing the number of facilities with minimum completeness standards and automated reports. Other strategies such as rewards and recognition may also have encouraged user uptake in the short term, yet their sustainability is questionable.

Studies conducted with frontline health workers prior to the integration of new technologies into their workflow have revealed high levels of acceptance and willingness to learn, despite the lack of experience with such tools [64, 68, 69]. In many cases, such interest is related to the appeal of innovative technologies as representative of modern medicine [64, 67]. Thus, efforts should be taken to capitalize on and preserve existing positive attitudes during the implementation of mobile health applications by ensuring the usability of new devices. Specifically, incurring higher upfront costs for more advanced mobile handsets may improve data accuracy and user adoption as compared to inexpensive, less user-friendly devices. MOTECH selected the Nokia 1680 model, in part, due to its lower cost (40 USD) [46] for use in Awutu Senya. Yet, as our participants concluded, the small-sized keypad was more problematic than anticipated. In later deployments of MOTECH in Gomoa West as well as the other regions not explored in this evaluation, the phone was upgraded to a more expensive, user-friendly Nokia Asha 200 [40]. The evolution of mobile phones used by MOTECH highlights the value of continually assessing user experiences and reevaluating the trade-offs inherent in each decision. As the participants noted, using larger tablets or laptops in the future may further improve client data management at facility and community levels.

Finally, greater global focus has been placed on ensuring the interoperability of mobile and digital health innovations [38]. The proliferation of multiple disconnected mHealth systems in many countries has led to calls to examine how systems operating in the same country can exchange information across multiple platforms. Systems like OpenHIE (https://ohie.org/) and similar "shared health record" alliances are being explored as a mechanism to allow smaller mHealth products to share connectivity to a central backbone of core information. In our evaluation, participants identified a lack of interoperability with the national DHIMS-2 as an important barrier to maximizing utility. Although often more expensive and time-consuming during development, the future benefits of building mobile applications to global health information standards quickly materialize with increased scale, through interoperability with other facility and national aggregate systems.

Limitations and Strengths. This evaluation was limited by the following factors. First, self-reported data is subject to social desirability bias, and thus participants may have exaggerated their positive reactions to the Client Data App. However, this bias may have been minimized by the fact that the interviewers were external consultants and not affiliated with MOTECH. Second, the transferability of the findings to other MOTECH districts may be limited by the unique situation of the Awutu Senya site. For example, the district health director from Awutu Senya was highly dedicated to and involved in project implementation, which may not be true in other settings. Nevertheless, by engaging with diverse user groups, this evaluation provided rich insights into the Client Data App's implementation challenges from multiple perspectives. The use of two types of qualitative methods further strengthened the credibility of the findings, as later-stage interviews and the focus groups were able to provide feedback on early analyses.

5. Conclusion

Mobile phones hold great promise for overcoming health disparities among rural populations by bridging the gap between access to client health information and service provision. MOTECH's Client Data App is a promising tool to aid health workers in collecting and tracking data across the health care continuum. Results of this evaluation may be used to guide future research on mHealth innovations to address challenges related to infrastructure, human resources, and technology before and during program deployment. Qualitative assessments of user perceptions should remain a priority in efforts to optimize the use of mobile data applications to alleviate barriers to maternal, neonatal, and child care in Ghana and beyond.

Competing Interests

The authors declare that there is no conflict of interests regarding the publication of this paper.

Authors' Contributions

Karen Romano is the principal investigator. Anitha Moorthy, Amnesty E. LeFevre, and Larissa Jennings conceived the aims of the evaluation with input from Fan Yang, Karen Romano, and David Hutchful. Data were collected by Fan Yang and analyzed by Jessica D. Rothstein and Larissa Jennings with contributions from Amnesty E. LeFevre, Fan Yang, and Lisa Gee. Jessica D. Rothstein wrote the first draft of this manuscript with input from Larissa Jennings and Amnesty E. LeFevre. All authors advised subsequent versions of the manuscript and read and approved the final paper.

Acknowledgments

The MOTECH Initiative in Ghana would not have been possible without the partnership with Ghana Health Service, and the authors would like to gratefully thank the leadership and support of national, regional, and district level teams, and staff and health workers in the pilot districts for their active engagement in the program. The authors also thank the participants in the evaluation, as their engagement and sharing of experiences made this research possible. The authors gratefully acknowledge Sena Dzokoto for his assistance during data collection. Funding for MOTECH was provided by the Bill and Melinda Gates Foundation, USAID's Saving Lives at Birth, and the United Nations Foundation. The second author's work on this manuscript was supported by the NIMH Grant no. K01MH107310. Additional support for the Johns Hopkins School of Public Health team came from the World Health Organization's Department of Reproductive Health and Research through the Innovation Working Group Catalytic mHealth Grant Mechanism, managed by the United Nations Foundation with funding from the Norwegian Agency for Development Cooperation (NORAD). This evaluation was conducted by the Grameen Foundation and the Johns Hopkins Bloomberg School of Public Health with support from the World Health Organization.

References

[1] World Health Organization (WHO), *Trends in Maternal Mortality: 1990 to 2015: Estimates by WHO, UNICEF, UNFPA, World Bank Group and the United Nations Population Division*, WHO, Geneva, Switzerland, 2015.

[2] UNICEF, *United Nations Inter-Agency Groups for Child Mortality Estimation (UN-IGME): Levels & Trends in Child Mortality: Report 2015*, UNICEF, New York, NY, USA, 2015.

[3] Ghana Statistical Service (GSS), *Millennium Development Goals in Ghana* , GSS, Accra, Ghana, 2013.

[4] Ghana Statistical Service (GSS), Ghana Health Service (GHS), and ICF International, *Ghana Demographic and Health Survey 2014*, GSS, GHS, and ICF International, Rockville, Md, USA, 2015.

[5] Z. A. Bhutta and R. E. Black, "Global maternal, newborn, and child health," *The New England journal of medicine*, vol. 370, no. 11, p. 1073, 2014.

[6] L. Liu, S. Oza, D. Hogan et al., "Global, regional, and national causes of child mortality in 2000-13, with projections to

inform post-2015 priorities: an updated systematic analysis," *The Lancet*, vol. 385, no. 9966, pp. 430–440, 2015.

[7] Z. A. Bhutta, "Global child survival: beyond numbers," *The Lancet*, vol. 379, no. 9832, pp. 2126–2128, 2012.

[8] P. Welaga, C. A. Moyer, R. Aborigo et al., "Why are babies dying in the first month after birth? A 7-year study of neonatal mortality in northern Ghana," *PLoS ONE*, vol. 8, no. 3, Article ID e58924, 2013.

[9] L. Say, D. Chou, A. Gemmill et al., "Global causes of maternal death: a WHO systematic analysis," *The Lancet Global Health*, vol. 2, no. 6, pp. e323–e333, 2014.

[10] K. J. Kerber, J. E. de Graft-Johnson, Z. A. Bhutta, P. Okong, A. Starrs, and J. E. Lawn, "Continuum of care for maternal, newborn, and child health: from slogan to service delivery," *The Lancet*, vol. 370, no. 9595, pp. 1358–1369, 2007.

[11] B. Ekman, I. Pathmanathan, and J. Liljestrand, "Integrating health interventions for women, newborn babies, and children: a framework for action," *The Lancet*, vol. 372, no. 9642, pp. 990–1000, 2008.

[12] Countdown to 2015, Health Metrics Network, and World Health Organization (WHO), *Monitoring Maternal, Newborn and Child Health: Understanding Key Progress Indicators*, WHO, Geneva, Switzerland, 2012.

[13] N. Puttkammer, J. G. Baseman, E. B. Devine et al., "An assessment of data quality in a multi-site electronic medical record system in Haiti," *International Journal of Medical Informatics*, vol. 86, pp. 104–116, 2016.

[14] V. Yazdi-Feyzabadi, M. Emami, and M. H. Mehrolhassani, "Health information system in primary health care: the challenges and barriers from local providers' perspective of an area in Iran," *International Journal of Preventive Medicine*, vol. 6, no. 1, p. 57, 2015.

[15] R. Bodavala, "Evaluation of Health Management Information System in India: Need for Computerized Databases in HMIS," 1998, https://cdn1.sph.harvard.edu/wp-content/uploads/sites/114/2012/10/rp176.pdf.

[16] A. B. Labrique, L. Vasudevan, E. Kochi, R. Fabricant, and G. Mehl, "mHealth innovations as health system strengthening tools: 12 common applications and a visual framework," *Global Health: Science and Practice*, vol. 1, no. 2, pp. 160–171, 2013.

[17] M. Mitchell, B. L. Hedt-Gauthier, D. Msellemu, M. Nkaka, and N. Lesh, "Using electronic technology to improve clinical care—results from a before-after cluster trial to evaluate assessment and classification of sick children according to Integrated Management of Childhood Illness (IMCI) protocol in Tanzania," *BMC Medical Informatics and Decision Making*, vol. 13, article 95, 2013.

[18] J. F. Florez-Arango, M. S. Iyengar, K. Dunn, and J. Zhang, "Performance factors of mobile rich media job aids for community health workers," *Journal of the American Medical Informatics Association*, vol. 18, no. 2, pp. 131–137, 2011.

[19] I. Mushamiri, C. Luo, C. Iiams-Hauser, and Y. Ben Amor, "Evaluation of the impact of a mobile health system on adherence to antenatal and postnatal care and prevention of mother-to-child transmission of HIV programs in Kenya," *BMC Public Health*, vol. 15, no. 1, article 102, 2015.

[20] W. C. Philbrick, *mHealth and MNCH: State of the Evidence*, mHealth Alliance, UN Foundation, Washington, DC, USA, 2012.

[21] A. Donabedian, "The quality of care. How can it be assessed?" *Journal of the American Medical Association*, vol. 260, no. 12, pp. 1743–1748, 1988.

[22] A. Blank, H. Prytherch, J. Kaltschmidt et al., "'Quality of prenatal and maternal care: bridging the know-do gap' (QUALMAT study): an electronic clinical decision support system for rural Sub-Saharan Africa," *BMC Medical Informatics and Decision Making*, vol. 13, article 44, 2013.

[23] F. Ngabo, J. Nguimfack, F. Nwaigwe et al., "Designing and implementing an innovative SMS-based alert system (RapidSMS-MCH) to monitor pregnancy and reduce maternal and child deaths in Rwanda," *The Pan African Medical Journal*, vol. 13, p. 31, 2012.

[24] B. DeRenzi, L. Findlater, J. Payne et al., "Improving community health worker performance through automated SMS," in *Proceedings of the 5th International Conference on Information and Communication Technologies and Development (ICTD '12)*, pp. 25–34, ACM, Atlanta, Ga, USA, March 2012.

[25] M. Alam, T. Khanam, and R. Khan, "Assessing the scope for use of mobile based solution to improve maternal and child health in Bangladesh: a case study," in *Proceedings of the 4th ACM/IEEE International Conference on Information and Communication Technologies and Development*, London, UK, December 2010.

[26] S. Agarwal, H. B. Perry, L.-A. Long, and A. B. Labrique, "Evidence on feasibility and effective use of mHealth strategies by frontline health workers in developing countries: systematic review," *Tropical Medicine and International Health*, vol. 20, no. 8, pp. 1003–1014, 2015.

[27] L. H. Nguyen, A. E. LeFevre, L. Jennings et al., "Perceptions of data processes in mobile-based versus paper-based health information systems for maternal, newborn and child health: a qualitative study in Andhra Pradesh, India," *BMJ Innovations*, vol. 1, no. 4, pp. 167–173, 2015.

[28] J. Finkelstein and E. M. Cha, "Using a mobile app to promote smoking cessation in hospitalized patients," *JMIR mHealth and uHealth*, vol. 4, no. 2, p. e59, 2016.

[29] A. D. Boyd, K. Moores, V. Shah et al., "My Interventional Drug-Eluting Stent Educational App (MyIDEA): patient-centered design methodology," *JMIR mHealth and uHealth*, vol. 3, no. 3, p. e74, 2015.

[30] B. C. Bock, R. K. Rosen, N. P. Barnett et al., "Translating behavioral interventions onto mHealth platforms: developing text message interventions for smoking and alcohol," *JMIR mHealth and uHealth*, vol. 3, no. 1, article e22, 2015.

[31] C. B. Aranda-Jan, N. Mohutsiwa-Dibe, and S. Loukanova, "Systematic review on what works, what does not work and why of implementation of mobile health (mHealth) projects in Africa," *BMC Public Health*, vol. 14, article 188, 2014.

[32] T. McCurdie, S. Taneva, M. Casselman et al., "mHealth consumer apps: the case for user-centered design," *Biomedical Instrumentation & Technology/Association for the Advancement of Medical Instrumentation*, pp. 49–56, 2012.

[33] C. K. Coursaris and D. J. Kim, "A meta-analytical review of empirical mobile usability studies," *Journal of Usability Studies*, vol. 6, pp. 117–171, 2011.

[34] A. Waugaman, "From principle to practice: implementing the principles for digital development," in *Proceedings of the Principles for Digital Development Working Group*, Washington, DC, USA, 2016.

[35] S. Mookherji, G. Mehl, N. Kaonga, and P. Mechael, "Unmet need: improving mHealth evaluation rigor to build the evidence base," *Journal of Health Communication*, vol. 20, no. 10, pp. 1224–1229, 2015.

[36] A. Labrique, L. Vasudevan, L. W. Chang, and G. Mehl, "H_pe for mHealth: more 'y' or 'o' on the horizon?" *International Journal of Medical Informatics*, vol. 82, no. 5, pp. 467–469, 2013.

[37] E. G. Guba and Y. S. Lincoln, "Competing paradigms in qualitative research," in *Handbook of Qualitative Research*, N. K. Denzin and Y. S. Lincoln, Eds., Sage, Thousand Oaks, Calif, USA, 1994.

[38] PLOS Medicine Editors, "A reality checkpoint for mobile health: three challenges to overcome," *PLoS Medicine*, vol. 10, no. 2, Article ID e1001395, 2013.

[39] K. Keisling, *Introduction to mHealth: How to Approach mHealth*, HealthEnabled, Cape Town, South Africa, 2015.

[40] Grameen Foundation, *Using Mobile Technology to Strengthen Maternal, Newborn, and Child Health: A Case Study of MOTECH's Five Years in Rural Ghana*, Grameen Foundation, Washington, DC, USA, 2015.

[41] Ghana Statistical Service (GSS), *2010 Population & Housing Census: Summary Report of Final Results*, GSS (Ghana Statistical Services), Accra, Ghana, 2012.

[42] Ghana Ministry of Health (MOH), *Holistic Assessment of the Health Sector Programme of Work 2014*, MOH, Accra, Ghana, 2015.

[43] C. A. Peterson, "The global impact of the nursing shortage," *Imprint*, vol. 51, no. 2, pp. 61–63, 2004.

[44] D. Dovlo, "Migration of nurses from Sub-Saharan Africa: a review of issues and challenges," *Health Services Research*, vol. 42, no. 3, pp. 1373–1388, 2007.

[45] J. Buchan and J. Sochalski, "The migration of nurses: trends and policies," *Bulletin of the World Health Organization*, vol. 82, no. 8, pp. 587–594, 2004.

[46] Grameen Foundation, *Mobile Technology for Community Health in Ghana: What It Is and What Grameen Foundation Has Learned So Far*, Grameen Foundation, Washington, DC, USA, 2012.

[47] K. N. Atuoye, J. Dixon, A. Rishworth, S. Z. Galaa, S. A. Boamah, and I. Luginaah, "Can she make it? transportation barriers to accessing maternal and child health care services in rural Ghana," *BMC Health Services Research*, vol. 15, article 333, 2015.

[48] B. B. MacLeod, J. Phillips, A. E. Stone, A. Walji, and J. K. Awoonor-Williams, "The architecture of a software system for supporting community-based primary health care with mobile technology: the Mobile Technology for Community Health (MoTeCH) initiative in Ghana," *Online Journal of Public Health Informatics*, vol. 4, no. 1, 2012.

[49] L. L. English, D. Dunsmuir, E. Kumbakumba et al., "The Paediatric Risk Assessment (PARA) mobile app to reduce postdischarge child mortality: design, usability, and feasibility for health care workers in Uganda," *JMIR mHealth and uHealth*, vol. 4, no. 1, p. e16, 2016.

[50] K. A. Babson, D. E. Ramo, L. Baldini, R. Vandrey, and M. O. Bonn-Miller, "Mobile app-delivered cognitive behavioral therapy for insomnia: feasibility and initial efficacy among veterans with cannabis use disorders," *JMIR Research Protocols*, vol. 4, article e87, 2015.

[51] B. Ploderer, W. Smith, J. Pearce, and R. Borland, "A mobile app offering distractions and tips to cope with cigarette craving: A Qualitative Study," *JMIR mHealth and uHealth*, vol. 2, no. 2, p. e23, 2014.

[52] G. O'Malley, G. Dowdall, A. Burls, I. J. Perry, and N. Curran, "Exploring the usability of a mobile app for adolescent obesity management," *Journal of Medical Internet Research*, vol. 2, no. 2, article e29, 2014.

[53] B. Sheehan and R. J. Lucero, "Initial usability and feasibility evaluation of a personal health record-based self-management system for older adults," *EGEMS*, vol. 3, no. 2, p. 1152, 2015.

[54] D. D. Luxton, M. C. Mishkind, R. M. Crumpton, T. D. Ayers, and V. Mysliwiec, "Usability and feasibility of smartphone video capabilities for telehealth care in the U.S. Military," *Telemedicine and e-Health*, vol. 18, no. 6, pp. 409–412, 2012.

[55] K. H. Chaiyachati, M. Loveday, S. Lorenz et al., "A pilot study of an mHealth application for healthcare workers: poor uptake despite high reported acceptability at a rural South African community-based MDR-TB treatment program," *PLoS ONE*, vol. 8, no. 5, Article ID e64662, 2013.

[56] M. Sandelowski, "Sample size in qualitative research," *Research in Nursing & Health*, vol. 18, no. 2, pp. 179–183, 1995.

[57] P. R. Ulin, *Qualitative Methods in Public Health: A Field Guide for Applied Research*, Josey-Bass, San Francisco, Calif, USA, 2005.

[58] T. A. Schwandt, *Dictionary of Qualitative Inquiry*, Sage, Thousand Oaks, Calif, USA, 2001.

[59] G. A. Tobin and C. M. Begley, "Methodological rigour within a qualitative framework," *Journal of Advanced Nursing*, vol. 48, no. 4, pp. 388–396, 2004.

[60] S. Agarwal, A. E. LeFevre, J. Lee et al., "Guidelines for reporting of health interventions using mobile phones: mobile health (mHealth) evidence reporting and assessment (mERA) checklist," *BMJ*, vol. 352, Article ID i1174, 2016.

[61] N. V. Lemay, T. Sullivan, B. Jumbe, and C. P. Perry, "Reaching remote health workers in Malawi: baseline assessment of a pilot mhealth intervention," *Journal of Health Communication*, vol. 17, supplement 1, pp. 105–117, 2012.

[62] N. Leon, H. Schneider, and E. Daviaud, "Applying a framework for assessing the health system challenges to scaling up mHealth in South Africa," *BMC Medical Informatics and Decision Making*, vol. 12, article 123, 2012.

[63] D. Opoku, P. Scott, and W. Quentin, "Healthcare professionals' perceptions of the benefits and challenges of a teleconsultation service in the amansie-west district of Ghana," *Telemedicine and e-Health*, vol. 21, no. 9, pp. 748–755, 2015.

[64] F. Sukums, N. Mensah, R. Mpembeni, J. Kaltschmidt, W. E. Haefeli, and A. Blank, "Health workers' knowledge of and attitudes towards computer applications in rural African health facilities," *Global Health Action*, vol. 7, no. 1, article no. 24534, 2014.

[65] J. E. Haberer, J. Kiwanuka, D. Nansera, I. B. Wilson, and D. R. Bangsberg, "Challenges in using mobile phones for collection of antiretroviral therapy adherence data in a resource-limited setting," *AIDS and Behavior*, vol. 14, no. 6, pp. 1294–1301, 2010.

[66] L. W. Chang, J. Kagaayi, H. Arem et al., "Impact of a mhealth intervention for peer health workers on AIDS care in rural Uganda: a mixed methods evaluation of a cluster-randomized trial," *AIDS and Behavior*, vol. 15, no. 8, pp. 1776–1784, 2011.

[67] A. S. Ginsburg, J. Delarosa, W. Brunette et al., "mPneumonia: development of an innovative mHealth application for diagnosing and treating childhood pneumonia and other childhood illnesses in low-resource settings," *PLoS ONE*, vol. 10, no. 10, Article ID e0139625, 2015.

[68] S. A. Zakane, L. L. Gustafsson, G. Tomson et al., "Guidelines for maternal and neonatal 'point of care': needs of and attitudes towards a computerized clinical decision support system in rural Burkina Faso," *International Journal of Medical Informatics*, vol. 83, no. 6, pp. 459–469, 2014.

[69] A. A. Medhanyie, A. Moser, M. Spigt et al., "Mobile health data collection at primary health care in Ethiopia: a feasible challenge," *Journal of Clinical Epidemiology*, vol. 68, no. 1, pp. 80–86, 2015.

20

Towards mHealth Systems for Support of Psychotherapeutic Practice: A Qualitative Study of Researcher-Clinician Collaboration in System Design and Evaluation

Karin Halje,[1] Toomas Timpka,[2,3,4] Joakim Ekberg,[2,3] Magnus Bång,[4] Anders Fröberg,[4] and Henrik Eriksson[4]

[1] *Young Adults Centre, Region Östergötland, 58185 Linköping, Sweden*
[2] *Department of Medical and Health Sciences, Linköping University, 58183 Linköping, Sweden*
[3] *Unit for Health Analysis, Centre for Healthcare Development, Region Östergötland, 58185 Linköping, Sweden*
[4] *Department of Computer and Information Science, Linköping University, 58183 Linköping, Sweden*

Correspondence should be addressed to Karin Halje; karin.halje@regionostergotland.se

Academic Editor: Aura Ganz

We examined clinicians' and researchers' experiences from participation in collaborative research on the introduction of Internet and mobile information systems (mHealth systems) in psychotherapeutic routines. The study used grounded theory methodology and was set in a collaboration that aimed to develop and evaluate mHealth support of psychotherapy provided to young people. Soundness of the central objects developed in the design phase (the collaboration contract, the trial protocol, and the system technology) was a necessary foundation for successful collaborative mHealth research; neglect of unanticipated organizational influences during the trial phase was a factor in collaboration failure. The experiences gained in this study can be used in settings where collaborative research on mHealth systems in mental health is planned.

1. Introduction

Various strategies have been proposed for strengthening the connection between intervention research and clinical practice in psychotherapy, for example, publication of treatment manuals supported by randomized controlled trials (RCTs) [1, 2]. Although these strategies contribute to evidence-based practice, many of them also reflect what has been called a "top-down" perspective on collecting and applying scientifically based information [3]. The widespread use of top-down methods for research-based intervention development has led to formulation of the "empirical imperialism" concept, which denotes a situation whereby researchers who themselves see few patients inform clinicians, who rarely participate in research design and therefore seldom influence what should be studied to improve psychotherapy [4]. The existence of a gap between intervention research and clinical practice is at present particularly worrisome in light of the rapid progress of Internet and mobile systems (mHealth systems) in mental health [5]. Less than two decades ago, the research-practice gap in health services meant that it could take up to 17 years before intervention research was translated into practice [6]. Although the situation is likely to have improved, the introduction of mHealth systems into psychotherapeutic practice risks being unnecessarily delayed by the research-practice gap if attention is not paid to the techniques used when these systems are adapted to clinical routines and the methods used when their effectiveness is evaluated [7].

The aim of this exploratory study is to examine clinicians' and researchers' experiences from participation in collaborative research on the introduction of an mHealth system in psychotherapeutic practice. The study is based on collection and analysis of qualitative data in accordance with the grounded theory methodology [8]. With this approach, models of social structures and processes are derived through an inductive process in which qualitative data are analysed to construct "local" theories that explain the data in the context in which they were gathered. The context where data were collected for the present study is a research collaboration aimed at developing and evaluating mHealth support of cognitive behavioural therapy (CBT) for young people with mental health problems.

Research Setting. In 2008, a research collaboration was initiated between the Young Adults Centre in Linköping, Sweden, and researchers at Linköping University. The Young Adults Centre provides psychological services to young adults (16–25 years of age) in Linköping, Åtvidaberg, and Kinda municipalities (combined population 145,000) in Östergötland County, Sweden [9]. The intervention programme follows a predefined structure with a basis in CBT, individually customized into one of four threads based on the client's mental health problems: (1) anxiety, (2) depression, (3) anxiety and depression combined, or (4) decreased well-being without specific anxiety or depression. It consists of six sessions, each lasting 45 minutes. Personalized homework tasks are also assigned to be completed before the next session. A report on the client's progress, including whether the client has expressed any suicidal intent, is routinely recorded. Clients receive whatever psychological treatment their therapist prescribes in parallel with other ongoing interventions, such as provision of practical or social assistance at the employment office, and further medical investigations. Clients continue to receive pharmacotherapy if previously prescribed by their physician. At the last session, a personalized postintervention knowledge and skills maintenance programme is outlined for each client to be used after discharge from the centre. The centre employs four psychotherapists with training in CBT. Self-referral by telephone is the only means for clients to contact the centre. Preliminary admission to the service is regulated by therapist triage by telephone. At the first session in the centre, the nature of the client's problems is evaluated. After this evaluation, clients are offered one of two alternatives: self-help instructions within the remaining session for clients with minor problems or a structured psychological intervention programme.

The aim of the research collaboration was to develop and evaluate mHealth support of CBT. The collaboration involved two research steps: meetings and workshops where the mHealth systems and trial design were conceived and the performance of the trial. The clinical trial was assessed and approved by the regional ethical review board in Linköping (Dnr. 111-09). For the first step, a PD approach was used whereby therapists, researchers, and information system developers worked together. The mHealth system was outlined in a series of design meetings with therapists and technically implemented as a smartphone application. The evaluation of the mHealth system was performed as an RCT [10]. The main aim of the trial was to examine whether mHealth systems can lead to improved treatment. A secondary goal was to study whether the mHealth technology aided treatment adherence. The inclusion criteria for the trial was that the client was 18–25 years of age and had scored seven points or higher on the anxiety subscale of the Hospital Anxiety Depression Scale (HADS) [11].

Background. A first basis for efficacious introduction of mHealth systems in psychotherapy is a reciprocal knowledge transfer between information system designers and clinical practitioners. Several approaches for human-centred information systems development have been reported, ranging from participatory design (PD) [12] to usability engineering [13] and contextual design [14]. PD was introduced for use in situations when social factors and work practice experiences were anticipated to be of particular importance for successful system implementation [15]. The first generation of PD methods, also denoted by collective systems design [16], was developed for industrial workplaces with support from trade unions, with the objective that the resulting IT-supported production systems should enhance workplace democracy and increase worker autonomy, skill set, and task variety. System users were given direct influence on the design through participation in design groups where they contributed with organizational and work task knowledge. The design methodology, based on techniques such as mock-up evaluations and future workshops [17], was straightforward to learn and put low demand on users' prior knowledge. A second generation of PD was characterized by a shift towards the commercial setting and by embracing teamwork and finding points of contact with the area of computer-supported cooperative work [18, 19]. However, several authors pointed out that even this generation of PD was seldom used in large, product-oriented projects and that, once it was applied, it resulted in only small-scale stand-alone IT applications [20, 21]. A third generation of PD emerged as a response to this criticism, providing means for adaptations to organizational trends, large organizations and projects, interorganizational collaboration, and networking, and with increased consideration of third parties (clients, customers) in the systems development process [22]. In parallel, design methods with their origin in PD have also been incorporated into general methods for the development of eHealth systems including those based on ubiquitous technologies [23].

Another basis for the introduction of mHealth systems in routine psychotherapy is a functional collaboration between clinical researchers and practicing psychotherapists [24]. For several decades, efforts have been made to reduce the research-practice gap in psychotherapy. An early attempt was presented in the Boulder model, a structure for scientist-practitioner collaboration that was developed in the 1950s [25]. However, before long, studies on psychological treatment in mental health practice showed that when the selective inclusion criteria used in experimental settings could no longer be applied, the observed effects on patients decreased [26]. Although a strong consensus that a scientific approach should permeate psychotherapeutic practices remains, it has repeatedly been suggested that experimental research can lead to unrealistic and overly optimistic beliefs about what evidence-based treatment can provide in everyday clinical practice [27]. Inspired by the work of Sobell [28], the Society of Clinical Psychology, Division 12 of the American

Psychological Association (APA), began therefore in 2010 an initiative to build a two-way bridge between research and practice [29]. A feedback mechanism was presented similar to that employed by the FDA; that is, after the introduction of an evidence-based treatment, practitioners can offer feedback based on their clinical experiences in using the treatment in practice. This two-way bridge model for obtaining feedback on the use of empirically supported therapies in practice was expanded in 2011 to become a collaborative effort together with the Division of Psychotherapy of the APA—Division 29. The practice research network (PRN) is another recent approach to facilitate integration between research and practice. A PRN is based on active collaboration between researchers and clinicians in the development of relevant clinical studies that are also profoundly scientific [1, 3]. This approach suggests that collaboration can help the psychotherapy field move beyond the efforts of building bridges between research and practice. Rather than conceiving the scientist-practitioner collaborations as links between two groups of individuals, creation of unified landscapes of knowledge is conceived where clinicians and therapists are working together on clinically actionable and scientifically rigorous studies. A concept closely related to the PRN approach is psychotherapy integration [30]. This notion highlights structural advances with regard to theoretical integration, technical eclectic, common factors, and assimilative integration and has been suggested for psychotherapy research and practice in areas such as harmful effects, therapist effects, practice-oriented research, and training.

2. Methods

The study was based on a cross-sectional design and used qualitative methods for data collection and analyses. According to Swedish legislation, the research did not require a separate review of ethical considerations.

2.1. Data Collection. Semistructured interviews took place with four psychotherapists and five researchers who had participated in the collaborative research at the Young Adults Centre. The interviews were conducted by a behavioural scientist who had not participated in the research study. The interview questions were aimed at uncovering what the clinicians and researchers had experienced when participating in the multidisciplinary research, as well as their recommendations for future studies [3]:

(A) What have you found to be most interesting and/or useful in your participation in the study?

(B) What have you found to be difficult and/or frustrating with your participation?

(C) What, if any, parts of this study have benefited and/or have entailed a risk to patients?

(D) What has been the most frequent and/or important obstacle to conduct the study? and

(E) If you confronted significant barriers when the study was conducted, what, if anything, has helped you to deal with these obstacles?

Further clarifying questions were posed when found necessary. The interviews lasted about 30 minutes and were transcribed from audio recordings. The transcribed data comprised about 30 printed pages of text.

2.2. Data Analysis. The data analysis based in the grounded theory methodology involved dividing the interview data into smaller units, conceptualization and coding of these units, and combining the labelled units into increasingly complex structures [8]. Initially, interview data were read thoroughly and notes were taken. At each step of the analysis, the data from two groups (researchers and clinicians) were analysed both separately and combined in order to allow comparisons. Three coding steps were performed: open coding, axial coding, and selective coding. These coding steps were performed iteratively, as they were revisited when categories or categorizations needed to be adjusted or added to. The open coding involved breaking down the interview data into smaller units, and iteratively examining, conceptualizing, comparing, and categorizing these units. Examples of typical codes applied at this level include "attitude-cooperation-researcher" and "experience-planning-clinician." In the axial coding, the categories of data units were related to each other by searching for associations between them. These associations were sought on the basis of, for instance, consequences, context, interactions, and influencing factors. At this level, the categories involved instances such as "cooperation endpoints," "surprising events," and "inspiring happenings." In the selective coding, the main (central) categories were selected and how they related to each other was tentatively described. For this categorization, the categories were divided into those associated with objects manufactured in the research process and social phenomena, respectively. Thereafter, the previous coding steps were revisited in order to identify categories that needed to be refined or added. Finally, a small-scale theory was formulated in terms of graphical models based on a conditional matrix, that is, charts that suggest causality and interactions between the different artefacts and phenomena identified in the analyses. The analyses were performed by the first author (Karin Halje). Preliminary results were then presented to the remaining authors. Adjustments were then made based on the feedback obtained. The procedure was repeated until no further significant comments emerged.

3. Results

Three manufactured objects and three social phenomena constituted the central concepts in the clinicians' and researchers' accounts of their experiences from the two phases of the collaborative research process (Table 1).

3.1. Participatory Design Phase. At the beginning of the PD phase, the researchers and the clinical system users jointly developed a structure for the collaborative research process. This structure was documented in the "participatory design contract." This contract defined the structure and process of this phase and included descriptions of, for instance, the frequency, length, content, and leadership of the joint

TABLE 1: Central concepts in the participants' accounts of their experiences from the collaborative research.

Manufactured objects	
A1	Participatory design contract: the document describing the mHealth system development process; that is, how the joint meetings were to be led, the frequency of meetings, the communications routines, and so forth
A2	Trial protocol: the document describing the procedures that were to be followed before and after a client had agreed to be included in the evaluation trial
A3	mHealth system technology: the software applications in smartphones and on the server, the clinicians' interface, and the data storage and communication infrastructure
Social phenomena	
SP1	Shared commitment: motivation and interest among the parties involved in the research
SP2	Organizational environment of the mHealth system: legislation, bureaucratic formalities, staff replacements, workload, and so forth
SP3	The clinician-client relationship: the relationship between the clinician and client during the treatment process and its quality with regard to factors such as alliance, adherence, homework completion, and so forth

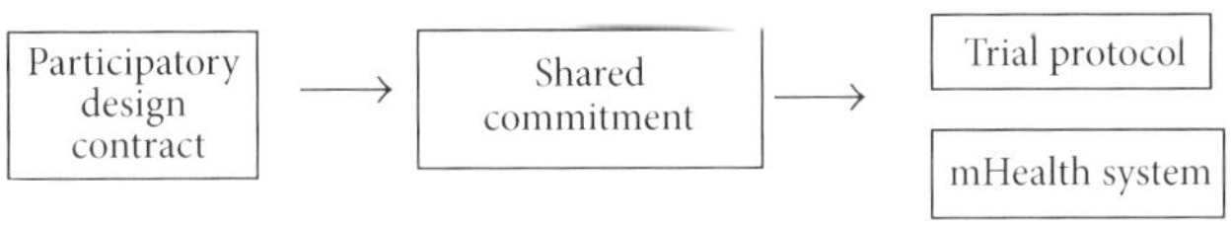

FIGURE 1: Model of the relationships identified in the analysis of the participatory design phase.

meetings that constituted the research process (Figure 1). One researcher expressed "It is important to have joint meetings at the beginning so that you really share what it's all about. And then go through the routines even more clearly" (Researcher 2). At these initial meetings, a shared foundation for the research was developed, including a mutual interest in each other's (researchers and clinicians) activities. This shared commitment to the foundations also included an openness to learn from each other, as expressed in the following quotes: "It has been interesting to have had the opportunity to understand how to plan research, because I have not been involved in such undertakings before" (Clinician 4). "... The most rewarding was the cooperation between the practitioners, technical researchers, and clinical researchers. I think this was interesting and fun" (Researcher 3). An interest in each other's work practices was noted among the clinicians, which provided them with motivation for increased involvement in the study. Another clinician expressed "... we could be more consistent in how we actually work" (Clinician 2). In this collaborative setting, the mHealth system and the trial protocol were elaborated. Implementation of the system based on the clinicians' preferences further increased the clinicians' commitment to the research. One of the clinicians stated that "It was interesting to be involved in designing an app that may help people cope with difficult situations when anxiety problems are encountered" (Clinician 4). Only a few negative experiences were reported from the PD phase. An example was when participating in the PD procedures interfered with and influenced the therapeutic process. A clinician explained that "... it was [sometimes] hard to decide if I really should squeeze in participation [in the PD process], because clients may have come with difficult problems and I could have been way behind my schedule already" (Clinician 4).

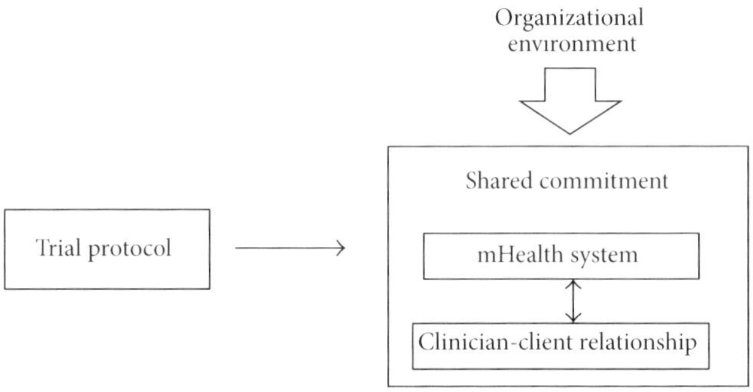

FIGURE 2: Model of the relationships identified in the analysis of the trial phase.

3.2. Trial Phase. In the trial phase of the collaborative research, organizational structures, systems, and processes that were not considered and controlled in the trial protocol were found to influence the research setting, and, in consequence, the shared foundations and commitment (Figure 2). At the start of this phase, the trial protocol that was jointly defined in the PD phase was approved by the regional research ethics committee and recorded in an international clinical trial registry (NCT01205191 at clinicaltrials.gov). In consequence, it was no longer possible to make substantial changes to the research process. However, a number of issues not addressed in the protocol were found to affect this process. One example of such external influence is that the legislation, procurement regulations, and bureaucracy associated with the payment of mobile network operator charges at times made the mHealth system unusable even though it was technically functional. One of the researchers explained that these influences were not easy to foresee: "I should have made sure I had enough research budget so I could solve these everyday problems without having to go through a lot of individuals to obtain permission to complete the payments and ensure that there was money in the account" (Researcher 3). Also, when they were encountered and comprehended as facts, problems with their origin outside the clinical and academic contexts in which the research was planned were not easy to solve: "... these mobile phone call payments were one of those things that caused problems. The regulations and procurement procedures made me to try to improvise a solution [outside the university routines] that worked with the actual network contracts" (Researcher 8). Another issue had its basis in the fact that the study was carried out at a small clinical unit with only four full-time positions. This situation meant that the trial was noticeably vulnerable to spells of absence in the clinician group. Throughout the study period, at least one of the regular staff members was on parental or sick leave. In parallel, three of the four regular clinicians were also absent part-time (30% each) for academic studies. Although replacements were employed, the unit was not adequately staffed at times in relation to client pressure. These problems were expressed by one of the researchers as follows: "... the clinic reflects working life of today. Employees are on sick leave or parental leave. New employees arrive and others disappear for good. These are not the kind of conditions you want to face when you are going to conduct a scientific evaluation, but the fact is reality. ... This turnover ... needs to be taken into account when [a trial] is organized. And also who is holding the responsibility for what should be decided" (Researcher 6). The replacements who were introduced into the trial received information individually about the study protocol by a member of the regular staff. Although each temporary staff member received individual instructions, their knowledge and commitment to the study were not at the same level as those of the regular staff. A clinician commented as follows: "Another thing that has been difficult and frustrating is the lack of continuity in the clinical staff presence ..., which has made it necessary to hire replacements .... This has had an impact on the trial" (Clinician 5).

Both the clinicians and the researchers perceived that organizational and bureaucratic factors with their origin outside the clinical and academic contexts in which the research was planned had come to influence the process and outcome of the clinical trial. However, although the clinicians believed that the unforeseen issues with the mHealth system, such as the problems with the smartphone payments, affected the treatment quality negatively, they also found that the system affected the treatment positively when it worked and brought a new dimension to the clinical practice. This stance with multiple perspectives is exemplified by the following statements: "I think that we have provided a better service via the app due to the fact that young people can use it to finish their homework assignments more easily than on paper. And they can more easily retrieve information to read about their problems .... [The system] also makes it easier for me to read about the homework I give them" (Clinician 4). The different organizational influences on the trial process thus made it hard for the clinicians themselves to recognize their original treatment-as-usual setting and whether the different experimental conditions involving the mHealth system had significantly improved or distorted clinical practice.

4. Discussion

The aim of this study was to explore clinicians' and researchers' experiences from participating in collaborative research on mHealth systems for support of psychotherapeutic practice. We identified objects manufactured in the research process (the PD contract, the trial protocol, and the mHealth technology) that constituted the reference points for the participants' experiences and observed consensus that, in the PD phase, mutual learning in regular meetings, shared commitment to the multidisciplinary design group, and daily communication between researchers and clinicians characterized the collaborative research. However, in the trial phase, organizational factors with their origin outside the setting in which the study was planned were found to have had a decisive influence on the experiences. In addition, in this phase, the researchers' and clinicians' experiences differed; the clinicians provided several post hoc examples of negative influences on clients from study participation, whereas the researchers explained that it was difficult to foresee such side effects in detail and they regarded these effects as a part of the knowledge obtained. Differences between researchers and clinicians have previously been explained by the fundamentals of their respective professions [31]; researchers strive for maintenance of controlled research conditions and clinicians focus on the best therapy for the client. These explanations are thus applicable to the present study. Nevertheless, despite these foundational differences, a shared perception of the collaborative research was created and sustained in the PD phase of the research by meetings where each other's "cultures/languages" were learnt and knowledge about each other's areas of activity was developed. Establishing interpersonal relationships, trust, and a shared culture/language has also been reported from other settings as essential factors for building sustainable collaborations between psychotherapists and researchers [32]. Yet, the prestudy differences in professional fundamentals became apparent again in the evaluation phase, when, according to the trial protocol, the clinicians were left to solve the problems that occurred independently. In consequence, as the technical-practical problems accumulated, the trial protocol was considered by the clinicians to interfere with the psychotherapy, and, in particular, introduced an adverse impact on creating alliances with clients. To minimize these effects, we infer that the ways that the evaluation procedures could affect clients should have been discussed in even greater detail in the design phase.

The results show that the PD approach seemingly was functional for the development of mHealth systems to support psychotherapeutic practice; obstacles to the collaborative research mainly surfaced in the trial phase. In the trial phase, uncontrolled influences from external social systems, such as legalization and staff management routines in the health service organization, had an impact on the trial performance, dedication to the collaborative research and, as perceived by the clinicians, the psychotherapeutic treatment. Thus it is important to identify and control possible external influences at the design phase in collaborations aiming to develop mHealth systems that support psychotherapeutic practice. The problems that arose with the smartphones in the present study can be seen as evidence of the need to ascertain that the planned mHealth system can be safely sustained over sufficient periods of time in the evaluation setting before the formal trial is initiated. In the present study, a pilot test involving three young adults, who not were clients, was performed over a 2- to 3-week period. This test was deemed successful and it was concluded that the trial could begin. What was not taken into account was that, in the RCT, smartphone use by one client could well extend to several months (which was a normal treatment time). This led to a need to introduce a way for a third party (the researchers) to pay for the clients' smartphone charges in the clinical setting over lengthy periods of time, yet not allowing abuse of the smartphone accounts. It is likely that if the pilot tests had been performed in a setting that more closely resembled the RCT conditions, including real clients over a longer period of time, these problems would have been detected and solved before the trial was initiated. This said, it is also probable that involvement of clients already in the PD phase of the collaborative research would have prevented at least some of the problems associated with phone use in practice. These experiences can be added to the recently published guidelines for evaluations of mobile mental health applications [33].

The present study has both strengths and limitations that need to be considered when interpreting the results. In the qualitative data analysis context, theoretical sensitivity means that professional experiences and personal life understandings can be utilized in data processing [8]. Theoretical sensitivity thus denotes an extended ability to recognize important data and meaningful interpretations in a particular context. A strength of the present study is that the theoretical sensitivity of the multiprofessional group analysing the data can be regarded as having covered all of the most important aspects of the study setting, that is, psychotherapeutic practice as well as clinical and informatics research. An associated potential limitation of the study is that the research was performed in a self-evaluation setting; all authors also participated in the collaborative research. Holme and Krohn Solvang [34] mentioned four elements that are crucial for avoiding bias when planning interviews and interpreting the collected data: (a) the interview themes (topics may be sensitive to discuss), (b) respondent roles (expectations on "correct" behaviour), (c) respondent competences (knowledge of interview topics), and (d) interview setting (the environment restricts data provision). To decrease the risk of interview topics being perceived as too sensitive to discuss, in this study, a behavioural scientist who did not participate in the collaborative research was appointed to conduct the interviews. Also, the behavioural scientist was asked to adjust each interview setting according to the respondent's requests. Five researchers, one technician, and four clinicians were interviewed, all of whom had participated in the research study from the beginning and should therefore have had sufficient competence to provide reliable data. Due to their lesser knowledge of the research process, the two replacements who participated for short periods of time were not interviewed; the administrative head of the Young Adults Clinic was also not interviewed. However, during the data analyses, it was found that interviews with these clinicians would probably have added further information. It is difficult to assess whether role behaviours influenced the results. The data provided in the interviews and the analysis may have been biased by prearranged positive or negative attitudes to the project or intentions to "save face" or point out scapegoats. However, during the initial analysis, the first author was careful not to let her own interests influence the process by constantly writing down notes and memos [8]. This process was repeated when the remaining authors iteratively reviewed the preliminary results and provided comments. Theoretical thoughts appearing during the course of the analysis were thus documented when moving from smaller units of analysis to broader categorization to ensure that the analysis was based on trustworthy and nonpartial interpretations of the data. We therefore trust that role behaviours had a minute or no influence on the results presented.

5. Conclusions

This study of clinicians' and researchers' experiences from participating in collaborative research on the introduction of an mHealth system in psychotherapeutic practice showed that the application of PD techniques narrowed the gap between researchers and clinicians in the initial system design phase, whereas maintenance of the collaboration during the trial phase was disturbed by unforeseen organizational and bureaucratic problems. The main lessons learnt are that the correctness and soundness of the central objects developed in the initial design phase (collaboration contract, trial protocol, and system components) constitute the necessary foundation for successful collaborative research; lack of preparedness for influences from unanticipated social influences during the trial phase is a factor in collaboration failure. Before the evaluative trial, the functions of the mHealth system and details of the trial protocol should be verified by extended pilot tests involving real clients in order to avoid negative influence on the therapist-client relationship, and, correspondingly, on the clinicians' commitment to participate in the research. The experiences gained in this study can be used in other settings in which collaborative research on mHealth systems in psychotherapeutic practice is planned.

References

[1] L. G. Castonguay, J. F. Boswell, S. E. Zack et al., "Helpful and hindering events in psychotherapy: a practice research network study," *Psychotherapy: Theory, Research, Practice, Training*, vol. 47, no. 3, pp. 327–344, 2010.

[2] G. C. Davison, "Being bolder with the boulder model: the challenge of education and training in empirically supported treatments," *Journal of Consulting and Clinical Psychology*, vol. 66, no. 1, pp. 163–167, 1998.

[3] L. G. Castonguay, D. L. Nelson, M. A. Boutselis et al., "Psychotherapists, researchers, or both? A qualitative analysis of psychotherapists' experiences in a practice research network," *Psychotherapy: Theory, Research, Practice, Training*, vol. 47, no. 3, pp. 345–354, 2010.

[4] G. K. Lampropoulos, M. R. Goldfried, L. G. Castonguay, M. J. Lambert, W. B. Stiles, and J. N. Nestoros, "What kind of research can we realistically expect from the practitioner?" *Journal of Clinical Psychology*, vol. 58, no. 10, pp. 1241–1264, 2002.

[5] Z. Hilvert-Bruce, P. J. Rossouw, N. Wong, M. Sunderland, and G. Andrews, "Adherence as a determinant of effectiveness of internet cognitive behavioural therapy for anxiety and depressive disorders," *Behaviour Research and Therapy*, vol. 50, no. 7-8, pp. 463–468, 2012.

[6] E. A. Balas, S. Weingarten, C. T. Garb, D. Blumenthal, S. A. Boren, and G. D. Brown, "Improving preventive care by prompting physicians," *Archives of Internal Medicine*, vol. 160, no. 3, pp. 301–308, 2000.

[7] D. A. Chambers, R. E. Glasgow, and K. C. Stange, "The dynamic sustainability framework: addressing the paradox of sustainment amid ongoing change," *Implementation Science*, vol. 8, article 117, 2013.

[8] A. Strauss and J. Corbin, *Basics of Qualitative Research. Grounded Theory Procedures and Techniques*, Sage, Newbury Park, Calif, USA, 1991.

[9] K. Halje, T. Timpka, P. Tylestedt et al., "Self-referral psychological treatment centre for young adults: two-year observational evaluation of routine practice before and after treatment," *BMJ Open*, vol. 5, no. 8, Article ID e008030, 2015.

[10] J. Ekberg, T. Timpka, M. Bång, A. Fröberg, K. Halje, and H. Eriksson, "Cell phone-supported cognitive behavioural therapy for anxiety disorders: a protocol for effectiveness studies in frontline settings," *BMC Medical Research Methodology*, vol. 11, article 3, 2011.

[11] I. Bjelland, A. A. Dahl, T. T. Haug, and D. Neckelmann, "The validity of the Hospital Anxiety and Depression Scale. An updated literature review," *Journal of Psychosomatic Research*, vol. 52, no. 2, pp. 69–77, 2002.

[12] J. Clemensen, S. B. Larsen, M. Kyng, and M. Kirkevold, "Participatory design in health sciences: using cooperative experimental methods in developing health services and computer technology," *Qualitative Health Research*, vol. 17, no. 1, pp. 122–130, 2007.

[13] A. W. Kushniruk and V. L. Patel, "Cognitive and usability engineering methods for the evaluation of clinical information systems," *Journal of Biomedical Informatics*, vol. 37, no. 1, pp. 56–76, 2004.

[14] J. L. Martin, E. Murphy, J. A. Crowe, and B. J. Norris, "Capturing user requirements in medical device development: the role of ergonomics," *Physiological Measurement*, vol. 27, no. 8, pp. R49–R62, 2006.

[15] C. Floyd, W.-M. Mehl, F.-M. Reisin, G. Schmidt, and G. Wolf, "Out of Scandinavia: alternative approaches to software design and system development," *Human-Computer Interaction*, vol. 4, no. 4, pp. 253–350, 1989.

[16] P. Ehn and M. Kyng, "The collective resource approach to systems design," in *Computers and Democracy—a Scandinavian Challenge*, G. Bjerknes, P. Ehn, and M. Kyng, Eds., pp. 17–58, Avebury, Aldershot, UK, 1987.

[17] P. Ehn and R. Badham, "Participatory design and the collective designer," in *Proceedings of the Participatory Design Conference*, T. Binder, J. Gregory, and I. Wagner, Eds., pp. 1–10, CPSR, Malmö, Sweden, June 2002.

[18] A. M. Oostveen and P. van den Besselar, "From small scale to large scale user participation: a case study of participatory design in Egovernment systems," in *Proceedings of the Participatory Design Conference*, pp. 173–182, CPSR, Palo Alto, Calif, USA, 2004.

[19] P. van den Besselar, "Democratizing technological change: limits to steering," in *Proceedings of the Participatory Design Conference*, R. Henderson Chatfield, S. Kuhn, and M. Muller, Eds., pp. 1–10, CPSR, Palo Alto, Calif, USA, 1998.

[20] J. Greenbaum, "Post modern times. Participation beyond the workplace," in *Proceedings of the Participatory Design Conference*, J. Blomberg, F. Kensing, and E. A. Dykstra-Erickson, Eds., pp. 65–72, CPSR, Palo Alto, Calif, USA, 1996.

[21] F. Kensing, "Participatory design in a commercial context—a conceptual framework," in *Proceedings of the Participatory Design Conference, Designing digital environments*, T. Chrekasky, J. Greenbaum, P. Mambrey, and J. Pors, Eds., New York, NY, USA, 2000.

[22] S. Pilemalm and T. Timpka, "Third generation participatory design in health informatics—making user participation applicable to large-scale information system projects," *Journal of Biomedical Informatics*, vol. 41, no. 2, pp. 327–339, 2008.

[23] M. van Limburg, J. E. W. C. van Gemert-Pijnen, N. Nijland, H. C. Ossebaard, R. M. G. Hendrix, and E. R. Seydel, "Why business modeling is crucial in the development of eHealth technologies," *Journal of Medical Internet Research*, vol. 13, no. 4, article e124, 2011.

[24] T. D. Borkovec, R. J. Echemendia, S. A. Ragusea, and M. Ruiz, "The Pennsylvania practice research network and future possibilities for clinically meaningful and scientifically rigorous psychotherapy effectiveness research," *Clinical Psychology: Science and Practice*, vol. 8, no. 2, pp. 155–167, 2001.

[25] C. Peterson and N. Park, "The enduring value of the Boulder model: 'upon this rock we will build'," *Journal of Clinical Psychology*, vol. 61, no. 9, pp. 1147–1150, 2005.

[26] B. E. Wampold, *The Great Psychotherapy Debate: Models, Methods, and Findings*, Lawrence Erlbaum, Mahwah, NJ, USA, 2001.

[27] D. Shapiro, "Renewing the scientist-practitioner model," *The Psychologist*, vol. 15, no. 5, pp. 232–233, 2002.

[28] L. C. Sobell, "Bridging the gap between scientists and practitioners: the challenge before us," *Behavior Therapy*, vol. 27, no. 3, pp. 297–320, 1996.

[29] M. R. Goldfried, M. G. Newman, L. G. Castonguay et al., "On the dissemination of clinical experiences in using empirically supported treatments," *Behavior Therapy*, vol. 45, no. 1, pp. 3–6, 2014.

[30] L. G. Castonguay, C. F. Eubanks, M. R. Goldfried, J. C. Muran, and W. Lutz, "Research on psychotherapy integration: building on the past, looking to the future," *Psychotherapy Research*, vol. 25, no. 3, pp. 365–382, 2015.

[31] B. E. Wolfe, "Healing the research-practice split: let's start with me," *Psychotherapy*, vol. 49, no. 2, pp. 101–108, 2012.

[32] A. F. Garland and L. Brookman-Frazee, "Therapists and researchers: advancing collaboration," *Psychotherapy Research*, vol. 25, no. 1, pp. 95–107, 2015.

[33] S. Chan, J. Torous, L. Hinton, and P. Yellowlees, "Towards a framework for evaluating mobile mental health apps," *Telemedicine and e-Health*, vol. 21, no. 12, pp. 1038–1041, 2015.

[34] M. I. Holme and B. K. Krohn Solvang, *Forskningsmetodik. Om Kvalitativa Och Kvantitativa Metoder*, Studentlitteratur, Lund, Sweden, 1991.

21

Ruling Out Brain CT Contraindications prior to Intravenous Thrombolysis: Diagnostic Equivalence between a Primary Interpretation Workstation and a Mobile Tablet Computer

Antonio J. Salazar,[1] Nicolás Useche,[2,3] Manuel Granja,[4] Aníbal J. Morillo,[2,3] and Sonia Bermúdez[2,3]

[1] *Electrophysiology and Telemedicine Laboratory, University of Los Andes, Carrera 1 Este No. 19A-40, Bogotá, Colombia*
[2] *Primary Stroke Center, University Hospital of Fundación Santa Fe de Bogotá, Calle 119 No. 7-75, Bogotá, Colombia*
[3] *School of Medicine, Universidad El Bosque, Av. Cra 9 No. 131A-02, Bogotá, Colombia*
[4] *Baptist Health, Lyerly Neurosurgery, 800 Prudential Drive, Jacksonville, FL 32207, USA*

Correspondence should be addressed to Antonio J. Salazar; ant-sala@uniandes.edu.co

Academic Editor: Malcolm Clarke

Objective. The aim of this study was to evaluate the equivalence of brain CT interpretations performed using a diagnostic workstation and a mobile tablet computer, in a telestroke service. *Materials and Methods*. The ethics committee of our institution approved this retrospective study. A factorial design with 1452 interpretations was used. The assessed variables were the type of stroke classification, the presence of contraindications to the tPA administration, the presence of a hyperdense intracranial artery sign (HMCA), and the Alberta Stroke Program Early CT Score (ASPECTS) score. These variables were evaluated to determine the effect that the reading system had on their magnitudes. *Results*. The achieved distribution of observed lesions using both the reading systems was not statistically different. The differences between the two reading systems to claim equivalence were 1.6% for hemorrhagic lesions, 4.5% for cases without lesion, and 5.2 for overall ischemic lesion. Equivalence was achieved at 2.1% for ASPECTS ≤ 6, 6.5% for the presence of imaging contraindication to the tPA administration, and 7.2% for the presence of HMCA. *Conclusion*. The diagnostic performance for detecting acute stroke is likely equivalent whether a tablet computer or a diagnostic workstation is used or not.

1. Introduction

A stroke is an acute neurologic dysfunction of vascular origin that involves focal areas in the brain and is a major cause of death and disability in developed [1–3] and developing countries [4] such as ours (Colombia) [5–7]. A stroke can be ischemic (near 87% of cases) or hemorrhagic, and both require different treatments and neurological and radiological expertise for diagnosis. For ischemic stroke, the early administration of tissue plasminogen activator (tPA) reduces disability, as measured by the modified Rankin scale (mRs) at 90 days, but only if it is administered before 4.5 hours [8]. However, even in countries such as the US, only 5% of eligible patients receive this treatment [8] due to geographic distances to primary stroke centers and the limited availability of vascular neurologists and neuroradiologist that after a complete neurological and radiological assessment define if a patient is eligible to receive this treatment. Noncontrast brain computed tomography (CT) is the most widely used method for the first imaging examination in patients with acute stroke symptoms [9].

The aim of this study was to evaluate the diagnostic equivalence of brain CT interpretations when using a primary diagnostic interpretation workstation and a mobile tablet computer in an emergency telestroke setting after providing radiologists with real clinical scenarios. The assessed variables were the distribution of the type of stroke classification, the detection of the presence of any imaging contraindication to the tPA administration for acute ischemic lesions, confidence in the presence of a hyperdense intracranial artery sign (HMCA), the Alberta Stroke Program Early CT Score (ASPECTS) [10], and the reading time. These variables were evaluated to determine the effect that the reading system had on their magnitudes as well as the variables' equivalence between the reading systems.

We were interested in evaluating mobile solutions to be used for telestroke at our hospital. By means of real clinical scenarios that included a complete clinical background, specific neurological symptoms, and the time of symptoms onset, we designed this study to perform image interpretations as closely and realistically as in routine clinical practice, using, first, emergency brain CT images instead of computer tomography angiography (CTA). We used the same radiologists who routinely read brain CT images in our hospital (i.e., neuroradiologists and neuroradiology fellows), and the same clinical information provided to radiologists in clinical practice (e.g., admission diagnosis, neurological symptoms, age, and sex). In addition, the same interpretation process was conducted, in which the type of stroke (i.e., hemorrhagic lesion, acute ischemic lesion, chronic ischemic lesion, or without lesion) was classified. Furthermore, according to the selected lesion type, the radiologist classified other variables: the presence of any imaging contraindication to the tPA administration; confidence in the presence of the hyperdense middle cerebral artery sign (HMCA); and the ASPECTS score (ranging from 1–10), which is a method for assessing the size of an infarct on CT scans in patients with acute stroke to determine when to administer the tPA treatment. Patients with ASPECTS scores less than or equal to six or with the presence of any other imaging contraindication for the tPA administration are not eligible to receive intravenous tPA; therefore, it is critical to detect these group of patients by means of brain CT scans. Although previous studies [9, 11–15] have evaluated the potential equivalence between diagnostic workstations and mobile tablet computers for the interpretation of stroke brain CT scans they lack the specific statistical methods used here along with the selected variables considered in our paper. Scoring variables like the ASPECTS were obtained after providing radiologists with a complete clinical background of anonymous patients and also considering common imaging CT contraindications for tPA administration. This whole approach resembles a real-life scenario just like the diagnostic process of any acute stroke patient.

No significant differences have been reported to support the null hypothesis that the performances of different reading methods are equal and because the power test was not reported, it is not clear if these studies failed to find significant differences given that failure to reject the null hypothesis does not mean this hypothesis is necessary true. In contrast, the present study was set to evaluate equivalence or noninferiority based on significant results. To establish the fact that the performances are equal or that one modality is noninferior to the other, the null hypothesis has to be that their performances are not equal or that one is inferior to the other. Only by rejecting such a hypothesis can it be concluded that the modalities under comparison are equivalent [16–19].

2. Materials and Methods

This retrospective study was approved by the ethics committee of our institution, and informed consent was not required. We employed a factorial design with repeated measures.

2.1. Sample. Patients with symptoms of acute stroke, who presented to the emergency room for acute stroke evaluation between 2013 and 2016 at the Blinded University Hospital (Blinded), were included in the study. Our hospital is a primary Joint Commission International- (JCI-) certified stroke center with endovascular treatment capabilities. The patients were randomly selected without repetition. Cases with image artifacts were excluded. The cases consisted of brain CT examinations stored in our hospital PACS, which were acquired using a General Electric LightSpeed 64 slice CT scanner (General Electric Healthcare, GE Medical Systems, Milwaukee, WI, USA), with 100 kV, 10 mAs, axial: 5 mm, sagittal: 3 mm, FOV: 26 cm, pixel spacing: 0.469, matrix: 512 × 512, and pitch: 0.984:1.

Based on a neuroradiologist routine primary diagnostic interpretation, the sample included patients without lesions (7) and those with hemorrhagic lesions (11), acute ischemic lesions (67), and chronic ischemic lesions (36). The ages ranged from 30 to 97 years, with a mean age of 70.8 years (standard deviation of 15.2). There were 59 males and 62 females.

2.2. Observers and Reading Observed Variables. Five neuroradiologists (three with more than ten years of experience) and one neuroradiology fellow were selected as observers. They were asked to classify the type of stroke (i.e., hemorrhagic lesion, acute ischemic lesion, chronic ischemic lesion, or without lesion). For acute ischemic lesions, the radiologists classified variables that included contraindications to the tPA administration for acute ischemic lesions (e.g., subacute ischemic stroke, intra-axial neoplasm, arteriovenous malformation, aneurysm, hemorrhagic transformation of an ischemic infarct, and hypodensity > 1/3 of the middle cerebral artery vascular territory) and the confidence in the presence of a hyperdense middle cerebral artery (HMCA) from the following scores: 0: definitely absent; 1: most likely absent; 2: cannot decide; 3: most likely present; and 4: definitely present. Finally, the ASPECTS score (ranged from 1 to 10) was recorded.

2.3. Display Monitors and Viewer Software. According to the American College of Radiology (ACR) guidelines for teleradiology [20], small matrix size images, such as CT, must be visualized on a monitor with a minimum of 512 × 512 matrix size at a minimum 8-bit pixel depth, for processing or manipulation with no loss of matrix size or bit depth at display. In addition, the Digital Imaging and Communications in Medicine (DICOM) standard recommends the use of monitors calibrated to a maximum luminance of 400–500 cd/m^2 and calibrated according to the DICOM grayscale standard display function (GSDF) [21]. Therefore, we used two displays with these specifications.

The routine system for CT readings in our hospital is a PACS workstation with a DICOM-compliant viewer software Agfa IMPAX 6.5 (AGFA HealthCare, Mortsel, Belgium). Images were displayed using an E-2620 BARCO monitor (BARCO N.V, Kortrijk, Belgium), which is a 2-megapixel (MPx) LCD medical grayscale display, DICOM-compliant, dot pitch of 0.249 mm, with a spatial resolution of 1600×1200 pixels, a maximum luminance of 700 cd/m^2, and an 8-bit grayscale. This system, hereafter referred to as MEDICAL-IMPAX, was used as the reference reading system in this study.

For the mobile option, an Apple iPad Pro 9.7 MLMN2CL/A (Apple Inc., Cupertino, CA, USA), with a "retina" display of 9.7 inches, dot pitch of 0.096 mm (264 dpi), with a spatial resolution of 1536×2048 pixels, and a maximum luminance of 500 cd/m^2 was selected. The viewer used on this tablet was the Agfa XERO Viewer 3.0 (Agfa HealthCare, Mortsel, Belgium) software, hereafter referred to as TABLET-XERO.

2.4. Procedure. Each radiologist read all cases using both the Medical-IMPAX and the Tablet-XERO systems. At each reading, the radiologist determined the variables mentioned in the section "observers and reading observed variables." The two reading software packages provided image manipulation tools to adjust window/level, zoom, and multiplanar reformation presentation. These tools were available for all images and could be used at the observer's discretion to improve the image interpretations. For each reading session, the radiologist verified the settings of the contrast and luminance of the display with the RP-133 pattern in a controlled illumination (ambient light of approximately 20 lux according to the American Association of Physicists in Medicine [AAPM] TG18 recommendations) [22].

The radiologists were blinded to the patient and examination identification, to the original interpretation, and to the type of lesion. To ensure that the radiologists were blinded, a junior radiology resident was in charge of uploading the images into the PACS workstation or tablet using the IMPAX or XERO viewer software. Data collection was performed using a web-based form, and the interpretations were stored in a database. This software presents the patients to be interpreted at random and guides the radiologist to complete the report, thus ensuring the integrity and completeness of data.

According to Mullins et al., the availability of a clinical history consistent with an early stroke significantly improves the sensitivity for detecting strokes on unenhanced brain CT. Thus, whenever possible, relevant clinical history should be made available to the physicians interpreting emergency CT scans of the head [23]. Therefore, the clinical history that is used in the standard protocol to interpret brain CT with suspicion of acute stroke was available to the radiologists, including the sex, age, main neurological symptoms, and relevant past medical history (e.g., diabetes, hypertension, headache, Parkinson, Alzheimer, sleep apnea/hypopnea syndrome, or cardiac arrhythmia). This was done to achieve a more realistic interpretation scenario. Hence, the only difference from the real practice was the reading system. All information was presented on a web-based collection form before beginning each image interpretation.

There was at least a five-month interval between the readings from the same patient by the same radiologist using the compared systems. The readings were performed over the course of ten months in two- or four-hour sessions by each radiologist, with no time limitations for each reading. The initial display used the default image window setting (WW = 174 and WL = 55), but the radiologists were free to select another window, such as a cerebral or a stroke window (WW = 80 and WL = 40, WW = 40 and WL = 40, resp.).

2.5. Data Analysis. Patients with an ASPECTS ≤ 6 were not eligible to receive the tPA treatment. Therefore, we dichotomized the ASPECTS score into two categories: 1 if the score ranged from 1 to 6 (a contraindication for tPA administration from the imaging point of view) and 0 if the score ranged from 7 to 10 (indicating eligibility for the administration of the tPA treatment from the imaging point of view). This variable was named "ASPECTS ≤ 6."

The variable confidence in the presence of a hyperdense middle cerebral artery (HMCA) was also dichotomized as follows: 0 if the score ranged 0–1 (HMCA not detected) and 1 if the score ranged from 2 to 4 (HMCA detected). This variable was named "presence of HMCA."

We evaluated the diagnostic equivalence between the reading systems based on (1) the distribution of type of stroke classification, (2) the "ASPECTS ≤ 6," (3) the detection of the presence of any imaging contraindication to the tPA administration for acute ischemic lesions, (4) the "presence of HMCA," and (5) the reading time.

These variables and the difference between the systems were evaluated using generalized estimating equations (GEE) with the IBM SPSS Statistics 19 software (IBM Corp., Armonk, NY, USA). To evaluate noninferiority and equivalence, the mean differences and their standard errors were obtained from the GEE analysis.

The hypothesis test for equivalence was as follows: the null hypothesis Ho was |Mean Difference $(I-J)| - \delta = 0$, and the alternative hypothesis Ha was |Mean Difference $(I-J)| - \delta < 0$, where I and J are the two reading systems compared and δ (delta) is the maximum allowable difference permitted to conclude equivalence or noninferiority, as suggested by several authors in recent years [16–19]. We calculated a $(1-2\alpha)\%$ confidence interval for all comparisons, which is a method to evaluate equivalence [18, 19]. The significance level was set to 5% (i.e., $\alpha = 0.05$), and δ was set to 0.1 (10%) for proportional variables and 15 seconds for reading time. Finally, we calculated the required value of δ to claim equivalence for each variable (named δ_{eq} in our result in Tables 2 and 4).

3. Results

3.1. Distribution of Type of Stroke Classification. The distribution of the type of stroke classification for each reading system and their comparisons are shown in Table 1. The observed category distribution of cases (i.e., without lesion, hemorrhagic lesion, acute ischemic lesion, and chronic ischemic lesion), using both Medical-IMPAX and Tablet-XERO, was not significantly different ($P = 0.332$). To compare the number of

TABLE 1: Comparison of the distribution of the type of stroke classification between the reading systems.

Lesion type	Reading system	Detected cases	Proportion (%)*	Std. error	95% Wald confidence		Wald chi-square	P value
					Lower	Upper		
Without lesion	Medical-IMPAX	214	29.5	0.032	0.23	0.36	2.024	0.155
	Tablet-XERO	229	31.5	0.032	0.25	0.38		
Hemorrhagic lesion	Medical-IMPAX	64	8.8	0.025	0.04	0.14	1.690	0.194
	Tablet-XERO	69	9.5	0.025	0.05	0.14		
Acute ischemic lesion	Medical-IMPAX	346	47.7	0.035	0.41	0.54	11.051	0.001
	Tablet-XERO	306	42.1	0.035	0.35	0.49		
Chronic ischemic lesion	Medical-IMPAX	102	14.0	0.022	0.10	0.18	6.183	0.013
	Tablet-XERO	122	16.8	0.024	0.12	0.22		
Overall ischemic lesion†	Medical-IMPAX	448	61.7	0.036	0.55	0.69	3.428	0.064
	Tablet-XERO	428	59.0	0.035	0.52	0.66		

*Each proportion was calculated from 726 readings (121 cases by 6 radiologists). Statistics were evaluated using generalized estimating equations (GEE) analysis. The overall Wald chi-square was 0.941 with a significance of 0.332. †Overall ischemic lesion was calculated as the aggregate values of acute and chronic ischemic lesions.

TABLE 2: Equivalence tests for the distribution on the type of stroke classification between reading systems.

Variable	δ (%)	Mean difference*	SE	$(1-2\alpha)$% CI for equivalence testing		z	P value ($P < -z$)	H	δ_{eq} (%)
				Lower	Upper				
Without lesion	10	−0.021	0.015	−0.045	0.003	−5.46	<0.001	Ha	4.5
Hemorrhagic lesion	10	−0.007	0.005	−0.016	0.002	−17.58	<0.001	Ha	1.6
Acute ischemic lesion	10	0.060	0.017	0.033	0.087	−2.41	0.0079	Ha	8.7
Chronic ischemic lesion	10	−0.030	0.011	−0.048	−0.012	−6.32	<0.001	Ha	4.8
Overall ischemic lesion	10	0.028	0.015	0.003	0.052	−4.87	0.0000	Ha	5.2

SE: standard error of the mean difference, CI: confidence interval; Ho: null hypothesis, Ha: alternative hypothesis for testing equivalence, α: significance of the test (0.05), δ: difference of the means allowed to achieve equivalence, z: test for difference of compared devices, that is, z = (|Mean Difference| − δ)/SE, H: retained hypothesis equivalence at δ level, "Ha" indicates equivalence achieved and " " indicates fail to reject Ho., δ_{eq}: δ required for equivalence (i.e., $P < \alpha$). Ho: |Difference $(I - J)$| − δ = 0; Ha: |Difference $(I - J)$| − δ < 0. *Each comparison was calculated by six radiologists and two devices.

cases detected by a reading system in each lesion category, nonsignificant differences were observed for hemorrhagic lesion ($P = 0.155$) and without lesions ($P = 0.194$). Although significant differences were observed for acute and chronic ischemic lesions, nonsignificant differences were noted for the overall ischemic lesions (combining acute and chronic ischemic lesions).

3.2. Equivalence Tests for the Distribution on the Type of Stroke Classification. Equivalence tests for the distribution on the type of stroke classification between the two reading systems are shown in Table 2. For δ (delta) values of equivalence of 0.1 (i.e., 10%) to claim equivalence, both reading systems were equivalent (all $P < 0.05$) for all individual type of stroke classification categories, even for chronic ischemic lesions.

In addition, we performed a sensitivity analysis for the equivalence δ value to determine the δ_{eq} value for which equivalence may be claimed with significant tests. In this analysis, Medical-IMPAX and Tablet-XERO achieved equivalence at 4.5% for the category without lesions, 1.6% for hemorrhagic lesion, 8.7% for acute ischemic lesion, and 4.8% for chronic ischemic lesion. In addition, a value of 5.2% for the overall ischemic lesion was observed.

3.3. Diagnostic Variables and Reading Time. The mean values and the comparisons for the proportions observed on the "ASPECTS ≤ 6," the presence of any imaging contraindication to the tPA administration for acute ischemic lesions, presence of HMCA, and reading time are presented in Table 3. The proportion of patients observed with an ASPECTS ≤ 6 was 0.14 for both reading systems, and nonsignificant differences were observed ($P = 0.855$). Similarly, nonsignificant differences were observed in the proportion of the presence of any imaging contraindication to the tPA administration for acute ischemic lesions ($P = 0.476$), with values of 0.32 on Medical-IMPAX and 0.34 on Tablet-XERO. However, the proportion of cases in which the presence of HMCA was detected using Medical-IMPAX and Tablet-XERO was 0.24 and 0.29, respectively, with significant differences observed ($P = 0.027$).

The reading times for the interpretations on Medical-IMPAX and Tablet-XERO were 126 s and 123 s, respectively, which were not significantly different ($P = 0.566$). The difference in the time to claim equivalence was 13.7 s ($P < 0.05$).

3.4. Equivalence Tests for Proportions on the Diagnostic Variables and Reading Time. Equivalence tests for the diagnostic

Table 3: Comparison of diagnostic variables and reading time between the reading systems.

Reading system	Readings	Mean*	Std. error	95% Wald confidence interval Lower	95% Wald confidence interval Upper	Wald chi-Square†	P value
ASPECTS ≤ 6							
Medical-IMPAX	81/586	0.14	0.027	0.09	0.19	0.034	0.855
Tablet-XERO	84/593	0.14	0.026	0.09	0.19		
Contraindication to the tPA administration for acute ischemic lesions							
Medical-IMPAX	112/346	0.32	0.038	0.25	0.40	0.508	0.476
Tablet-XERO	105/306	0.34	0.039	0.27	0.42		
Presence of HMCA							
Medical-IMPAX	123/505	0.24	0.029	0.19	0.30	4.912	0.027
Tablet-XERO	141/492	0.29	0.034	0.22	0.35		
Reading time							
Medical-IMPAX	726	126.0	4.47	117.1	134.9	0.332	0.566
Tablet-XERO	726	122.5	5.28	112.0	132.9		

ASPECTS = Alberta Stroke Early CT Scan score; HMCA = hyperdense middle cerebral artery; *For ASPECTS ≤ 6, presence of imaging contraindications to the tPA administration, and the presence of HMCA, the mean proportion was calculated from the detected cases on each variable over the number of readings. Statistics were obtained using generalized estimating equations (GEE) analysis; †For the reading time the F statistic for ANOVA analysis was used.

Table 4: Equivalence tests for the diagnostic variables and reading time.

Variable	δ	Mean difference[a]	SE	$(1-2\alpha)$% CI for equivalence testing Lower	$(1-2\alpha)$% CI for equivalence testing Upper	z	P value ($P < -z$)	H	δ_{eq}
ASPECTS ≤ 6	10.0%	−0.002	0.011	−0.021	0.017	−8.59	<0.001	Ha	2.1%
Presence of imaging contraindications to the tPA administration	10.0%	0.020	0.028	−0.026	0.065	−2.90	0.0018	Ha	6.5%
Presence of HMCA	10.0%	−0.040	0.019	−0.072	−0.008	−3.09	0.0010	Ha	7.2%
Reading time	15 s	3.6 s	6.2	−6.6	13.7	−1.85	0.0318	Ha	13.7 s

SE: Standard error of the mean difference, CI: confidence Interval; Ho: null hypothesis, Ha: alternative hypothesis for testing equivalence, α: significance of the test (0.05), δ: difference of the means allowed to achieve equivalence, z: test for difference of compared devices, that is, $z = (|\text{Mean Difference}| - \delta)/\text{SE}$, H: retained hypothesis equivalence at δ level, "Ha" indicates equivalence achieved and "–" indicates fail to reject Ho., $\delta_{eq} = \delta$ required for equivalence (i.e., $P < \alpha$); Ho: $|\text{Difference } (I - J)| - \delta = 0$; Ha: $|\text{Difference } (I - J)| - \delta < 0$. [a]Each comparison was calculated for six radiologists and two devices.

variables and reading time are shown in Table 4. The average reading times for the interpretations on the Medical-IMPAX and Tablet-XERO were 126 s and 123 s, respectively, with no significant difference ($P = 0.566$). For δ (delta) values of equivalence of 0.1 (i.e., 10%) to claim equivalence on the diagnostic variables and 15 s on the reading time, both reading systems were equivalent (all $P < 0.05$). In addition, we performed a sensitivity analysis of the equivalence δ (delta) value to determine the δ value for which equivalence may be claimed with significant values (δ_{eq}). In this analysis, Medical-IMPAX and Tablet-XERO achieved equivalence at 2.1% for "ASPECTS ≤ 6," 6.5% for acute ischemic lesion without contraindications, 7.2% for "presence of HMCA," and 13.7 s for the reading time.

4. Discussion

The distribution of observed lesions using both the Medical-IMPAX and the Tablet-XERO was not significantly different. For hemorrhagic lesions and the without lesion categories, differences were also not significantly different. Equivalence for the two reading systems can be claimed for differences of 1.6% for the hemorrhagic lesions. These results for hemorrhagic lesions in our study are in line with those from other studies that reported high agreement and accuracy for identifying hemorrhagic lesions [9, 11, 12]. For overall ischemic lesion (combining acute and chronic ischemic lesions), nonsignificant differences were noted between the two reading systems. The equivalence of the two reading systems can be claimed for differences of 5.2%.

Previous studies have reported nonsignificant differences in the detection of overall ischemic lesion and acute hemorrhage between mobile solutions and PACS workstations [9, 12, 14, 15]. Although the variables and evaluation methods used in these studies were different than those used in ours, this study agrees with the previous works in that the reading system does not affect the detection of hemorrhagic lesions or the overall ischemic lesion.

The results of our study indicate that patients with an ASPECTS ≤ 6 were well detected using both reading systems when the interpretations were performed by experienced radiologists and that the equivalence of the two reading systems may be claimed for low differences (2.1%). When detecting the presence of a HMCA, we observed significant differences. Nevertheless, equivalence was confirmed at differences lower than 10%. Besides, the actual difference achieved to claim equivalence was 7.2%. This assessment was designed to evaluate the equivalence of the magnitudes of the related variables, rather than to find differences or to show that they are equal. In addition, this evaluation is not an accuracy assessment (as the results are not compared to the gold standard). Therefore, it is not possible, at present, to declare which of the two magnitudes is the most accurate. Although more cases with HMCA were detected using the tablet, this does not mean that the tablet was better to detect the HMCA. If the difference is due to true positives, this is a rare result as the tablet has the lower contrast. On the other hand, the difference may be due to false positives, but this is not possible to state at present in the absence of the gold standard, which we will set further.

These findings are consistent with those described by McLaughlin et al., who used the same kind of tablet to determine the interpretations of senior radiologists [9]. To our knowledge, however, no study has described the performance of observers when detecting the presence of any imaging contraindication to the tPA administration for acute ischemic lesions that should not receive tPA treatment. In our study, nonsignificant differences were noted, and equivalence was confirmed at 10%. In addition, the equivalence of the two reading systems may be claimed for differences of 6.5%.

The approach used to perform the interpretations, the assessment process, the variables evaluated, especially, for ruling out brain CT contraindications prior to intravenous thrombolysis, and the statistical methods used to analyze them are the principal differences between our study and previous ones [9, 11–15], which focused on evaluating accuracy or reliability. In contrast, our study was set to evaluate the equivalence of the reading systems on the diagnostic variables (i.e., the distribution of type of stroke classification, the ASPECTS score, the detection of acute ischemic lesions without contraindications, and the confidence in the presence of a hyperdense middle cerebral artery) and on the reading time. In this sense, our study agrees with previous studies in terms of which nonsignificant differences were observed between the reading systems, but, from another perspective, our study investigates the effects of reading systems and the equivalence of the variables assessed. Hence, our study is a complement to the previous studies without statistical type II errors.

At present, we are evaluating other mobile alternatives, such as a smartphone with a high-resolution display and a portable computer, for use by the same observers and in the same sample used in this study. Our three neuroradiologists with more than ten years of experience will develop, by consensus, the reference gold standard for our sample. Nevertheless, to avoid bias, these neuroradiologists will complete all readings before establishing the gold standard. For these reasons, this study is not an accuracy evaluation. Further, when the reference standard is available, we will be able to evaluate the accuracy.

One limitation of this study centers on the illumination conditions. Readings using the Medical-IMPAX system were performed in diagnostic reading stations in which the ambient light levels were controlled according to the AAPM TG18 recommendations (i.e., 15–60 lux) [22]. In contrast, readings using the TABLET-XERO system were performed without controlling ambient light levels. Nevertheless, this situation is more realistic for a telestroke system in which a radiologist is asked to read the brain CT as soon as possible wherever he is located and may reproduce a situation in which a Medical-IMPAX system is not available. The reading time difference was not a concern in this study.

The results of this study provide reassurance to radiologists who interpret brain CTs using the TABLET-XERO system that their performance is likely equivalent to their performance when using the Medical-IMPAX system. To the best of our knowledge, this is the first study that uses nonequivalence or noninferiority statistical methods to identify potential diagnostic differences between a primary diagnostic workstation and a mobile tablet computer in the process of ruling out imaging contraindications prior to intravenous thrombolysis.

In conclusion, the results of the present study show that, even after challenging radiologists with real clinical scenarios of acute stroke patients, mobile solutions with high-resolution displays, such as the "retina" display of the iPAD 3, may provide useful telestroke solutions.

Acknowledgments

The authors thank the radiologists who carried out the interpretations. The authors thank their institutions and the National Department of Science, Technology and Innovation of Colombia for funding this study (Grant 1204-744-55680).

References

[1] WHO, "WHO Task Force on Stroke and other Cerebrovascular Disorders: stroke Recommendations on stroke prevention, diagnosis and therapy," *Stroke*, vol. 20, no. 10, pp. 1407–1431, 1989.

[2] T. N. Taylor, P. H. Davis, J. C. Torner, J. Holmes, J. W. Meyer, and M. F. Jacobson, "Lifetime cost of stroke in the United States," *Stroke*, vol. 27, no. 9, pp. 1459–1466, 1996.

[3] R. Bonita, "Epidemiology of stroke," *The Lancet*, vol. 339, no. 8789, pp. 342–344, 1992.

[4] G. Saposnik and O. H. Del Brutto, "Stroke in South America: a systematic review of incidence, prevalence, and stroke subtypes," *Stroke*, vol. 34, no. 9, pp. 2103–2107, 2003.

[5] F. A. Silva, J. G. Zarruk, C. Quintero et al., "Enfermedad cerebrovascular en Colombia," *Revista Colombiana de Cardiología*, vol. 13, pp. 85–89, 2006.

[6] R. Díaz Cabezas and M. I. Ruano Restrepo, "Conocimiento de síntomas y factores de riesgo de enfermedad cerebro vascular en una población urbana colombiana," *Acta Neurológica Colombiana*, vol. 27, pp. 195–204, 2011.

[7] F. Silva-Sieger, W. Arenas-Borda, J. G. Zarruk et al., "Factores asociados al tiempo de consulta en pacientes con enfermedad cerebrovascular isquémica," *Revista De Neurologia*, vol. 44, no. 05, pp. 0259–0264, 2007.

[8] M. Kulcsar, S. Gilchrist, and M. G. George, "Improving stroke outcomes in rural areas through telestroke programs: an examination of barriers, facilitators, and state policies," *Telemedicine journal and e-health : the official journal of the American Telemedicine Association*, vol. 20, no. 1, pp. 3–10, 2014.

[9] P. D. McLaughlin, F. Moloney, S. B. O'Neill et al., "CT of the head for acute stroke: Diagnostic performance of a tablet computer prior to intravenous thrombolysis," *Journal of Medical Imaging and Radiation Oncology*, vol. 61, no. 3, pp. 334–338, 2017.

[10] J. H. W. Pexman, P. A. Barber, M. D. Hill et al., "Use of the Alberta Stroke Program Early CT Score (ASPECTS) for assessing CT scans in patients with acute stroke," *American Journal of Neuroradiology*, vol. 22, no. 8, pp. 1534–1542, 2001.

[11] S. Panughpath, S. Kumar, and A. Kalyanpur, "Utility of mobile devices in the computerized tomography evaluation of intracranial hemorrhage," *Indian Journal of Radiology and Imaging*, vol. 23, no. 1, pp. 4–7, 2013.

[12] S. Tewes, T. Rodt, S. Marquardt, E. Evangelidou, F. K. Wacker, and C. Von Falck, "Evaluation of the use of a tablet computer with a high-resolution display for interpreting emergency CT scans," *RöFo - Fortschritte auf dem Gebiet der Röntgenstrahlen und der bildgebenden Verfahren*, vol. 185, no. 11, pp. 1063–1069, 2013.

[13] J. B. Park, H. J. Choi, J. H. Lee, and B. S. Kang, "An assessment of the iPad 2 as a CT teleradiology tool using brain CT with subtle intracranial hemorrhage under conventional illumination," *Journal of Digital Imaging*, vol. 26, no. 4, pp. 683–690, 2013.

[14] K. Yoshimura, T. Nihashi, M. Ikeda et al., "Comparison of liquid crystal display monitors calibrated with gray-scale standard display function and with γ 2.2 and ipad: Observer performance in detection of cerebral infarction on brain ct," *American Journal of Roentgenology*, vol. 200, no. 6, pp. 1304–1309, 2013.

[15] A. Bhatia, S. Patel, G. Pantol, Y. Wu, M. Plitnikas, and C. Hancock, "Intra and Inter-Observer Reliability of Mobile Tablet PACS Viewer System vs. Standard PACS Viewing Station-Diagnosis of Acute Central Nervous System Events," *Open Journal of Radiology*, vol. 03, no. 02, pp. 91–98, 2013.

[16] W. Chen, N. A. Petrick, and B. Sahiner, "Hypothesis testing in noninferiority and equivalence MRMC ROC studies," *Academic Radiology*, vol. 19, no. 9, pp. 1158–1165, 2012.

[17] H. Jin and Y. Lu, "A non-inferiority test of areas under two parametric ROC curves," *Contemporary Clinical Trials*, vol. 30, no. 4, pp. 375–379, 2009.

[18] J.-P. Liu, M.-C. Ma, C.-y. Wu, and J.-Y. Tai, "Tests of equivalence and non-inferiority for diagnostic accuracy based on the paired areas under ROC curves," *Statistics in Medicine*, vol. 25, no. 7, pp. 1219–1238, 2006.

[19] N. A. Obuchowski, "Testing for equivalence of diagnostic tests," *American Journal of Roentgenology*, vol. 168, no. 1, pp. 13–17, 1997.

[20] ACR, "American College of Radiology Standard for Teleradiology," vol. Res. 35, ed: ACR, 1998.

[21] NEMA, "Digital imaging and communications in medicine," in *Part 14: Grayscale Standrad Display Function*, National Electrical Manufacturer's Association, Rosslyn, Va, USA, 2001.

[22] E. Samei, A. Badano, D. Chakraborty et al., "Assessment of display performance for medical imaging systems: Executive summary of AAPM TG18 report," *Medical Physics*, vol. 32, no. 4, pp. 1205–1225, 2005.

[23] M. E. Mullins, M. H. Lev, D. Schellingerhout, W. J. Koroshetz, and R. G. Gonzalez, "Influence of availability of clinical history on detection of early stroke using unenhanced CT and diffusion-weighted MR imaging," *American Journal of Roentgenology*, vol. 179, no. 1, pp. 223–228, 2002.

Clinical Decision Support Systems for Comorbidity: Architecture, Algorithms, and Applications

Aihua Fan,[1] Di Lin,[2] and Yu Tang[2]

[1]*Xi'an Polytechnic University, Shaanxi, China*
[2]*University of Electronic Science and Technology of China, Sichuan, China*

Correspondence should be addressed to Di Lin; di.lin2@mail.mcgill.ca

Academic Editor: Manolis Tsiknakis

In this paper, we present the design of a clinical decision support system (CDSS) for monitoring comorbid conditions. Specifically, we address the architecture of a CDSS by characterizing it from three layers and discuss the algorithms in each layer. Also we address the applications of CDSSs in a few real scenarios and analyze the accuracy of a CDSS in consideration of the potential conflicts when using multiple clinical practice guidelines concurrently. Finally, we compare the system performance in our design with that in the other design schemes. Our study shows that our proposed design can achieve a clinical decision in a shorter time than the other designs, while ensuring a high level of system accuracy.

1. Introduction

A clinical decision support system (CDSS) is designed for ubiquitous health monitoring, which provides mobile health service in order to help physicians and doctors monitor patients' conditions anytime and anywhere with the aid of wireless networks [1]. In such an ubiquitous health monitoring system, building on the biosignal data of patients, a CDSS can assess their conditions with a certain algorithm and inform physicians and doctors immediately when an emergency case occurs, being able to reduce the delay for medical treatment of a critical patient [2].

Most work in the design of CDSS has focused on making clinical decisions on one type of disease, either following the clinical guidelines of this specific disease or employing various data mining schemes to extract clinical rules from numerous biosignal data of patients [3–10]. The primary algorithms include k-nearest neighbors based algorithms (k-NN), artificial neural networks based algorithms (ANN), decision trees based algorithms (DTs), fuzzy logic based algorithms (FL), and the extension of these algorithms by merging them.

(a) K-Nearest Neighbors Based Algorithms. A k-nearest neighbors based algorithm is a method for classifying cases by referring to the closest training cases in the feature space. A typical k-NN algorithm runs as follows [10]: cases in question are firstly mixed with the other known cases to constitute a case set. Next, all these cases in this set are mapped into a finite-dimension feature space. A dimension in this space characterizes a feature of cases, so a point in this space uniquely represents a case. Finally, all the points in this space are classified into k disjoint subsets, and each subset represents one type of cases. The type of cases in question is assigned by the type of known cases which are within the same subset.

(b) Artificial Neural Network Based Algorithms. Quite similar to the structure of a human brain, an ANN based algorithm is composed of a few interconnected layers of neurons and extracts the exact way of connecting layers by training the historical data of patients. Based on the different training schemes, numerous ANN methods are presented in the literature. In the context of wireless health, two main ANN based algorithms are widely employed in a CDSS [9], including clustering, self-organizing map: clustering based training scheme is implemented by extracting a few critical features of cases and then mapping these features into the structure of an ANN [8]; self-organizing map alters the structure of an

ANN by adding necessary neurons and deleting unnecessary neurons [7].

(c) Decision Tree Based Algorithms. Generally, a decision tree based algorithm makes a decision through a series of question and answer sessions. Firstly, the tree based algorithm starts with a root node, which represents the most significant feature in determining the condition of a patient. Then, cases with different states of this feature are split into two or more branches. If all the cases fall into one branch, the branch can be denoted as a leaf. The process of splitting is repeated until all the branches are denoted as leaves [5].

(d) Fuzzy Logic Based Systems. The application of fuzzy models into decision support systems is motivated by the uncertainty of thresholds to make a decision on the patient condition [4]. For example, if the normal range of heart rate is 80–90 times/min, a heart rate of 79 or 91 times/min should not be certainly determined as abnormal [3]. Instead, the result should be determined as normal with a certain probability. In general, the fuzzy process is composed of three procedures: (1) Fuzzification, which is characterized as mapping crisp inputs into fuzzy variables by acquiring the membership values of these crisp inputs, the membership functions can take different shapes, and the simplest but quite widely employed is trapezoidal function; (2) inference based on some rules; (3) defuzzification, which is characterized as converting fuzzy variables into crisp outputs with various mapping methods, and one typical defuzzification method is the centroid of area (COA) method.

Also a few CDSSs are designed to implement in the scenario of making clinical decisions on a comorbid patient (e.g., a patient with Atrial Fibrillation in the setting of Wolff Parkinson's White Syndrome), and in such scenarios the decisions on the treatment of multiple diseases might be in conflict with each other. Such a need is especially clear for elderly patients: several studies have shown that about half of people above 65 years old have a comorbid condition [11]. Boyd et al. in [12] discuss the employment of multiple clinical practice guidelines (CPG) to the care of patients in a comorbid condition. By analyzing various hypothetical clinical scenarios of typical clinical diseases and their associated CPGs, the authors conclude that a blind combination of individual CPGs in the presence of comorbid condition may negatively impact a clinical decision due to the potential mutual conflicts between guidelines. They explain this situation by the fact that a CPG is developed by a specialty-dominated committee and thus is not designed to provide help with regard to evaluating and managing comorbid patients. The conclusion in [12] motivates the research on how to develop a computing algorithm in the design of CDSS for making clinical decisions on the patients in a comorbid condition. Research in the stream of computing algorithms in the design of CDSS for patients in a comorbid condition, despite its importance, seems to be in its infancy. Riaño et al. in [13] advocate using an ontological model for guideline personalization. Unfortunately, the development of this model needs to be conducted manually by physicians using a specialized clinical guideline editor instead of automatically by a computer. In [14], the authors propose a methodology as well as its specific implementation for automatically combining multiple clinical guidelines; however, the data of patients need to be manually entered by physicians.

1.1. Motivation. All these above-mentioned papers do not address how to establish a system which can automatically extract the patient data and offer a decision for clinical practice. Also all the aforementioned research focuses on the level of algorithms and do not mention the design of a CDSS at the system level. The importance of designing a CDSS for comorbidity monitoring as well as the lack of efficient design in the system level motivates us to investigate how to design a CDSS for monitoring comorbid patients by merging the clinical guidelines as well as how to assess the system performance.

1.2. Main Contributions. In this paper, we present the design of a CDSS for monitoring comorbid conditions, specifically from the perspectives of the architecture, the algorithms, and the applications of a CDSS. Also we address how to analyze the accuracy of a CDSS in consideration of the potential conflicts when using multiple clinical practice guidelines concurrently.

The primary contributions of this paper rest at the following issues:

(i) address the architecture, the algorithms in the design of a CDSS for comorbidity;
(ii) present the implementation process of a CDSS for comorbidity;
(iii) assess the system accuracy of a CDSS for comorbidity.

2. Architecture of CDSS for Comorbidity Monitoring

In this section, we address the architecture of a CDSS in our design for comorbidity monitoring, and it is shown in Figure 1. As shown in Figure 1, the architecture of a CDSS is composed of three layers: physical layer, data layer, and application layer.

In the physical layer, the system needs to extract data from various data sources. The primary data source in clinical scenarios is hospital information systems (HIS), which are located in hospitals or medical centers. Also the medical data may be from a few medical sensors, including the medical sensors attached to or even embedded into the body of a patient, for example, Holter and blood pressure sensors. As shown in Figure 2, data from different sources might be in different formats, and we employ a front end processor (FEP) to do the data extraction, transformation, and loading (ETL) process and also convert data into XML or JSON. In consideration of the security issues, we add a virtual private network (VPN) connection into the system, and also we use a firewall and web service server at the end of data center, to ensure that the data center is not directly connected to public networks for security issues.

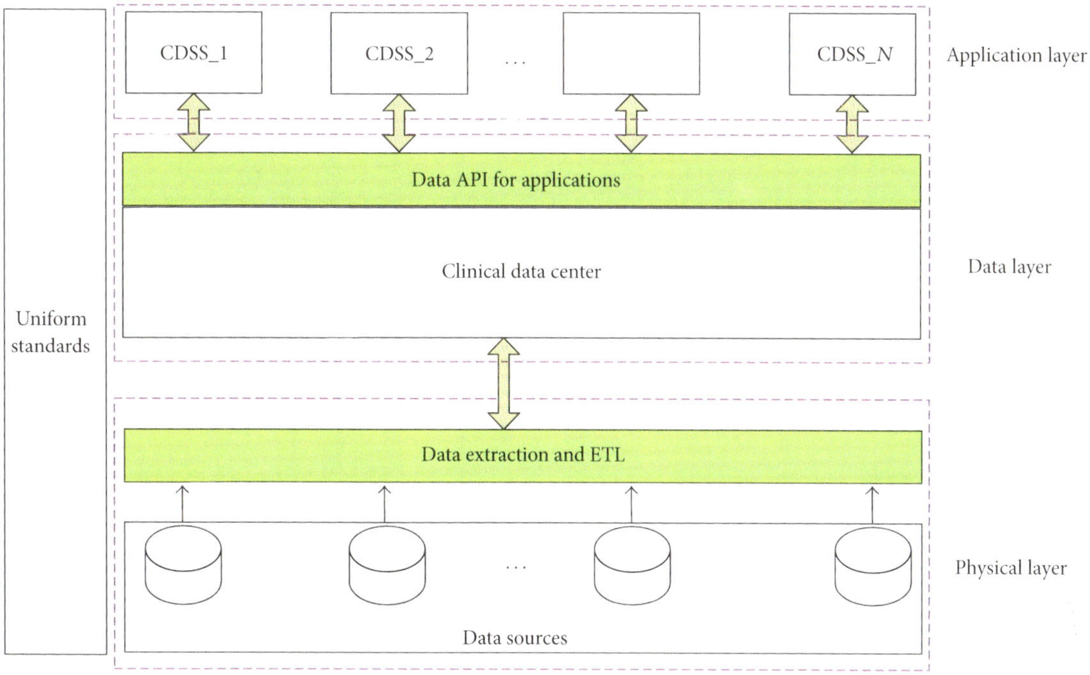

FIGURE 1: Architecture of a CDSS for comorbidity monitoring.

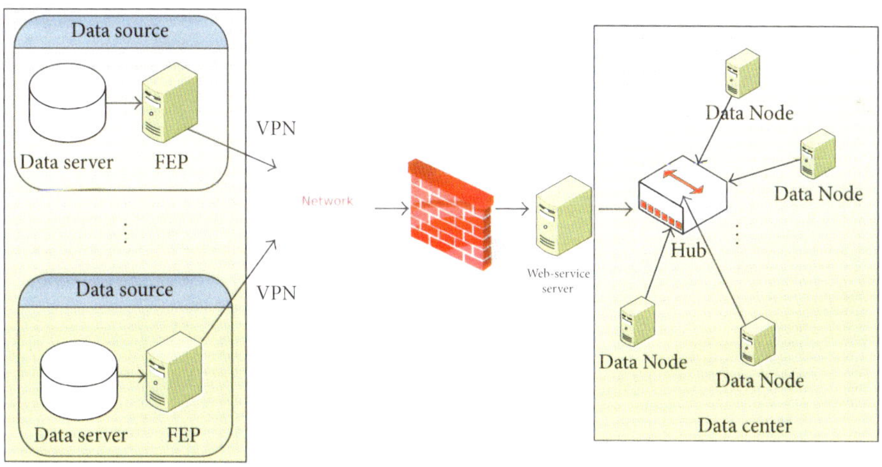

FIGURE 2: Physical layer of a CDSS.

In the data layer, with the dramatic increase of clinical data, the traditional data processing applications are inadequate to process such a large set of data, so we employ a Hadoop/Hbase based server cluster to store and process data. The data stored in the data center are prepared to offer data APIs to the application layer, and we use a few off-the-shelf tools of Hadoop to achieve the data APIs [15]. The detailed Hadoop ecosystem is shown in Figure 3. Specifically, we employ Pig and Hive to support the application layer by combining them with Hbase [16] and also Sqoop to connect with the traditional relational databases.

In the application layer, the system can support the CDSS for specific clinical diagnosis, and we focus on the diagnosis on the comorbid patients. The CDSS for comorbidity diagnosis needs to merge clinical practice guidelines (CPG) and detect and mitigate the potential conflicts between CPGs. After mitigating all the conflicts, the system can achieve a final decision on the clinical practice. In the design of an application layer, we use a constraint logic programming model to represent all the CPGs and detect the potential conflicts. The detailed algorithms are illustrated in Sections 3 and 4.

Additionally, the issue of security is critical in the application of healthcare, and generally the security issues in Hadoop involve three aspects: authentication, authorization, and network encryption. We can employ a few off-the-shelf

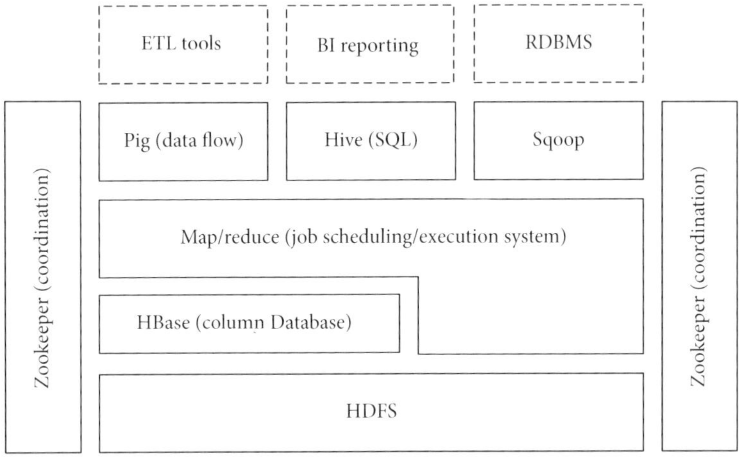

FIGURE 3: Hadoop ecosystem.

security solutions in the architecture of Hadoop. A summary of security solutions in the Hadoop for security is presented as follows.

(1) Authentication. Kerberos is a secret-key based authentication system, which can provide authentication and Single-Sign-On (SSO) of users and servers in a network. Hadoop uses the Kerberos protocol to authenticate users to Hadoop and to authenticate Hadoop services to each other.

(2) Authorization. Hadoop provides authorization controls to authenticated users with the aid of HDFS file permissions and service-level authorization. Each of the files is associated with a group and has associated permissions of read and write. Based on such file permissions, HDFS controls access to reads and writes to the distributed file system. Service-level authorization is used by a cluster to control the permission of users to submit jobs.

(3) Network Encryption. If a few sensitive data are exchanged in a network, then we need to protect the cluster from eavesdroppers and network sniffers by encrypting these data.

3. Algorithms of CDSS for Comorbidity Monitoring

As shown in Figure 1, the architecture of a CDSS is composed of three layers: physical layer, data layer, and application layer. In this section, we present the specific algorithms in each of the layers.

3.1. Physical Layer. In the physical layer, the CDSS extracts data from various data sources and runs the ETL on raw data in order to load the processed data (clean data) into the data center. The detailed algorithm in the physical layer is in Figure 4. The CDSS firstly accesses the data from data sources and extracts data, does the data cleaning, and standardizes the data into the XML or JSON format. Data cleaning includes data transformation, duplication elimination, replacing missing data, and removing outliers. Of course, the process of data cleaning refers to a standard, for example, HL7, and thus the system supports HL7 to transform the data from different sources (in different formats) into the data in a uniform format. Then, the CDSS calls a web service, and once the connection is successfully built up, the formatted clean data would be transmitted to the data center. Usually, the data are transmitted in bulk, so the data transmission would finish

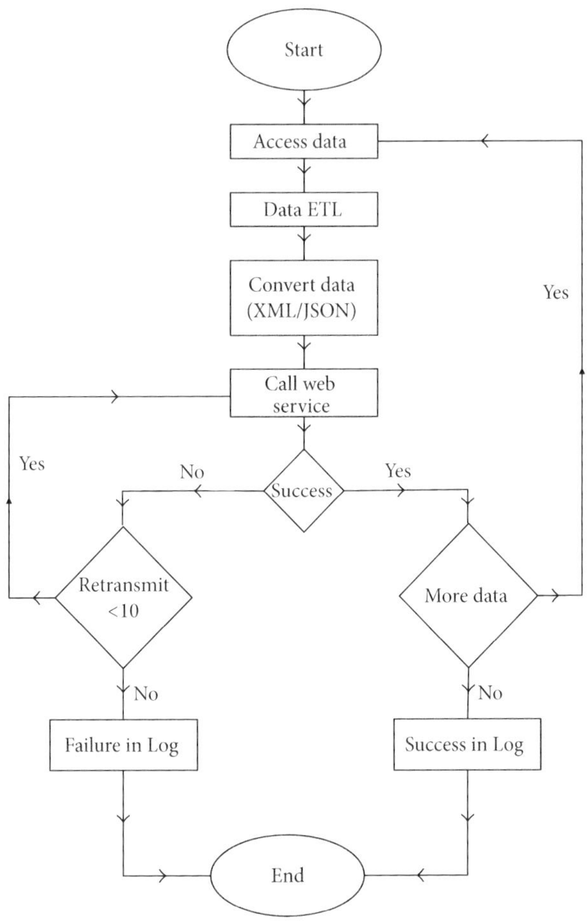

FIGURE 4: Algorithms in physical layer.

Table 1: Design of table in Hbase.

Row key	Time stamp	ColumnFamily	
		PersonBasicInfo	PersonExternalInfo
*_11112222_*	T9	Name = "Peter"	National = "Canada"
	T8	IDNumber = "11112222"	FamilyDisease = "None"
	T7	Address = "Ottawa"	Allergen = "None"
*_22223333_*	T6	Name = "Steven"	National = "USA"
	T5	IDNumber = "22223333"	FamilyDisease = "Diabetes"
	T4	Sex = "Male"	Allergen = "Sea food"
*_33334444_*	T3	Name = "Lee"	National = "China"
	T2	IDNumber = "33334444"	FamilyDisease = "None"
	T1	Sex = "Male"	Allergen = "Peanut"
⋮	⋮	⋮	⋮

until all of the bulks of data are transmitted. When calling the web service, if the connection is failed, the CDSS would recall the web service 10 times and write the results into the Log if none of 10 tries succeeds. Otherwise, when the connection succeeds, the CDSS would extract more data and repeat the above-mentioned procedures.

3.2. Data Layer. In the data layer, the clinical data are stored in Hbase tables, the design of which is shown in Table 1. In the CDSS applications, we consider the big data computation architecture and thus employ Hadoop architecture. Hbase is the native database of Hadoop and is well compatible with the tools of Hadoop ecosystem. In comparison with the relational database, Hbase can improve the computation performance, that is, running efficiency. As shown in Table 1, Hbase tables are composed of row keys, time stamps, and column families. A row key is the unique key in a Hbase table and it can be used for indexing in the Hbase table. In the scenario of clinical data, a row key is represented by the patient ID. Time stamps are automatically generated by Hbase, and they denote the time of data entry. Column families are usually a set of columns, and one column represents a property of patients. For example, in the first row, the row key "11112222" represents the identification (ID) of such a row. The time stamps "T7," "T8," and "T9" represent the time of data entry. Specifically, the entry of "Name = Peter" in the column "PersonBasicInfo" and the entry of "National = Canada" in the column "PersonExternalInfo" occur at the time stamp of "T9"; the entry of "IDNumber = 11112222" in the column "PersonBasicInfo" and the entry of "FamilyDisease = None" in the column "PersonExternalInfo" occur at the time stamp of "T8"; the entry of "Address = Ottawa" in the column "PersonBasicInfo" and the entry of "Allergen = None" in the column "PersonExternalInfo" occur at the time stamp of "T7."

3.3. Application Layer. In the application layer, the algorithms of our CDSS are developed with CLP-CPG models. A CLP-CPG model refers to the development of a combined clinical practice guideline for a specific patient with the aid of constraint logic programming (CLP) [14]. The CLP-CPG model is motivated by the fact that the diagnosis and treatment plan for a specific patient may not be made in consideration of only one CPG; instead, the consideration of combining multiple CPGs is necessary to develop a treatment for patients, especially for those with comorbidity [17].

However, the challenge of combining multiple CPGs is the possible conflicts among multiple CPGs, these conflicts constituting a point of contention (POC) [18]. The CLP-CPG model attempts to mitigate all the POCs by modifying the details of a CPG with the approval of physicians, and the modification of CPGs leads to a modified CLP-CPG model. The modified CLP-CPG model can provide a complete diagnosis and treatment plan to physicians if all the POCs are mitigated. Otherwise, physicians can achieve the conflicts between the CPGs, and they will manually make a complete plan based on the information offered by the model. The work flow of a CLP-CPG model can be shown in Figure 5, given that N CPGs are considered.

In the following, we show the detailed process of establishing a CDSS for comorbidity monitoring by providing the example of CDSS for both hypertension (HTN) and deep vein thrombosis (DVT), but our design of CDSS for comorbidity is applicable to the monitoring of comorbid patients with other diseases. The work flow is composed of 3 steps (see details in Section 4): (1) For each of CPGs (in the format of text or graph), the system can establish a corresponding CPG-CLP model to represent the specific CPG. (2) Usually, the CDSS for comorbidity requires multiple CPGs, which might be in conflict with each other. Thus, the second step is to combine each of the CPG-CLP models which are relevant to the comorbid patient and investigate the potential conflicts. (3) When any conflict exists, the CDSS needs to find a solution which can mitigate the conflict. If no conflict exists, the CDSS can output the final plan of making diagnosis decisions on the patient; if all the possible solutions are tried, but cannot mitigate all the conflicts, the CDSS needs to report the conflicts to the physicians. Then, the physicians need to manually make a plan, and the CDSS memorizes the solution by the physicians for future decision making.

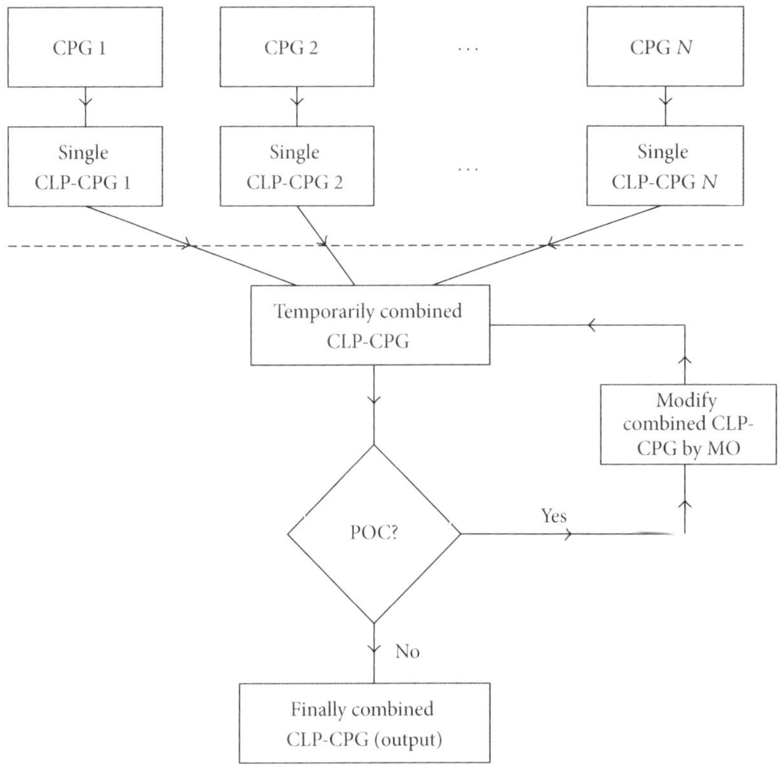

FIGURE 5: Flow chart of a CPG-CLP model given N CPGs to combine (CLP = constant logic programming, CPG = clinical practice guideline, POC = point of contention, and MO = mitigation operator).

4. Applications of CDSS for Comorbidity Monitoring

In this section we present how to use a CLP-CPG model in a clinical scenario for comorbidity monitoring. Specifically, we take the scenario of a patient suffering from both hypertension (HTN) and deep vein thrombosis (DVT) as an example. In such example, we use anonymized patient data transcribed from a public data source [19]. Please note that the design of a CDSS for HTN/DVT monitoring can also be applied to the monitoring of the other diseases.

4.1. Clinical Guideline. The clinical guidelines for a patient who has both HTN and DVT are illustrated in Figure 6. Based on the clinical guideline of DVT, the patient would be inquired whether he or she has a history of severe bleeding tendency (sbt). If so, a physician would recommend this patient to use an inferior vena cava filter (ivcf). Otherwise, this patient would be inquired whether he or she has a history of heparin-induced thrombocytopenia (hit). If so, this patient would be required to use anticoagulant agents (ana), and otherwise this patient would be recommended to take warfarin (wa). Finally, after this patient uses ivcf or ana or wa, the physician would transfer this patient to his or her family doctor to follow up (fdfu).

Based on the clinical guideline of HTN, a patient would be checked to confirm that the hypertension he or she suffers is controlled (htnc) or uncontrolled (htnuc). If the type of hypertension is in the type of controlled, the patient would be directly transferred to his or her family doctor to follow up. If the type of hypertension is uncontrolled, the patient would be further checked to confirm whether this patient's hypertension is in urgency (htnur) or emergency (htnem). If the patient is in the status of htnur, the patient would be required to take oral antihypertensive agents (oaa) and otherwise to take the IV antihypertensive agents (iaa). Finally, the patient would be transferred to his or her family doctor to follow up. For a patient with both HTN and DVT, he/she must follow the guidelines of both. An adverse interaction between guidelines for HTN and DVT is that a patient who suffers urgency hypertension (htnur) cannot take warfarin (wa) or anticoagulant agents (ana), since wa and ana have negative impact on the treatment of hypertension. In such a case, physicians must replace the wa or ana with the other types of treatment, that is, intra-vena cava filter.

4.2. Work Flow of a CDSS for Comorbidity Monitoring. In this section, we would like to address the detailed design of a CDSS, and usually a CDSS is embedded in a patient device. As the primary component of a patient device, a CDSS is designed by referring to clinical guidelines and can output the diagnosis on patient conditions. The first procedure of designing a CDSS is to combine multiple clinical guidelines by translating each of the clinical guidelines into a logic expression. A clinical guideline is composed of a few clinical rules, and each of the rules can be represented by a logic

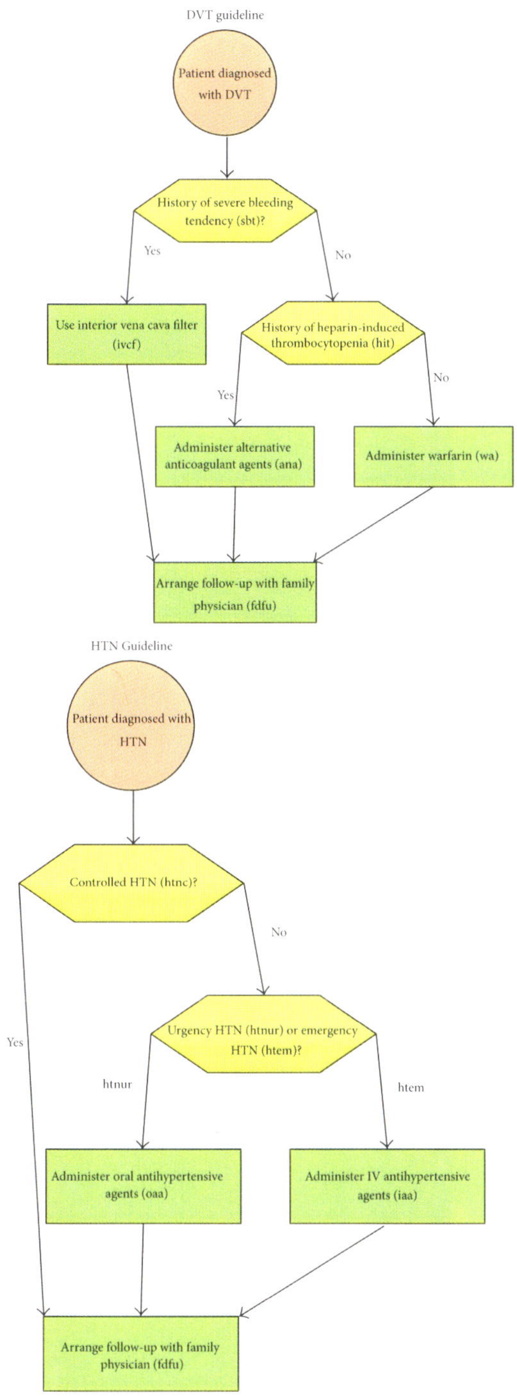

Figure 6: Clinical guidelines for HTN and DVT [17].

programming expression. Thus, we can use the constraint logic programming to combine clinical practice guidelines by following the 3 steps: (1) Translating the rules of each clinical guideline into a few logic expressions; (2) combing the logic expressions of multiple guidelines together; (3) transforming the constraints between all of the guidelines into logic expressions.

Table 2: CLP model for combining clinical guidelines.

Transform	CLP expression
Paths (DVT)	sbt ∧ ivcf ∧ fdfu, not (sbt) ∧ hit ∧ ana ∧ fdfu, not (sbt) ∧ not (hit) ∧ wa ∧ fdfu.
Paths (HTN)	htnc ∧ fdfu, htnuc ∧ htnur ∧ oaa ∧ fdfu, htnuc ∧ htnem ∧ iaa ∧ fdfu.
Constraints	not (htnur ∧ wa) not (htnur ∧ ana).

(1) Transform Rules in the Clinical Guidelines. A clinical guideline consists of multiple clinical rules. For each rule in a clinical guideline, we can denote it in the form of a logic expression. For example, we can transform the rule of sbt → ivcf → fdfu into the logic expression of sbt ∧ ivcf ∧ fdfu; we can transform the rule of htnc → fdfu into the logic expression of htnc ∧ fdfu. Similarly, we can transform all of the rules in clinical guidelines into logic expressions.

(2) Transform Constraints between Guidelines. Taking warfarin (wa) or anticoagulant agents (ana) could result in negative impacts on an urgency hypertension patient. Thus, we need to set a constraint of htnur for the combination of guidelines of HTN and DVT. In this paper, we assume that the constraints are manually analyzed and set by a few physicians. In the future, when all these constraints, that is, the conflicts between clinical guidelines, can be analyzed and stored in a repository, the CDSS can automatically detect the potential conflicts by searching in the repository. This constraint is not presented in any individual clinical guideline but appears when we need to combine multiple guidelines together for the diagnosis on a comorbid patient. In the form of logic expressions, we can denote this constraint as not (htnur∧wa) and not (htnur ∧ ana). When this constraint is violated, that is, in the setting of htnur ∧ wa, the clinicians must adjust the regular treatment plan for this patient.

4.3. Establish a Constraint Logic Programming Model. Based on Sections 4.1 and 4.2, we can establish a constraint logic programming (CLP) model by transforming rules as well as the constraints between multiple clinical guidelines. Consequently, the problem of designing a CDSS can be characterized as a CLP model, and the detailed model is shown in Table 2. In the CLP model, we can capture the clinical decision by ensuring that at least one of the logic expressions which represent the rules of HTN and DVT is "true."

In the stage of implementation, we employ an ECLiPSe platform [20] to represent the above-mentioned CLP model which is established by referring to Table 2. ECLiPSe is a platform designed to support a CLP modelling language—Zinc, which is high-level enough to well characterize most CLP problems and also low-level enough to be easily compatible with many CLP solvers. Also the ECLiPSe offers a special library (called repair) to capture any violations of constraints between CLP expressions. When a constraint in the CLP expressions leads to a conflict, it can be captured by the repair library.

In the following, we present a few sample ECLiPSe codes for capturing the violations of constraints between clinical guidelines:

$$\begin{aligned}&\text{Constraint1 (htnur, wa) r\_conflict cs1,}\\&\text{Constraint2 (htnur, ana) r\_conflict cs2,}\\&\text{conflict\_constraints (cs1, Conflicts),}\\&\text{conflict\_constraints (cs2, Conflicts),}\\&\text{Constraint1 (htnur, wa): (htnur and wa) \$ = 0,}\\&\text{Constraint2 (htnur, ana): (htnur and ana) \$ = 0.}\end{aligned}$$

To illustrate the results of the above-mentioned ECLiPSe sample codes running on the platform, we consider the following clinical scenario: a patient takes both htnur and wa; then ECLiPSe will return the results

$$\text{Conflicts} = [\text{Constraint1}\ (1, 1)].$$

As expected, ECLiPSe captures the violation of constraint Constraint1 (htnur, wa) between clinical guidelines. Then, the CDSS would find a few solutions in order to mitigate the violation of constraints, for example, replacing a few types of medicine by the others. If a CDSS cannot find any solutions, the results would be reported to the physicians who will manually handle the problem.

5. Analysis on the System Accuracy of a CDSS

The nodes in a CLP-CPG model of a CDSS are composed of decision nodes (i.e., the yellow hexagon box in Figure 6) and process nodes (i.e., the green rectangle box in Figure 6). The errors of a CDSS can only occur at the decision nodes when the physicians make a mistake in diagnosis or recording the testing results. In such a case, the final decision made by a CDSS might also be incorrect. In this section we analyze the system accuracy of a CDSS to investigate the performance of our design of system architecture.

The system accuracy (ACC) refers to the probability of correct decision results of both HTN and DVT, and its value equals the multiplication of P_{HTN} and P_{DVT}:

$$\text{ACC} = P_{\text{HTN}} \times P_{\text{DVT}}, \tag{1}$$

where P_{HTN} represents the probability that the decision for HTN is correct, while P_{DVT} represents the probability that the decision for DVT is correct. Given that

$$\begin{aligned}P_{\text{DVT}} &= P\left(\text{sbt} = 1, \widehat{\text{sbt}} = 1\right)\\&\quad + P\left(\text{sbt} = 0, \widehat{\text{sbt}} = 0\right) P\left(\text{hit} = 1, \widehat{\text{hit}} = 1\right)\\&\quad + P\left(\text{sbt} = 0, \widehat{\text{sbt}} = 0\right) P\left(\text{hit} = 0, \widehat{\text{hit}} = 0\right),\end{aligned} \tag{2}$$

where sbt $=$ 1 and sbt $=$ 0 denote that the patient has a history of severe bleeding tendency or not (refer to Figure 6), respectively, while $\widehat{\text{sbt}} = 1$ and $\widehat{\text{sbt}} = 0$ denote that the physicians record that the patient has a history of severe bleeding tendency or not, respectively. Similarly, hit $=$ 1 and hit $=$ 0 denote that the patient has a history of heparin-induced thrombocytopenia or not (refer to Figure 6), respectively, while $\widehat{\text{hit}} = 1$ and $\widehat{\text{hit}} = 0$ denote that the physicians record that the patient has a history of heparin-induced thrombocytopenia or not, respectively.

$$\begin{aligned}P_{\text{HTN}} &= P\left(\text{htnc} = 1, \widehat{\text{htnc}} = 1\right)\\&\quad + P\left(\text{htnuc} = 1, \widehat{\text{htnuc}} = 1\right)\\&\quad \cdot P\left(\text{htnur} = 1, \widehat{\text{htnur}} = 1\right)\\&\quad + P\left(\text{htnuc} = 1, \widehat{\text{htnuc}} = 1\right)\\&\quad \cdot P\left(\text{htnem} = 1, \widehat{\text{htnem}} = 1\right),\end{aligned} \tag{3}$$

where htnc $=$ 1 denotes that the patient actually suffers the controlled hypertension, and $\widehat{\text{htnc}} = 1$ denotes that the patient is diagnosed to suffer the controlled hypertension (refer to Figure 6). Similarly, htnuc $=$ 1 denotes that the patient actually suffers the urgency hypertension, and $\widehat{\text{htnuc}} = 1$ denotes that the patient is diagnosed to suffer the urgency hypertension (refer to Figure 6), respectively. htnem $=$ 1 denotes that the patient actually suffers the emergency hypertension, and $\widehat{\text{htnem}} = 1$ denotes that the patient is diagnosed to suffer the emergency hypertension, respectively.

The rationale for (2) and (3) is calculating the probability of correct decisions on each rule of Table 2.

6. Simulation and Results

In consideration of the errors in the clinical diagnosis, we investigate the system accuracy of a CDSS. Also we compare the average running time of achieving a clinical decision by the CDSS in our design with that in the other designs. In the comparison, we employ anonymized patient data transcribed from a public data source [19]. MIT-BIH database is a well-known standard ECG database, which is used universally for ECG analysis purpose. ECG signals in the database have normal sinus rhythm with a sample rate of 128 Hz and have uniform intervals of 7.8125 ms. We employ all the samples in the above-mentioned database as the dataset to analyze the performance of various systems.

6.1. Accuracy of a CDSS. Based on (1), the accuracy has been assessed both analytically and through Monte-Carlo simulations. In the Monte-Carlo simulations, both the actual patient status and the diagnosed patient status are generated. If the clinical decision results with both the actual status and the diagnosed status match well, then, we increase the number of correct clinical decisions by 1; otherwise, we increase the number of incorrect clinical decisions by 1. Such a process is repeated 10^5 times. Finally, the numbers of both correct and incorrect clinical decisions are recorded. Also we can compute the accuracy of a CDSS by dividing the

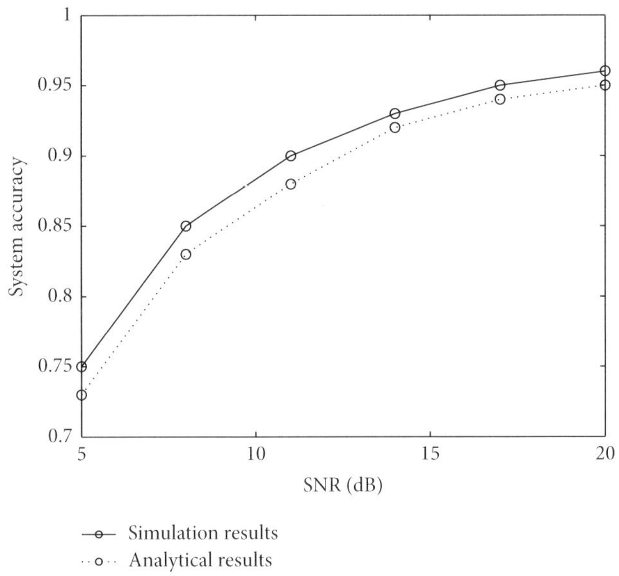

FIGURE 7: Average system accuracy versus SNR.

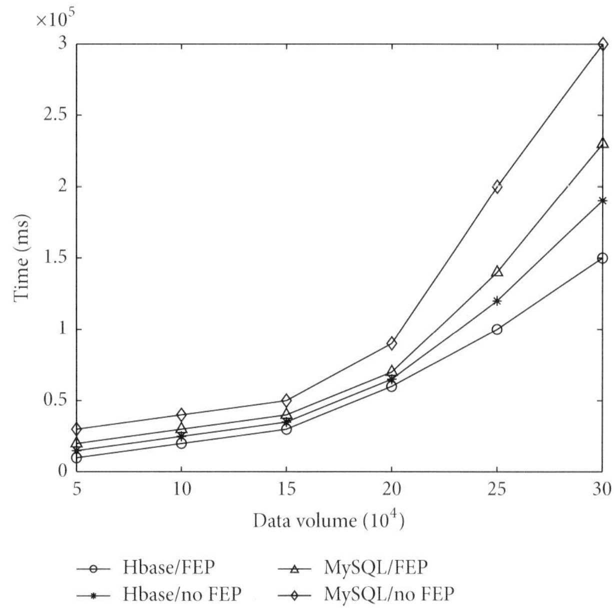

FIGURE 8: Running time of CDSS in various designs.

number of correct clinical decisions by that of all clinical decisions (both correct and incorrect decisions). For both analytical and simulation results, we define SNR $= P(x = \hat{x})/P(x \neq \hat{x})$ in the following simulation, where $x =$ sbt, hit, htnc, htnuc, htnur. A large value of SNR represents a small number of errors in the clinical diagnosis.

Figure 7 illustrates that both analytical results and simulation results of the average accuracy of a CDSS match well, verifying the accuracy of our analytical results. Also Figure 7 illustrates that our designed system can achieve a 95% of accuracy when the level of SNR reaches 20 dB or above (i.e., the average probability of diagnosis errors is around 1% or below).

As expected, we can find that the system accuracy increases with the values of SNRs. However, when the SNR is increasing, the cost of system may also increase, because it takes cost (both in time and in money) to help physicians or clinical staff reduce their errors in the diagnosis or recording the testing results. Given an acceptable level of system performance, we should search for a necessary SNR to guarantee the performance of a CDSS. For instance, we need to design a CDSS with an acceptable level of system accuracy as 95%; we must guarantee the SNR higher than 20 dB (SNR depends on the communication channel conditions between the transmitter and the receiver. In the simulation, we analyze the accuracy with the change of SNR in order to investigate the accuracy of a system under various channel conditions. However, the level of SNR cannot be manually adjusted.). Such a rule of system design can partially determine whether clinical staff or physicians need to be trained. Thus, the analysis on system accuracy can not only help healthcare staff estimate the accuracy of a system, but enable the administrator of a hospital or medical center to make the plan of training their staff.

6.2. Running Time of a CDSS. In this section, we compare the running time of a CDSS in our design with that in a few current designs. The running time is primarily determined by the design in the physical layer and data layer. More specifically, we investigate the impact of FEP (FEP versus no FEP) in the physical layer as well as Hbase (Hbase versus MySQL) in the data layer on the running time of a CDSS.

Figure 8 shows that the running time of a CDSS with Hbase and FEP can dramatically decrease in comparison with that without Hbase and FEP. When the data volume reaches 300000 entries (data volume refers to the number of entries in the data table. The number of entries does not mean the number of users, since a user usually has multiple entries; e.g., a patient may visit a clinic multiple times and therefore have multiple entries of clinical records. Thus, 300000 entries are possible in the real world), the running time of a CDSS with Hbase and FEP is just around a half of that of a CDSS without Hbase and FEP. Also we investigate the proportion of contributions made by the use of Hbase and FEP on the decrease of running time. Figure 8 shows that the design of Hbase in the data layer is the primary contributor, while the design of FEP makes less contributions on reducing running time than the design of Hbase. When the data volume reaches 300000 entries, the use of Hbase can achieve an 8×10^4 decrease of running time, while the use of FEP can only attain a 4×10^4 decrease of running time.

7. Discussion and Conclusion

In this paper, we present the detailed design of a CDSS for monitoring comorbid conditions from the perspectives of architecture, algorithms, and applications. Specifically, we establish the architecture of a CDSS with three layers, that is, physical layer, data layer, and application layer, and discuss the detailed algorithms in each of the layers. Also we address the application of our CDSS in a real scenario of monitoring comorbid patients with both DVT and HTN and analyze the system accuracy of a CDSS. Finally, we compare the running time of making a clinical decision in our design with that in the other designs. The results are that our proposed design of CDSS can achieve a clinical decision faster than the other designs, while ensuring a 90%–95% of the system accuracy.

Using typical clinical scenarios, we have shown how our scheme can process two clinical guidelines by developing a computable model to identify the adverse interactions between clinical guidelines. Such a scheme can support the concurrent application of clinical guidelines, and it is an important step in the process of building up an automated CDSS for the management of comorbid patients.

In the following, we present a few open issues we will work on: (1) Expanding our proposed scheme to process more than two CPGs at a time: while the proposed scheme is general enough, the increased complexity in the operations on multiple guidelines requires substantial modifications to the proposed scheme; (2) allowing for dosages of medications for a detailed description of adverse interactions: this requires revisiting definitions of logical models in our proposed scheme; (3) allowing for the automatic extraction of clinical knowledge from diversified sources to update the scheme of processing multiple clinical guidelines.

Acknowledgments

This work was partially supported by the National Natural Science Foundation of China (no. 61601082) and partially supported by the Fundamental Research Funds for the Central Universities (no. ZYGX2015J071).

References

[1] D. He, C. Chen, S. Chan, J. Bu, and A. V. Vasilakos, "ReTrust: attack-resistant and lightweight trust management for medical sensor networks," *IEEE Transactions on Information Technology in Biomedicine*, vol. 16, no. 4, pp. 623–632, 2012.

[2] N. Xiong, A. Vasilakos, L. Yang et al., "Comparative analysis of quality of service and memory usage for adaptive failure detectors in healthcare systems," *IEEE Journal on Selected Areas in Communications*, vol. 27, no. 4, pp. 495–509, 2009.

[3] S. Agarwal, A. Joshi, T. Finin, Y. Yesha, and T. Ganous, "A pervasive computing system for the operating room of the future," *Mobile Networks and Applications*, vol. 12, no. 2-3, pp. 215–228, 2007.

[4] M. Mahfouf, M. F. Abbod, and D. A. Linkens, "A survey of fuzzy logic monitoring and control utilisation in medicine," *Artificial Intelligence in Medicine*, vol. 21, no. 1–3, pp. 27–42, 2001.

[5] H. Deng, G. Runger, and E. Tuv, "Bias of importance measures for multivalued attributes and solutions," in *Proceedings of the 21st International Conference on Artificial Neural Networks (ICANN '11)*, Espoo, Finland, June 2011.

[6] H. Shin and M. K. Markey, "A machine learning perspective on the development of clinical decision support systems utilizing mass spectra of blood samples," *Journal of Biomedical Informatics*, vol. 39, no. 2, pp. 227–248, 2006.

[7] M. T. Taner, J. D. Walls, M. Smith, G. Taylor, M. B. Carr, and D. Dumas, "Reservoir characterization by calibration of self organized map clusters," SEG Technical Program Expanded Abstracts 1552C1555, 2011.

[8] W. Yao and A. Kumar, "CONFlexFlow: integrating flexible clinical pathways into clinical decision support systems using context and rules," *Decision Support Systems*, vol. 55, no. 2, pp. 499–515, 2013.

[9] P. Musiat, P. Goldstone, and N. Tarrier, "Understanding the acceptability of e-mental health—attitudes and expectations towards computerised self-help treatments for mental health problems," *BMC Psychiatry*, vol. 14, no. 1, article no. 109, 2014.

[10] B. Tang and H. He, "ENN: Extended Nearest Neighbor method for pattern recognition," *IEEE Computational Intelligence Magazine*, vol. 10, no. 3, pp. 52–60, 2015.

[11] H. Medjahed, D. Istrate, J. Boudy, and B. Dorizzi, "Human activities of daily living recognition using fuzzy logic for elderly home monitoring," in *Proceedings of the IEEE International Conference on Fuzzy Systems*, pp. 2001–2006, August 2009.

[12] C. M. Boyd, J. Darer, C. Boult, L. P. Fried, L. Boult, and A. W. Wu, "Clinical practice guidelines and quality of care for older patients with multiple comorbid diseases: implications for pay for performance," *Journal of the American Medical Association*, vol. 294, no. 6, pp. 716–724, 2005.

[13] D. Riaño, F. Real, J. A. López-Vallverdú et al., "An ontology-based personalization of health-care knowledge to support clinical decisions for chronically ill patients," *Journal of Biomedical Informatics*, vol. 45, no. 3, pp. 429–446, 2012.

[14] M. Michalowski, M. Mainegra Hing, S. Wilk, W. Michalowski, and K. Farion, "A constraint logic programming approach to identifying inconsistencies in clinical practice guidelines for patients with comorbidity," in *Proceedings of the 13th Conference on Artificial Intelligence in Medicine (AIME '11)*, M. Peleg, N. Lavrač, and C. Combi, Eds., pp. 296–301, Bled, Slovenia, July 2011.

[15] The hadoop software package, http://hadoop.apache.org/.

[16] The hbase software package, http://hbase.apache.org/.

[17] S. Wilk, W. Michalowski, M. Michalowski, K. Farion, M. M. Hing, and S. Mohapatra, "Mitigation of adverse interactions in pairs of clinical practice guidelines using constraint logic programming," *Journal of Biomedical Informatics*, vol. 46, no. 2, pp. 341–353, 2013.

[18] S. Z. Wilk, M. Michalowski, W. Michalowski, M. Mainegra Hing, and K. Farion, "Reconciling pairs of concurrently used clinical practice guidelines using constraint logic programming," in *Proceedings of the AMIA Annual Symposium. Improving Health: Informatics and IT Changing the World*, pp. 944–953, Washington, DC, USA, October 2011.

[19] The MIT-BIH Sinus Rhythm database, http://www.physionet.org/physiobank/database/nsrdb/.

[20] The ECLiPSe software package, http://www.eclipseclp.org/.

23

Managing Emergencies in Rural North Queensland: The Feasibility of Teletraining

Tarsh Pandit,[1] **Robin A. Ray**,[1] **and Sabe Sabesan**[1,2]

[1]*College of Medicine and Dentistry, James Cook University, Townsville, QLD, Australia*
[2]*Tropical Centre for Telehealth Practice and Research, Townsville Hospital and Health Services, Townsville, QLD, Australia*

Correspondence should be addressed to Tarsh Pandit; pandittarsh@gmail.com

Academic Editor: Vincenzo Della Mea

Introduction. Historically, the use of videoconference technologies in emergency medicine training has been limited. Whilst there are anecdotal reports of the use of teletraining for emergency medicine by rural doctors in Australia, minimal evidence exists in the literature. This paper aimed to explore the use of teletraining in the context of managing emergency presentations in rural hospitals. *Methods.* Using a qualitative approach, a mixture of junior and senior doctors were invited to participate in semistructured interviews. Data were transcribed and analysed line by line. Applying the grounded theory principles of open and axial coding, themes and subthemes were generated. *Results.* A total of 20 interviews were conducted with rural doctors, rural doctors who are medical educators, and emergency medicine specialists. Two major themes—(1) teletraining as education and (2) personal considerations—and ten subthemes were evident from the data. Most participants had some previous experience with teletraining. Access to peer teaching over videoconference was requested by rural generalist registrars. There was a preference for interactive training sessions, over didactic lectures with little mention of technical barriers to engagement. The ability of teletraining to reduce professional isolation was a major benefit for doctors practicing in remote locations. *Discussion.* For these rural doctors, teletraining is a feasible method of education delivery. Wider application of teletraining such as its use in peer teaching needs to be explored. The benefits of teletraining suggest that teletraining models need to be core business for health services and training providers, including specialist colleges.

1. Introduction

Addressing the rural workforce shortages in Australia has been a challenge for the Australian Government for over 20 years [1]. Issues such as lack of professional contact with colleagues, specialist backup in emergencies, and remoteness from families have been well described in the literature as reasons for doctors leaving rural practice [2]. Further training has also been linked with promoting retention of rural doctors [3]. Given the vast distances in Australia, it is not feasible for doctors to regularly travel to larger centres for upskilling. Whilst some rural sites have sufficient medical staff to conduct regular on-site teaching, this is not feasible for smaller hospitals.

The use of videoconference technologies for medical education (teletraining) has been described in the literature from as early as 1996 [4]. It has successfully been used for paediatric cardiology and surgical education including practical training in laparoscopic procedures [5–7]. In oncology, telesupervision and teleeducation for remote administration of chemotherapy have been successfully implemented in rural Australia [8]. However the application for videoconferencing for emergency medicine (EM) education has been limited [9]. Encouragingly a recent Canadian study demonstrated that videoconference technologies can be successfully used to teach the internationally recognized Advanced Trauma Life Support course [10].

A state-wide roll-out of telehealth services by Queensland's Department of Health has resulted in rural doctors having access to high quality videoconferencing technology [11]. Both web based applications and traditional high-end videoconferencing capabilities have been installed in many rural hospitals as part of this state-wide agenda. Anecdotal evidence suggests that videoconferencing is regularly used for

EM training in North Queensland, such as the Rural Grand Round and lectures delivered by the Emergency Medicine Education and Training (EMET) team. However, the literature is limited in many aspects of teletraining including description of training models and needs of the rural doctors.

This study aimed to evaluate the training needs of rural doctors and explore the use of teletraining in the context of managing emergency presentations. For the purposes of the paper, only the findings relevant to the use of teletraining have been reported.

2. Methods

2.1. Recruitment. Using purposive and theoretical sampling, doctors with range of practice years were invited by telephone, email, and professional encounters to participate in the study.

2.2. Participants. The inclusion criteria were doctors working in North Queensland with (a) current/recent work in a rural area that involved managing emergencies, (b) involvement with rural medical education, or (c) Fellowship of the Australasian College of Emergency Medicine and working in a tertiary referral centre. Rurality was defined as working in a Modified Monash (MM) category greater than 3. The seven Modified Monash Model categories are a revised version of the previous Australian Standard Geographic Classification-Remoteness Areas (ASGC-RA) which add an extra dimension of population size: (1) metropolitan; (2) regional > 50,000; (3) large rural 15,000–50,000; (4) medium rural 5000–15,000; (5) small rural < 5000; (6) remote; (7) very remote [12, 13].

Roughly equal numbers of junior and senior doctors were recruited. Senior doctors were defined as those who had obtained full fellowship of their respective college, and junior doctors were defined as any doctor yet to meet this criterion. (Fellowship of the Australasian College of Emergency Medicine requires a minimum of 5 years of postgraduate training and satisfactory progression through required assessments. Fellowship of the Australian College of Rural and Remote Medicine or Royal Australian College of General Practitioners requires a minimum of 4 years of postgraduate training and satisfactory progression through required assessments.)

2.3. Interview Guide. Adopting a descriptive qualitative approach, an interview guide based on current literature was developed by the research team and revised after discussion with three rural doctors and the approving Human Research Ethics Committee (HREC) [14]. The guide was piloted and refined for data collection. Semistructured interviews covering topics such as practice demographics, experience with video-conferenced based technologies, positive and negative aspects of teletraining, and feasibility of teletraining were conducted by the first author.

2.4. Data Analysis. Data analysis occurred concurrently with data collection. Interviews were audiorecorded, transcribed, and analysed line by line in NVivo data management software version 11©. To improve analytical rigour a selected number of interviews were descriptively coded independently by two investigators. The codes were compared to ensure consistency and any disagreements between coding were resolved by consensus. As new themes arose from the analysis, the interview guide was amended enabling a process of participant validation to further enhance the validity of the data. Applying the grounded theory principles of open and axial coding, themes and subthemes were generated. Data saturation was achieved when no new themes emerged in the last four interviews. Relationships between themes were explored using mind-mapping. Demographic information such as position, qualification, and MM category was incorporated into the analysis. Ethical approval to conduct the study was granted by Queensland Health and James Cook University.

3. Results

A total of 20 interviews averaging 28 minutes were conducted with doctors from various rural hospitals in North Queensland. Junior doctors were two rural relievers, two GP registrars working as primary house officers, one non-hospital based GP registrar, and six provisional fellows. Senior doctors were seven rural generalists and two emergency medicine specialists (see Table 1 for participant characteristics).

Ten interviews were conducted in person, nine were conducted via telephone and one was conducted over videoconference. During one interview the participant withdrew midinterview due to a clinical emergency. Attempts were made to reschedule, but this was not feasible due to the participant's work schedule.

Two Major Themes. Teletraining as education and personal considerations alongside ten subthemes arose from the data.

3.1. Teletraining as Education

3.1.1. Previous Experiences with Teletraining. Most participants reported previous experience with teletraining. These experiences included tutorials provided by GP training organisations, lectures by EMET, and training on nonemergency topics such as sexual and mental health in primary care. Two participants mentioned undertaking further academic studies that used videoconference for lectures.

All participants exposed to teletraining talked about its use in positive terms. In particular the Rural Grand Round, a video-conferenced presentation between multiple rural sites, was rated highly by a number of participants. The ability for further education with specialists of the region was also beneficial to rural doctors (see Table 2).

However, some participants described negative experiences in relation to relevance of presentations to current working conditions, sessions lacking interaction, or presentation skills of the presenter. Interestingly, those who described negative experiences continued to recognize it as an acceptable mode of education delivery.

Table 1: Demographics.

	Junior (11)	Senior (9)
MMM		
1-2	-	3
3	-	-
4	6	4
5	1	1
6	2	1
7	2	-
Postgraduate years/years of fellowship		
0-1	-	2
2	2	-
3	2	1
4	1	1
5	3	
>5	3	5
Advanced skill*		
Emergency	1	3
Others	4	4
N/A	6	4
Others		
Medical superintendent	-	1
Involved with training	-	2

*Some doctors had more than one advanced skill.

3.1.2. Face-to-Face versus Videoconference Learning. Overall participants perceived teletraining to be a good adjunct to traditional forms of teaching for staff of all levels. The ability to have regular, ongoing education without significant travel was a key factor for doctors, particularly in high MM categories (6 and 7). Participants with significant previous experience with teletraining viewed it as a regular part of continuing education. Whilst some participants mentioned that it was not as good as face-to-face training, they agreed that it was preferable to no training at all.

3.1.3. Peer Teaching. Peer teaching using videoconference was supported by a number of provisional fellows and rural generalists. It was suggested that this teaching should be an interactive, case-based small group discussion facilitated by a senior doctor. The ability to share different approaches relevant to rural settings, formalising conversations that already occur informally, and having training targeted to the participant's level were cited as positive reasons to provide peer teaching.

3.1.4. Teaching Skills Using Videoconference. Concerns about teaching skills over videoconference ranged from technological challenges such as insufficient camera angles to correct technique and the notion that teletraining should only be used for static forms of learning and that certain skills could only be learnt by feeling the anatomy.

However, of the 20 doctors, only one participant reported learning skills in a setting similar to videoconferencing where a colonoscopy was broadcast on a screen to viewers outside the procedure room. The participant suggested that similar demonstrations may be useful.

In terms of learning new skills, participants varied in their opinions about which skills could be successfully taught over videoconference. For example, some doctors stated advanced airways skills could not be taught over videoconference, whilst others suggested it would be achievable if combined with simulation training. There was further disagreement between some junior and senior doctors about the addition of videoconferencing to simulations. The senior doctors argued that technologically intensive simulations detracted from the learning experience; therefore local staff should be trained to run the simulations. However, the suggested benefit of the addition of videoconference to simulations was organisation by an experienced external source, thus making training less likely to be missed.

For brushing up on previous learnt skills, teletraining was not seen to be useful, due to the availability of online resources such as YouTube™ or Life in the Fast lane©. The ability to use resources anytime, when required, was preferable to real-time videoconference education.

3.1.5. Didactic versus Interactive Sessions. Having an interactive component, particularly the ability to have a back-forth discussion is an important aspect of learning via teletraining. Whilst some participants agreed that didactic sessions could be useful in certain scenarios such as major updates, this information could also be provided through online sources. The overwhelming preference was for interactive sessions with increased engagement in discussion sessions.

Table 2: Teletraining as education.

Subtheme	Quote
Previous experiences with teletraining	"What I actually find more useful [in Rural Grand Rounds] is quite often he gets paediatricians, emergency medicine from [bigger regional centres], from everywhere who actually do speeches and talks" [PF 4] "So yeah, that lack of physical-ness about the situation means often you can get apathetic and sometimes just be a bit blasé about it all and sign on just because you have to sign on" [PF 3] "Oh, I think it serves a purpose. So these people are spread off all over North Queensland and the distances that are involved are prohibitive for everyone together on a really regular basis" [PF 3]
Face to Face versus videoconference learning	"I think any access to any teaching would be appropriate and even if you do not pick up at come place like do not pick up as much from face to face teaching. . .Sometimes telehealth teaching can teach you maybe if you do pick up 50% of it just because it's ongoing" [PF 5] "I think tele-training is the way of the future especially for people in our area that more and more of us are going out to rural sites" [RR 2]
Peer teaching	"The best benefit is you get to experience different thinking outside the box and different ways of doing things that apply to rural areas, rather than the textbook stuff that does not always apply" [PF 6] "I enjoy catching up with people that are in a similar role and have a chance to debrief and have a chance to learn from each other and that is not really a lot of opportunity for that, and the peer education, just people in the same situation and learning from things they have seen and done before, that is probably the only thing I have noticed as a difference" [PF 1]
Teaching skills using videoconference	"I think though that there are certain skills that you need to do person - face-to-face and have immediate feedback on" [RG 2] "Unfortunately the technology is what people take away from those learning opportunities; they do not take away the actual message of simulation" [RG 6] "There is no reason why they cannot create a resus with a mannequin, put a dress on it and bring it to the ED and run their own simulation. We all have inherent skills and knowledge. Doing simple stuff, it does not need to be complex" [RG 6] "The biggest issue with rural is that often you plan to do something every week . . .then it just falls off the radar. . . I think you'd need to have a bunch of passionate people at a centralised location to really push it to happen every week" [PF 4] "I do not see why you would need someone to teach a practical skill online as a teleconference when you can use YouTube, pause it and revisit all of the steps" [PF 6]
Didactic versus interactive sessions	"Interactive, I definitely prefer, but sometimes in the early years of GP training, a lot of the stuff was a bit didactic, but I did not mind that, I found it to be quiet useful" [GPRNH] "There would be scope for that as long as it's not didactic lectures, as long as there can be interaction and the facilitators have a skill in that and the people who are being educated, the students, are prepared enough to interact. . .it would have to be an interactive thing otherwise you can get that from a YouTube, cannot you?" [RG 3]

[RR] rural reliever; [PHO] GP Registrar Primary House Officer; [GPRNH] non-hospital based GP registrar; [PF] provisional fellow; [FACEM] Fellow of Australasian College of Emergency Medicine; [RG] rural generalist.

3.2. Personal Considerations

3.2.1. Technological Issues. Interestingly many participants reported minimal issues with Internet connections. Of the doctors who mentioned issues with Internet connections, most described it as a potential challenge rather than a continual problem or only in relation to home Internet. However one doctor did report a number of experiences

TABLE 3: Personal considerations.

Subtheme	Quote
Technological issues	"You could say in theory talk about technological glitches but really they were hardly there in my experience. There is so much support, there's hardly any technological problem" [RG 7] I've been to lots of courses where - or video conferences that are halfway through and it's cut out and then they come back and you get a bit of it, and then you've lost the rest of it. So you just end up chatting and not really engaging" [PF 2]
Interacting with the technology	"Places like [Health Service A], Tele-health is what we did. Everyone knew how to work the machines, everyone knew what the limitations of the technologies were. I am not convinced that in [Health Service B] that is the case yet. I think we can still do a little more work to improve our access to utilisation of videoconferencing as a medium of education. I think if you compared the people from [A] and people from [B], I think you would get very different answers. [A] is more tele-health engaged then [B] is" [RG 6] "That's something that really frustrates us as people who are really adept at using technology, that they're using platforms that are really not user friendly" [PF 3]
Work hours versus out of work hours	"I find it very hard to imagine squeezing anything into workhours here, because we are so flat out" [PF 6] "I've got three kids so often when I come home from work; I am home from work" [PF 4] The referral hospital sends an emergency consultant up once every few months to do training. But if it is busy, or you are in theatre you cannot go. So you miss out on that. [PF 1] "People tend to make the time [for EMET] because it is such a valuable learning experience" [PF 4]
Paid time versus own time	"Then you've got issues then is that paid or unpaid time, because it's work-related or not work-related. . .So do you then do extra hours at the hospital, do your kind of video conference and not being paid for them. You know, that that becomes a big thing" [PF 2] "SMOs get paid incredible well, they have all these bonuses which I think as long as it is not every night, doing it once a week or once a fortnight they should suck it up" [PF 6]
Reducing professional isolation	"The fact that is keeps you connected with equivalent peers in the region, has been really good" [GPRNH] "They are very helpful because more so when you are working in a remote area it's so easy to feel isolated. . . At least you know that there are other people out there in a similar situation as you. It is really good and it is quite effective". . .I think their welfare is important in terms of professional and personal health [RG 7]

[RR] rural reliever; [PHO] GP Registrar Primary House Officer; [GPRNH] non-hospital based GP registrar; [PF] Provisional Fellow; [FACEM] Fellow of Australasian College of Emergency Medicine; [RG] rural generalist.

of technological issues that detracted from the learning experience (see Table 3).

3.2.2. Interacting with the Technology. One rural generalist suggested that the overall acceptance of telehealth in health services was directly linked to acceptance of teletraining. The increased usage by certain sites meant staff were more comfortable using the technology for other services. Participants from MM 6 locations appeared to have more experience with teletraining and telehealth.

However, for doctors familiar with videoconference technologies, the negative experiences may be dependent on user platforms. Certain platforms were reported to be more successful in facilitating interactive discussion and reducing frustration in terms of logging in. The frustration with using non-user friendly platforms may be amplified because the users are aware of the capabilities of better platforms. Frustrations also arose from limitations to preparation for education sessions, such as availability of PowerPoint presentations ahead of time or testing web links before dissemination.

3.2.3. Work Hours versus Out of Work Hours. A number of doctors mentioned that whilst further education is important and necessary, finding appropriate timings for sessions would be a significant barrier. The main arguments for having training scheduled afterhours were from participants working in hospitals without adequate staff to cover training time absences. Participants who preferred to avoid afterhours training cited reasons such as family commitments and exhaustion after work.

Finding protected time to attend training activities was an ongoing challenge. Participants described similar issues when EM specialists visited for face-to-face training. Interestingly two participants mentioned that if the learning experience is valuable enough, most doctors would reorganise schedules to attend. Yet, both participants worked in a town with a Modified Monash Category of 4, in relatively well-staffed hospitals.

3.2.4. Paid Time versus Own Time. Remuneration for training undertaken outside work time is also an issue. Unfortunately remuneration negotiations are beyond the scope of this paper but may need to be considered if emergency teletraining activities were offered.

3.2.5. Reducing Professional Isolation. Remote participants mentioned that the use of teletraining is an effective strategy for improving professional connection and reducing professional isolation. Seeing colleagues in a similar situation over videoconference enabled participants to feel connected and improved the overall wellbeing of rural doctors.

4. Discussion

Most participants in this study had some form of experience with teletraining and identified it as a feasible model of delivering EM education to rural doctors. Of particular note was the Rural Grand Round delivered by video conference for the past seven years, which demonstrates the overall acceptability of this method of training delivery.

Similar to previous studies, some participants agreed that whilst teletraining was not as good as traditional forms of teaching, the ability to have regular education without significant travel made it a useful tool for rural doctors [15, 16].

The findings of this study indicate that rural doctors would like access to peer teaching. Other authors have demonstrated successful use of small group learning via videoconference for medical education, a strategy that would support peer learning [15]. Furthermore its small size would mean logistical considerations such as timings could be overcome by tailoring it to individual rosters. In relation to this study's findings on training needs (reported elsewhere), peer teaching would help rural doctors manage emergencies in the context of limitations specific to rural sites as well as support new provisional fellows taking up senior positions. Furthermore, peer teaching combines both videoconferencing and continued medical education. Both of these factors have been shown to reduce professional isolation and improve retention of rural doctors [8, 17]. However the practicalities in the application of peer teaching require further research.

The doctors in this study raised concerns regarding the use of teletraining for nonstatic forms of learning, unaware that teaching of surgical and EM skills over videoconference has been previously demonstrated [5, 10]. Determining which emergency skills can successfully be taught is an area for future research. However, based on this study's training needs research, procedural skills were not identified as a major training need; therefore skills training via videoconference may not be required. In contrast regular in-house simulations were requested by rural doctors. The possibility of incorporating videoconferencing to simulations was raised by some doctors and rejected by others. A potential avenue that overcomes divided opinion may be a low-fidelity simulation organised via videoconference. Consequently, the technology would not detract from the learning experience and external motivation would ensure it does not get forgotten. However this would require an external organisation to set up such a system. More research would be required before feasibility of simulations with videoconferencing can be confirmed.

Contrary to older studies, technological glitches such as Internet connection were not perceived to be a major concern [4]. This study reaffirms another recent paper on videoconference technologies in North Queensland, suggesting that over time the technology has improved [8]. Instead doctors who were less familiar with videoconferencing were those more resistant to teletraining. Previous studies have found overcoming scepticism and doctors not understanding the value of the technology as important barriers to teleconferencing technology [18]. For some experienced users of teletraining negative experiences may be driven by the inability of the user-platform to meet their expectations.

Opinion was divided about timings for teletraining opportunities. Judging by this variability, perhaps a better approach would be to book teletraining in consultation with the individual site, considering relevant rosters and the personal preference of the doctors. Other logistical concerns such as remuneration were beyond the scope of this paper but may be relevant to training providers/organisational bodies intending to offer teletraining opportunities.

It is of interest that when discussing the limitations of teletraining, participants also discussed the skills of the presenter separate to the technology itself. The successful utilisation of this technology requires alternative teaching styles in comparison to traditional models of lecturing. As mentioned above, interactive sessions are not offered by local training providers, despite having access to the technology. Therefore the feasibility of teletraining may be underreported as training providers are not using the technology to its full capabilities.

5. Limitations

The study was limited in its evaluation of the use of videoconferencing to teach EM skills, as most participants had no prior experiences with this learning. Consequently the study's findings are based on participant's assumptions regarding its capabilities.

6. Conclusion

Teletraining for management of emergency condition is welcomed and appreciated by rural doctors in North Queensland. For these rural doctors it is a feasible mode of delivering education to rural sites. Among the benefits of teletraining, reducing professional isolation is an important factor for sustaining rural practice. Therefore teletraining models need to be established as core business for health services and training providers including specialist colleges.

Acknowledgments

Funding for this study was provided by the James Cook University Honours program and used solely for transcription of the interviews. The researchers and participants received no monetary compensation for their work.

References

[1] J. S. Humphreys, "Health and the 1999 Regional Australia Summit," *Australian Journal of Rural Health*, vol. 8, no. 1, pp. 52–57, 2000.

[2] R. B. Hays, P. C. Veitch, B. Cheers, and L. Crossland, "Why doctors leave rural practice.," *Australian Journal of Rural Health*, vol. 5, no. 4, pp. 198–203, 1997.

[3] C. Alexander and J. D. Fraser, "Education, training and support needs of Australian trained doctors and international medical graduates in rural Australia: a case of special needs?" *Rural and Remote Health*, vol. 7, no. 2, p. 681, 2007.

[4] P. W. Callas, M. A. Ricci, and M. P. Caputo, "Improved rural provider access to continuing medical education through interactive videoconferencing," *Telemedicine and e-Health*, vol. 6, no. 4, pp. 393–399, 2000.

[5] K. M. Augestad and R. O. Lindsetmo, "Overcoming distance: Video-conferencing as a clinical and educational tool among surgeons," *World Journal of Surgery*, vol. 33, no. 7, pp. 1356–1365, 2009.

[6] E. M. Bogen, K. M. Augestad, H. R. Patel, and R. O. Lindsetmo, "Telementoring in education of laparoscopic surgeons: An emerging technology," *World Journal of Gastrointestinal Endoscopy*, vol. 6, no. 5, pp. 148–155, 2014.

[7] J. P. Finley, M. J. Beland, C. Boutin et al., "A national network for the tele-education of Canadian residents in pediatric cardiology.," *Cardiology in the Young*, vol. 11, no. 5, pp. 526–531, 2001.

[8] M. Cameron, R. Ray, and S. Sabesan, "Remote supervision of medical training via videoconference in northern Australia: a qualitative study of the perspectives of supervisors and trainees," *BMJ Open*, vol. 5, no. 3, p. e006444, 2015.

[9] S. Binks and J. Benger, "Tele-education in emergency care," *Emergency Medicine Journal*, vol. 24, no. 11, pp. 782–784, 2007.

[10] J. Ali, A. Sorvari, S. Camera, M. Kinach, S. Mohammed, and A. Pandya, "Telemedicine as a potential medium for teaching the advanced trauma life support (ATLS) course," *Journal of Surgical Education*, vol. 70, no. 2, pp. 258–264, 2013.

[11] S. Sabesan, S. Larkins, R. Evans et al., "Telemedicine for rural cancer care in North Queensland: Bringing cancer care home," *Australian Journal of Rural Health*, vol. 20, no. 5, pp. 259–264, 2012.

[12] D. J. Russell and M. R. McGrail, "How does the workload and work activities of procedural GPs compare to non-procedural GPs?" *Australian Journal of Rural Health*, vol. 25, no. 4, pp. 219–226, 2017.

[13] J. Mason, *Review of Australian Government Health Workforce Programs*, The Department of Health, 2013.

[14] T. Pandit, R. Ray, and S. Sabesan, "Review article: Managing medical emergencies in rural Australia: A systematic review of the training needs," *Emergency Medicine Australasia*, 2018.

[15] M. Allen, J. Sargeant, K. Mann, M. Fleming, and J. Premi, "Videoconferencing for practice-based small-group continuing medical education: feasibility, acceptability, effectiveness, and cost.," *The Journal of Continuing Education in the Health Professions*, vol. 23, no. 1, pp. 38–47, 2003.

[16] M. P. L. Cameron, R. Ray, and S. Sabesan, "Physicians' perceptions of clinical supervision and educational support via videoconference: A systematic review," *Journal of Telemedicine and Telecare*, vol. 20, no. 5, pp. 272–281, 2014.

[17] C. D. White, K. Willett, C. Mitchell, and S. Constantine, "Making a difference: education and training retains and supports rural and remote doctors in Queensland.," *Rural and Remote Health*, vol. 7, no. 2, p. 700, 2007.

[18] M. A. Ricci, M. Caputo, J. Amour et al., "Telemedicine reduces discrepancies in rural trauma care," *Telemedicine and e-Health*, vol. 9, no. 1, pp. 3–11, 2003.

24

A Multiple-Classifier Framework for Parkinson's Disease Detection Based on Various Vocal Tests

Mahnaz Behroozi and Ashkan Sami

Department of CSE and IT, School of Electrical Engineering and Computer Science, Shiraz University, Shiraz 71348-51154, Iran

Correspondence should be addressed to Ashkan Sami; sami@shirazu.ac.ir

Academic Editor: Aura Ganz

Recently, speech pattern analysis applications in building predictive telediagnosis and telemonitoring models for diagnosing Parkinson's disease (PD) have attracted many researchers. For this purpose, several datasets of voice samples exist; the UCI dataset named "*Parkinson Speech Dataset with Multiple Types of Sound Recordings*" has a variety of vocal tests, which include sustained vowels, words, numbers, and short sentences compiled from a set of speaking exercises for healthy and people with Parkinson's disease (PWP). Some researchers claim that summarizing the multiple recordings of each subject with the central tendency and dispersion metrics is an efficient strategy in building a predictive model for PD. However, they have overlooked the point that a PD patient may show more difficulty in pronouncing certain terms than the other terms. Thus, summarizing the vocal tests may lead into loss of valuable information. In order to address this issue, the classification setting must take *what* has been said into account. As a solution, we introduced a new framework that applies an independent classifier for each vocal test. The final classification result would be a majority vote from all of the classifiers. When our methodology comes with filter-based feature selection, it enhances classification accuracy up to *15%*.

1. Introduction

Parkinson's disease was first introduced in 1817 by Doctor James Parkinson as "shaking palsy" [1]. It is the second common neurological disease coming afterwards Alzheimer and is mostly common among elders [2, 3]. PD is a kind of progressive disease in which an area of brain becomes damaged over the years. It causes various signs and symptoms. From one perspective, these signs and symptoms can be grouped into two major categories: motor symptoms and nonmotor symptoms. Motor symptoms are those that affect movement and muscles and nonmotor symptoms include neurobehavioral and cognitive problems, sleep problems, sensory problems, and autonomic neuropathy (dysautonomia) [4].

Speech disturbance is one of the most common motor problems of PD [4]. Research has shown that about 90% of PWP are affected with motor problems, especially speech impairment [5, 6]. In addition to the prevalence of vocal impairments in PD patients, gathering speech samples and doing signal processing of their voice has low cost and it is appropriate for telemonitoring and telediagnosis systems [7, 8]. Therefore, PD diagnosis from speech impairments is becoming more widespread.

In Parkinsonism patients, speech disorders result from neurologic impairments which are associated with weakness, slowness, or incoordination of the muscles used to produce speech [9, 10]. Speech disturbance usually occurs in the following forms: *hypophonia*, which is soft speech that results from weakness in the vocal musculature, *monotonic speech*, which deals with speech quality in the cases that are soft, hoarse, and monotonous, and *festination speech*, which is when the speech becomes excessively rapid, soft, breathy, and poorly intelligible [4].

Many approaches have been proposed in order to find the severity of each speech impairment sign. There are two types of the best known vocal tests for this purpose: *sustained phonation* [11, 12] and *running speech* [12] tests. In sustained phonation, the patient is asked to say a single vowel, while holding its pitch as constant and long as possible.

In running speech, the patient says a standard sentence which includes representative linguistic units that can show possible impairment signs of vocal disorder. The main focus of this research is on the latter problem statement. Previous researches had two main flaws: (a) all the voice samples were classified by a single classifier; (b) the vocal samples of each subject were summarized with the help of statistical metrics irrespective of discriminating ability of each vocal test.

Since most studies in the area of PD detections based on speech are done on datasets gathered on just one or a few types of vocal tests, we have brought our attention to a dataset with multiple sound recordings. The main contributions of this study are twofold: (1) to suggest a new distinctive classification framework which proposes to apply a unique classifier to vocal samples of *each type*, for example, have a classifier just for vowel "a," rather than applying a single classifier for all vocals and (2) to present which vocal tests are more representative and to indirectly omit less discriminating vocal tests by embedding majority voting in our proposed method.

The rest of the paper is organized as follows. Section 2 reviews previous studies of this domain. In Section 3, a brief description of the dataset, evaluation metrics, and the proposed method can be found. Section 4 demonstrates the results of this work and, finally, Section 5 presents the conclusion of this study.

2. Related Work

In recent years the detection of vocal disorders with the help of machine learning turned into a hot topic. Various research papers have attempted to solve this problem by considering acoustic measurements of dysphonia as effective features to distinguish normal (control) from disordered cases [7, 8, 13, 14]. Studies in this field can be categorized into two main groups: (1) those that attempt to find the most effective vocal features and produce new datasets [8, 13, 15] and (2) those that try to find more effective features from existing datasets and concentrate on enhancing classification accuracy [14, 16–26].

Some studies focused on how to produce new datasets based on their research findings. Little et al. in [8] aimed to analyze the effectiveness of nonstandard measurements. Their work led to the introduction of a new dysphonia measurement named as PPE (pitch period entropy). In their study, they had collected sustained vowel "a" phonations from 31 subjects of which 23 were PD patients and they reached the classification accuracy of 91.4%. In [13], Sakar et al. presented a dataset of 40 subjects including 20 PD. Each individual was trained to say a set of 26 distinct disorder representative terms consisting of sustained vowels, words, numbers, and short sentences. This dataset is the focus of current work. They applied *summarized leave-one-out* (s-LOO) validation technique in which all the voice samples of each individual will be summarized using central tendency and dispersion metrics such as median, mean, standard deviation, trimmed mean, interquartile range, and mean absolute deviation. Their approach obtained 77.5% of classification accuracy. Tsanas et al. in [15] focused on monitoring the PD progression with the help of extracted features using signal processing techniques applied on a huge dataset of about 6000 voice samples from 42 patients with early-stage PD. They have attempted to estimate the unified Parkinson's disease rating scale (UPDRS) using linear and nonlinear regression. Their results show the accuracy of about 7.5-point difference from clinical UPDRS estimations. These three datasets are the main publicly available datasets of PD speech-based area of study.

Other studies tried to improve the PD detection rate using the existing datasets. For instance, Tsanas et al. in [14] computed 132 dysphonia new measurements using an existing dataset consisting of 263 vowels "ahh..." phonations from 43 cases by applying feature selection techniques. They obtained 99% overall classification accuracy. In another work, Sakar and Kursun [16] tried to assess the relevance and correlation between the features and PD score by applying mutual information-based selection algorithm with permutation test and feed the data with selected features ranked based on maximum-relevance-minimum-redundancy (mRMR) into an SVM classifier. They used leave-one-subject-out (LOSO) as the cross validation technique of their model in order to avoid bias. In LOSO validation scheme, all the voice samples of an individual which is the candidate of being the testing sample will be left out from the rest of the data. Their approach gained 92.75% classification accuracy [8]. Shahbaba and Neal [17] presented a nonlinear model based on Dirichlet mixtures and obtained the classification accuracy of 87.7%. Das [18] conducted a comparative study of neural networks (NN), DMneural, regression, and decision trees for PD diagnosis; their study resulted in classification performance of 92.9% based on NN. Guo et al. [19] applied a combination of genetic programming and the expectation maximization (EM) and obtained a classification accuracy of 93.1%. Luukka [20] proposed a method that used fuzzy entropy measures and similarity classifier and resulted in the mean accuracy of 85.03%. Li et al. [21] introduced a fuzzy-based nonlinear transformation approach combined with SVM; their best classification accuracy was 93.47%. Ozcift and Gulten [22] proposed classifier ensemble construction with a rotation forest approach which got classification accuracy of 87.13%. Åström and Koker [23] achieved the classification accuracy of 91.2% by using a parallel neural network model. Polat [24] applied the fuzzy C-means clustering feature weighting together with the k-nearest neighbor classifier; their best obtained classification accuracy was 97.93%. Chen et al. [25] proposed a model which combined PCA and the fuzzy k-nearest neighbor method; their classification approach achieved an accuracy of 96.07%. Zuo et al. [26] used a diagnosis model based on particle swarm optimization (PSO) to strengthen the fuzzy k-nearest neighbor classifier which resulted in mean classification accuracy of 97.47%.

In most of the studies, SVM was used as the base classifier to distinguish healthy subjects from PWP [8, 14, 27] and the success of the diagnostic system is measured with ROC curves, AUC, and reporting True Positive and False Positive rates [28].

The speech datasets used in the field of PD diagnosis consist of multiple speech recordings per subject [29]. These datasets can be grouped into two categories: (1) those that

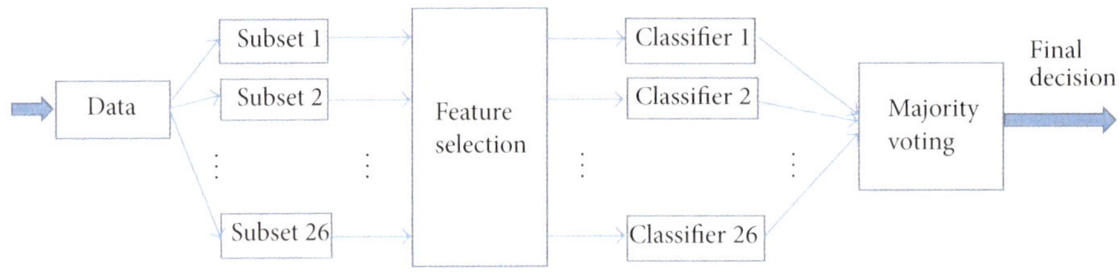

FIGURE 1: An illustration of the proposed method.

contain the repetition of one term and (2) those that consist of *different* vocal terms. The majority of datasets go to the first category. Hence, most of the studies on PD diagnosis are conducted on these datasets [14, 16–26]; however, none of them could obtain 100% classification accuracy. The most popular and available datasets of this type are "*Parkinson's Data Set*" [7] and "*Parkinson's Telemonitoring Data Set*" [15], both accessible from *UCI Machine Learning Repository*. The only dataset of the second category that is available in the form of processed data matrix was produced by Sakar et al. [13]. Less research has been conducted on this type of datasets; also, corresponding classification accuracies are not promising up to this time. The aim of this study is to show that this type of data collection can lead to high PD detection rates just by altering the classification strategy.

3. Materials and Methods

3.1. Data. In this work we used *Parkinson Speech Dataset with Multiple Types of Sound Recordings* [13], which is available on the University of California, Irvine (UCI) machine learning dataset repository website. This dataset consists of 40 subjects, including 20 PD patients and 20 control subjects. For each subject, 26 different sound recordings have been gathered, consisting of three sustained vowels, numbers one through 10, nine words, and four short sentences. There are 26 features extracted from these recordings. Table 1 lists the features gathered in Sakar et al.'s work and their corresponding groups (see [13] for more details).

TABLE 1: Time-frequency based features presented in Parkinson speech dataset with multiple types of sound recordings [13].

Feature number	Feature name	Group
1	Jitter (local)	*Frequency parameter*
2	Jitter (local, absolute)	
3	Jitter (rap)	
4	Jitter (ppq5)	
5	Jitter (ddp)	
6	Number of pulses	*Pulse parameters*
7	Number of periods	
8	Mean period	
9	Standard deviation of period	
10	Shimmer (local)	*Amplitude parameters*
11	Shimmer (local, dB)	
12	Shimmer (apq3)	
13	Shimmer (apq5)	
14	Shimmer (apq11)	
15	Shimmer (dda)	
16	Fraction of locally unvoiced frames	*Voicing parameters*
17	Number of voice breaks	
18	Degree of voice breaks	
19	Median pitch	*Pitch parameters*
20	Mean pitch	
21	Standard deviation	
22	Minimum pitch	
23	Maximum pitch	
24	Autocorrelation	*Harmonicity parameters*
25	Noise-to-harmonic	
26	Harmonic-to-noise	

3.2. Overview of the Proposed Method. The aim of this paper is to propose a classification framework which focuses on the discriminating values of each vocal test. Unlike the conventional LOSO cross validation technique and s-LOO, the proposed methodology considers that all the recordings in the setting of the dataset are not necessarily discriminating and not every PD patient demonstrates distinguishable vocal disorders in all vocal tests. The overall view of the proposed method can be seen in Figure 1.

The four steps of the proposed methodology are (1) separating the dataset based on the types of sounds recorded, (2) applying feature selection with Pearson Correlation Coefficient, we called the two approaches we took as follows: (a) *Multiple-Classifier with Feature Selection* (MCFS) and (b) *Adjusted Multiple-Classifier with Feature Selection* (A-MCFS) which will be introduced shortly, (3) applying a classifier on each subset, and finally (4) fusing the results of all classifiers to obtain the final decision by means of majority voting.

(1) Data Separation. Each subset of the dataset includes all the vocal tests of the same type; for instance, all the recorded vowel sounds of type "a" go to the first subset and those of "o" go to the second subset. Thus, considering the present dataset, there are 26 subsets, each containing 40 samples. Separation has been done since the mixture of all the voice samples of an individual diminishes the discriminating effect

of more descriptive tests and it will affect the classification results negatively.

(2) Pearson Correlation Coefficient Feature Selection. For feature selection phase, a filter-based feature selection technique based on Pearson Correlation Coefficient [30–32] was used to find highly correlated features to the class label. A more precise definition of this feature selection is as follows: suppose that each feature consists of $\{x_1, x_2, \ldots, x_n\}$ values for samples 1 through n (in this study n is equal to 40) in vector $\mathbf{X}$ and the corresponding class labels are $\{y_1, y_2, \ldots, y_n\}$ stored in vector $\mathbf{Y}$. So the Pearson Correlation Coefficient of each feature can be calculated as

$$r = r_{\mathrm{XY}} = \frac{\sum_{i=1}^{n}(x_i - \overline{x})(y_i - \overline{y})}{\sqrt{\sum_{i=1}^{n}(x_i - \overline{x})^2}\sqrt{\sum_{i=1}^{n}(y_i - \overline{y})^2}}, \quad (1)$$

where $\overline{x} = (1/n)\sum_{i=1}^{n} x_i$ and similarly $\overline{y} = (1/n)\sum_{i=1}^{n} y_i$. This equation gives a value between −1 and +1, where +1 is maximum positive correlation, 0 is no correlation, and −1 is the strongest negative correlation.

The p values were calculated using Student's t-distribution for a transformation of the correlation. Those features in the correlation coefficient matrix with p values less than 0.05 were selected.

(3) MCFS and A-MCFS. When the Pearson Correlation Coefficient feature selection is applied, some vocal tests may remain with no relevant features. We call those vocal tests as *unsuccessful vocal tests*. Two approaches for dealing with those unsuccessful vocal tests are taken in this study. The first is the MCFS approach; the vocal tests are used in the analysis only based on the prevalent features of other vocal tests. Table 2 shows each vocal test and its corresponding correlated features after applying feature selection and Figure 2 shows the frequency of each feature. Features 2 and 4 with frequency of six and five were, respectively, the most frequent selected features. The third most frequent was shared by features 25 and 26 with frequency of four. The most four frequent features were used in MCFS as selected features for unsuccessful vocal tests. The other methodology, A-MCFS, is to simply omit unsuccessful vocal tests.

(4) Classification and Majority Voting. After doing feature selection on each subset, for each of them, a classifier is built. Since we have 26 vocal tests, 26 classifiers are built. Each of these classifiers will predict the class label of its own subset. *Leave-one-out* cross validation technique was used for all of these classifiers. Since each subject has only one record in each subset, we do not have to worry about how to treat each subject for doing cross validation as it was the case in LOSO or previous approaches.

The majority vote of classifiers decides which class the person belongs to. Each classifier votes whether the subject has PD or not. Then, the subject whom the majority of the classifiers have voted to be a PD patient will be labeled as "1" showing the presence of PD and "0" otherwise.

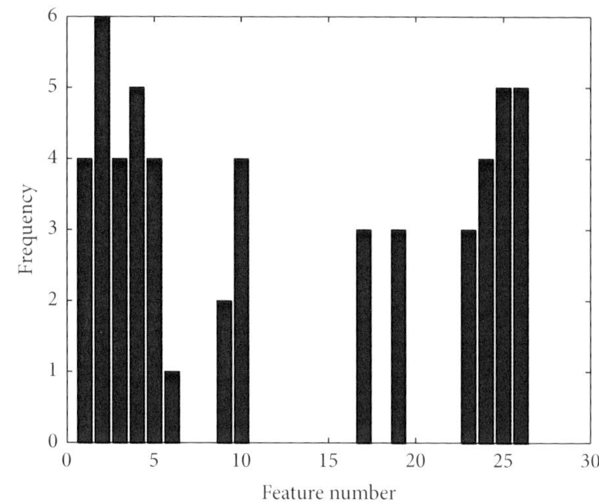

Figure 2: Frequency of each selected feature as relevant feature of a vocal test.

Table 2: Each vocal test and its related features after applying filter-based feature selection.

ID	Vocal test	Related features
1	Vowel "a"	None
2	Vowel "o"	24
3	Vowel "u"	None
4	Number 1	1, 2, 3, 4, 5, 24
5	Number 2	2, 9, 10
6	Number 3	17, 19, 23, 25, 26
7	Number 4	1, 2, 3, 4, 5, 10
8	Number 5	24
9	Number 6	None
10	Number 7	None
11	Number 8	9
12	Number 9	26
13	Number 10	None
14	Short sentence 1	None
15	Short sentence 2	25, 26
16	Short sentence 3	4, 10, 25, 26
17	Short sentence 4	1, 2, 3, 4, 5, 10, 26
18	Word 1	2
19	Word 2	None
20	Word 3	17, 19, 23, 25
21	Word 4	None
22	Word 5	None
23	Word 6	None
24	Word 7	None
25	Word 8	1, 2, 3, 4, 5, 6, 17, 19, 23, 25
26	Word 9	24

3.3. Evaluation Metrics. The evaluation metrics used to show the effectiveness of the proposed methodology are accuracy, sensitivity, specificity, and Matthew's correlation coefficient score (MCC). The definitions of these metrics are as follows:

$$\text{accuracy} = \frac{\text{TP} + \text{TN}}{\text{TP} + \text{TN} + \text{FP} + \text{FN}}, \tag{2}$$

where TP (True Positive) is the number of PD patients who are correctly classified as Parkinsonism patients by the model, TN (True Negative) is the number of control subjects who are labeled as healthy by the model, FN (False Negative) is the number of patients that the model falsely labeled them as healthy, and finally FP (False Positive) is the number of healthy cases who are incorrectly labeled as having PD by the classifier. It simply shows that the accuracy is the ratio of the correctly classified samples to the total number of instances:

$$\text{sensitivity} = \frac{\text{TP}}{\text{TP} + \text{FN}}$$
$$\text{specificity} = \frac{\text{TN}}{\text{TN} + \text{FP}}. \tag{3}$$

A well-known metric in machine learning which can be used for evaluating the quality of a binary classifier is MCC. This metric is reliable since it takes TP, TN, FN, and FP into account and this makes it stable even if classes are of very different sizes. Actually, MCC is a correlation coefficient between observed (actual) labels of the samples and those predicted by the binary classifier:

$$\text{MCC} = \frac{(\text{TP} \times \text{TN}) - (\text{FP} \times \text{FN})}{\sqrt{(\text{TP} + \text{FP})(\text{TP} + \text{FN})(\text{TN} + \text{FP})(\text{TN} + \text{FN})}}. \tag{4}$$

This equation returns a value between −1 and +1. A coefficient of +1 shows a perfect prediction, 0 represents the fact that the classifier is not better than random guessing, and finally −1 indicates a complete disagreement between the actual values and the predicted ones.

4. Results and Discussions

After separating the data into subsets, the z-score normalization process was applied on each subset. In other words, after transformation, mean is equal to zero and standard deviation changes to one. Then the proposed framework was applied on the refined data.

Four classifiers including k-NN, SVM, discriminant analysis, and Naïve Bayes were applied to the preprocessed data. Distance metric used for the k-NN classifier was Euclidean distance and k with values of 1, 3, 5, and 7 was used. SVM classifier was applied using linear and radial basis kernels (RBF) with scaling factor (sigma) of 3 and penalty parameter (C) of 1. Table 3 includes the accuracy, sensitivity, specificity, and MCC obtained from applying mentioned classifiers under LOSO, s-LOO, and the proposed frameworks. The results reveal that k-NN classifier performance is almost analogous to random guessing when it is used with LOSO cross validation technique. Besides that, s-LOO could not perform much better than LOSO when it comes to k-NN since its best overall accuracy and MCC are 65.00% and 0.3062, respectively. Results show that A-MCFS outperforms s-LOO's best result with overall accuracy of 77.50%, which is a **12.5**% improvement and MCC of 0.5507.

When k is 1, 3, and 5, MCFS results are better than s-LOO at least for 5% and at most 12.5%, but its accuracy is 2.5% lower than s-LOO when k is 7.

Sensitivity is another important factor, especially in biomedical sciences, which should be investigated closely in the results. As the results show, A-MCFS also has improved the sensitivity up to 80.00% and its lowest sensitivity (70.00%) is still better than that of LOSO and s-LOO when k-NN is used. k-NN achieved its best results when A-MCFS was applied; besides this, LOSO and s-LOO could not reach MCFS's results except for $k = 7$.

In addition, the best classification accuracy obtained by applying A-MCFS is 87.5% which is a 10% accuracy enhancement in comparison to the best accuracy obtained by s-LOO.

Figure 3 gives a better demonstration of classification accuracies obtained by different methods.

In order to examine the correctness of our approach toward finding less discriminating vocal tests, we have reported the classification accuracy of each vocal test prior to the majority voting phase. The results are shown in Table 4. Comparing the results shown in Tables 2 and 4 reveals that the features which were excluded in A-MCFS are those that achieved a mean accuracy of below 55%. This shows the reason of the superiority of A-MCFS over MCFS. As a result, a closer investigation toward finding more effective vocal tests is necessary.

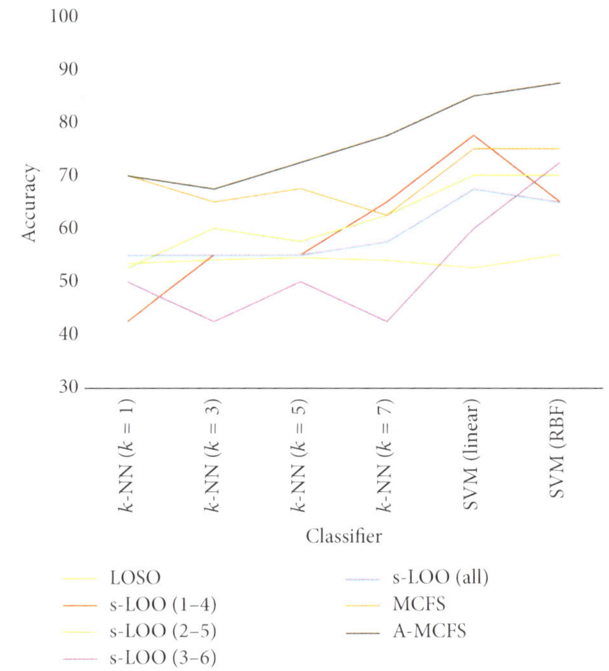

FIGURE 3: Obtained accuracies based on the reported results in Table 3.

TABLE 3: Results obtained from applying different methods and classifiers.

Classifier	Method	Accuracy (%)	Sensitivity (%)	Specificity (%)	MCC
k-NN ($k = 1$)	LOSO	53.37	49.62	57.12	0.0007
	s-LOO (1–4)	42.50	30.00	55.00	0.0015
	s-LOO (2–5)	52.50	45.00	60.00	0.0005
	s-LOO (3–6)	50.00	55.00	45.00	0.0000
	s-LOO (all)	55.00	55.00	55.00	0.1000
	MCFS	67.50	75.00	60.00	0.3549
	A-MCFS	**70.00**	**80.00**	**60.00**	**0.4082**
k-NN ($k = 3$)	LOSO	54.04	53.27	54.81	0.0008
	s-LOO (1–4)	55.00	45.00	65.00	0.1021
	s-LOO (2–5)	60.00	55.00	65.00	0.2010
	s-LOO (3–6)	42.50	55.00	30.00	0.0015
	s-LOO (all)	55.00	55.00	55.00	0.1000
	MCFS	65.00	60.00	70.00	0.3015
	A-MCFS	**67.50**	**75.00**	**60.00**	**0.3540**
k-NN ($k = 5$)	LOSO	54.42	53.65	55.19	0.0009
	s-LOO (1–4)	55.00	45.00	65.00	0.1201
	s-LOO (2–5)	57.50	65.00	50.00	0.1517
	s-LOO (3–6)	50.00	70.00	30.00	0.0000
	s-LOO (all)	55.00	70.00	40.00	0.1048
	MCFS	67.5	60.00	75.00	0.3540
	A-MCFS	**72.50**	**70.00**	**75.00**	**0.4506**
k-NN ($k = 7$)	LOSO	53.94	54.04	53.85	0.0008
	s-LOO (1–4)	65.00	55.00	75.00	0.3062
	s-LOO (2–5)	62.50	60.00	65.00	0.2503
	s-LOO (3–6)	42.50	65.00	20.00	0.0017
	s-LOO (all)	57.50	65.00	50.00	0.1517
	MCFS	62.5	65.00	60.00	0.2503
	A-MCFS	**77.50**	**80.00**	**75.00**	**0.5507**
SVM (linear kernel)	LOSO	52.50	52.50	52.50	0.0006
	s-LOO (1–4)	77.50	80.00	75.00	0.5507
	s-LOO (2–5)	70.00	80.00	60.00	0.4082
	s-LOO (3–6)	60.00	65.00	45.00	0.2000
	s-LOO (all)	67.50	70.00	65.00	0.3504
	MCFS	75.00	75.00	75.00	0.5000
	A-MCFS	**85.00**	**85.00**	**85.00**	**0.6000**
SVM (RBF kernel)	LOSO	55.00	60.00	50.00	0.1005
	s-LOO (1–4)	65.00	60.00	70.00	0.3015
	s-LOO (2–5)	70.00	70.00	70.00	0.4000
	s-LOO (3–6)	72.50	70.00	75.00	0.4506
	s-LOO (all)	65.00	70.00	60.00	0.3015
	MCFS	75.00	80.00	70.00	0.5025
	A-MCFS	**87.50**	**90.00**	**85.00**	**0.7509**
Naïve Bayes	MCFS	75.00	90.00	60.00	0.5241
	A-MCFS	**80.00**	**80.00**	**80.00**	**0.6000**
Discriminant analysis	MCFS	72.50	75.00	70.00	0.4506
	A-MCFS	**82.50**	**80.00**	**85.00**	**0.6508**

Central tendency metrics used in s-LOO method: 1: mean, 2: median, and 3: trimmed mean (25% removed).
Dispersion metrics used in s-LOO method: 4: standard deviation, 5: mean absolute deviation, and 6: interquartile range.

TABLE 4: Prediction ability of each vocal test, based on their obtained classification accuracy.

Vocal test ID	Classification accuracy (%)								
	k-NN ($k = 1$)	k-NN ($k = 3$)	k-NN ($k = 5$)	k-NN ($k = 7$)	SVM (linear kernel)	SVM (RBF kernel)	Naïve Bayes	DA	Mean accuracy ± standard deviation
1	42.5	35	27.5	27.5	47.5	25	52.5	37.5	**36.9 ± 10**
2	57.5	67.5	70	70	62.5	62.5	60	70	65 ± 5
3	40	42.5	60	55	27.5	50	50	47.5	**46.56 ± 10**
4	67.5	70	75	67.5	60	65	65	62.5	66.6 ± 4.6
5	67.5	57.5	60	65	67.5	67.5	67.5	65	64.7 ± 3.9
6	62.5	67.5	67.5	72.5	62.5	72.5	72.5	65	67.8 ± 4.3
7	52.5	60	57.5	55	67.5	67.5	70	50	60 ± 7.6
8	57.5	62.5	62.5	70	65	67.5	65	62.5	64 ± 3.8
9	47.5	62.5	65	50	60	50	55	57.5	55.9 ± 6.4
10	62.5	62.5	65	55	55	55	57.5	55	58.4 ± 4.2
11	42.5	60	72.5	72.5	75	72.5	70	72.5	67.2 ± 11
12	50	45	42.5	57.5	65	65	65	65	56.9 ± 9.7
13	40	45	57.5	57.5	52.5	60	60	45	**52.2 ± 7.8**
14	52.5	60	55	55	50	60	45	55	**54.1 ± 5**
15	57.5	60	62.5	65	72.5	72.5	65	72.5	65.9 ± 6
16	50	55	62.5	65	72.5	72.5	65	72.5	64.4 ± 8.4
17	60	57.5	57.5	65	72.5	60	72.5	67.5	64.1 ± 6.3
18	45	45	55	65	67.5	67.5	65	67.5	59.7 ± 9.9
19	40	37.5	45	35	40	40	22.5	42.5	**37.8 ± 6.9**
20	52.5	55	55	47.5	60	62.5	65	62.5	57.5 ± 6
21	47.5	40	40	27.5	45	55	52.5	52.5	**45 ± 9**
22	42.5	35	52.5	52.5	67.5	55	55	65	**53.1 ± 10.7**
23	47.5	55	55	47.5	62.5	60	60	50	**54.7 ± 5.9**
24	35	35	22.5	35	42.5	42.5	37.5	50	**37.5 ± 8**
25	62.5	62.5	67.5	67.5	62.5	67.5	65	62.5	64.7 ± 2.5
26	55	62.5	57.5	62.5	57.5	57.5	55	55	57.8 ± 3.1

5. Conclusion

PWP detection based on vocal samples has been an attractive area of research. Finding a solution toward discriminating PD patients from the healthy people based on different vocal tests had been less accurate since all the vocal terms were treated by a single classifier. The proposed method treated each vocal test separately and used majority voting to resolve any potential confusion. Obtained results from this research showed that more accurate PD detection based on multiple vocal tests is achievable.

Another important result, achieved from this study, was that the discriminating ability of all the vocal terms is not the same, even some of those vocal terms that have been considered to be discriminating in the literature, such as vowel "a," failed to be successful. As a result, our study may encourage other researchers to conduct further studies on different vocal terms from the proposed perspective.

As the future work, we plan to devise a laboratory setting to collect data from PWP and healthy subjects with several vocal tests from various languages and extend our results to other languages.

Competing Interests

The authors declare that they have no competing interests.

References

[1] J. W. Langston, "Parkinson's disease: current and future challenges," *NeuroToxicology*, vol. 23, no. 4-5, pp. 443–450, 2002.

[2] L. M. de Lau and M. M. Breteler, "Epidemiology of Parkinson's disease," *The Lancet Neurology*, vol. 5, no. 6, pp. 525–535, 2006.

[3] M. C. de Rijk, L. J. Launer, K. Berger et al., "Prevalence of Parkinson's disease in Europe: a collaborative study of population-based cohorts," *Neurology*, vol. 54, no. 11, supplemen 5, pp. S21–S23, 2000.

[4] J. Jankovic, "Parkinson's disease: clinical features and diagnosis," *Journal of Neurology, Neurosurgery and Psychiatry*, vol. 79, no. 4, pp. 368–376, 2007.

[5] A. K. Ho, R. Iansek, C. Marigliani, J. L. Bradshaw, and S. Gates, "Speech impairment in a large sample of patients with Parkinson's disease," *Behavioural Neurology*, vol. 11, no. 3, pp. 131–137, 1998.

[6] J. A. Logemann, H. B. Fisher, B. Boshes, and E. R. Blonsky, "Frequency and cooccurrence of vocal tract dysfunctions in the speech of a large sample of Parkinson patients," *Journal of Speech and Hearing Disorders*, vol. 43, no. 1, pp. 47–57, 1978.

[7] M. A. Little, P. E. McSharry, S. J. Roberts, D. A. E. Costello, and I. M. Moroz, "Exploiting nonlinear recurrence and fractal scaling properties for voice disorder detection," *BioMedical Engineering OnLine*, vol. 6, article 23, 2007.

[8] M. A. Little, P. E. McSharry, E. J. Hunter, J. Spielman, and L. O. Ramig, "Suitability of dysphonia measurements for telemonitoring of Parkinson's disease," *IEEE Transactions on Biomedical Engineering*, vol. 56, no. 4, pp. 1015–1022, 2009.

[9] J. Duffy, *Motor Speech Disorders: Substrates, Differential Diagnosis, and Management*, Mosby, St. Louis, Mo, USA, 3rd edition, 2012.

[10] M. McNeil, *Clinical Management of Sensorimotor Speech Disorders*, Thieme, Stuttgart, Germany, 2nd edition, 2008.

[11] R. J. Baken and R. F. Orlikoff, *Clinical Measurement of Speech and Voice*, Cengage Learning, 2nd edition, 1999.

[12] P. H. Dejonckere, P. Bradley, P. Clemente et al., "A basic protocol for functional assessment of voice pathology, especially for investigating the efficacy of (phonosurgical) treatments and evaluating new assessment techniques: guideline elaborated by the Committee on Phoniatrics of the European Laryngological Society (ELS)," *European Archives of Oto-Rhino-Laryngology*, vol. 258, no. 2, pp. 77–82, 2001.

[13] B. E. Sakar, M. E. Isenkul, C. O. Sakar et al., "Collection and analysis of a Parkinson speech dataset with multiple types of sound recordings," *IEEE Journal of Biomedical and Health Informatics*, vol. 17, no. 4, pp. 828–834, 2013.

[14] A. Tsanas, M. A. Little, P. E. McSharry, J. Spielman, and L. O. Ramig, "Novel speech signal processing algorithms for high-accuracy classification of Parkinsons disease," *IEEE Transactions on Biomedical Engineering*, vol. 59, no. 5, pp. 1264–1271, 2012.

[15] A. Tsanas, M. A. Little, P. E. McSharry, and L. O. Ramig, "Accurate telemonitoring of Parkinson's disease progression by non-invasive speech tests," *IEEE Transactions on Biomedical Engineering*, vol. 57, no. 4, pp. 884–893, 2010.

[16] C. O. Sakar and O. Kursun, "Telediagnosis of parkinson's disease using measurements of dysphonia," *Journal of Medical Systems*, vol. 34, no. 4, pp. 591–599, 2010.

[17] B. Shahbaba and R. Neal, "Nonlinear models using dirichlet process mixtures," *Journal of Machine Learning Research*, vol. 10, pp. 1829–1850, 2009.

[18] R. Das, "A comparison of multiple classification methods for diagnosis of Parkinson disease," *Expert Systems with Applications*, vol. 37, no. 2, pp. 1568–1572, 2010.

[19] P.-F. Guo, P. Bhattacharya, and N. Kharma, "Advances in detecting Parkinson's disease," in *Medical Biometrics*, vol. 6165 of *Lecture Notes in Computer Science*, pp. 306–314, Springer, Berlin, Germany, 2010.

[20] P. Luukka, "Feature selection using fuzzy entropy measures with similarity classifier," *Expert Systems with Applications*, vol. 38, no. 4, pp. 4600–4607, 2011.

[21] D.-C. Li, C.-W. Liu, and S. C. Hu, "A fuzzy-based data transformation for feature extraction to increase classification performance with small medical data sets," *Artificial Intelligence in Medicine*, vol. 52, no. 1, pp. 45–52, 2011.

[22] A. Ozcift and A. Gulten, "Classifier ensemble construction with rotation forest to improve medical diagnosis performance of machine learning algorithms," *Computer Methods and Programs in Biomedicine*, vol. 104, no. 3, pp. 443–451, 2011.

[23] F. Åström and R. Koker, "A parallel neural network approach to prediction of Parkinson's Disease," *Expert Systems with Applications*, vol. 38, no. 10, pp. 12470–12474, 2011.

[24] K. Polat, "Classification of Parkinson's disease using feature weighting method on the basis of fuzzy C-means clustering," *International Journal of Systems Science*, vol. 43, no. 4, pp. 597–609, 2012.

[25] H.-L. Chen, C.-C. Huang, X.-G. Yu et al., "An efficient diagnosis system for detection of Parkinson's disease using fuzzy k-nearest neighbor approach," *Expert Systems with Applications*, vol. 40, no. 1, pp. 263–271, 2013.

[26] W.-L. Zuo, Z.-Y. Wang, T. Liu, and H.-L. Chen, "Effective detection of Parkinson's disease using an adaptive fuzzy k-nearest neighbor approach," *Biomedical Signal Processing and Control*, vol. 8, no. 4, pp. 364–373, 2013.

[27] O. Kursun, E. Gumus, A. Sertbas, and O. V. Favorov, "Selection of vocal features for Parkinson's Disease diagnosis," *International Journal of Data Mining and Bioinformatics*, vol. 6, no. 2, pp. 144–161, 2012.

[28] I. Bhattacharya and M. Bhatia, "SVM classification to distinguish Parkinson disease patients," in *Proceedings of the 1st Amrita ACM-W Celebration on Women in Computing in India (A2CWiC '10)*, New Delhi, India, 2010.

[29] L. O. Ramig, S. Sapir, C. Fox, and S. Countryman, "Changes in vocal loudness following intensive voice treatment (LSVT®) in individuals with Parkinson's disease: a comparison with untreated patients and normal age-matched controls," *Movement Disorders*, vol. 16, no. 1, pp. 79–83, 2001.

[30] J. Gibbons, *Nonparametric Statistical Inference*, Chapman & Hall/CRC, 5th edition, 2010.

[31] M. Hollander and D. A. Wolfe, *Nonparametric Statistical Methods*, John Wiley & Sons, New York, NY, USA, 3rd edition, 2013.

[32] M. M. Kendall, *Rank Correlation Methods*, Griffin, London, UK, 5th edition, 1990.

25

Patients' and Healthcare Personnel's Experiences of Health Coaching with Online Self-Management in the Renewing Health Project

Inger Lindberg,[1] Birgitta Lindberg,[1] and Siv Söderberg[2]

[1]*Division of Nursing, Department of Health Science, Luleå University of Technology, 971 87 Luleå, Sweden*
[2]*Department of Nursing Sciences, Mid Sweden University, 83125 Östersund, Sweden*

Correspondence should be addressed to Inger Lindberg; inger.lindberg@ltu.se

Academic Editor: Velio Macellari

Background. Telehealth applications have shown positive effects for people with chronic conditions and their awareness of health. *Objective.* To describe patients' and healthcare personnel's experiences of using health coaching with online self-management in primary health care. *Method.* A pragmatic randomised controlled trial was conducted. Patients in the intervention group measured and reported medical parameters such as blood pressure, blood glucose, prothrombin complex (PK) values, and 2-channel ECG. Data were collected through a questionnaire, individual interviews with patients, and focus group discussions with healthcare personnel. The questionnaire was analysed using statistics; texts from interviews and focus groups were analysed using content analysis. *Findings.* Patients were satisfied and believed that the intervention had enhanced their care and increased accessibility without causing concerns about privacy. Although being positive, patients commented the lack of support and feedback from healthcare personnel. Healthcare personnel regarded the intervention valuable for the patients' abilities to perform self-management healthcare tasks but preferred that patients did so without them supporting the patients. *Conclusion.* Patients expressed satisfaction and acceptance regarding the use of the application. It seems that healthcare personnel are convinced about the benefits for patients and the potential for the intervention but are not convinced about its benefits for healthcare organisations.

1. Introduction

The world prevalence of diabetes among adults (ages 20–79 years) is estimated to be 8.8 percent, affecting 415 million adults in 2015. This is expected to increase to 10.4 percent and 642 million people by 2040 [1]. It is estimated that more than 59.8 million people in the European region have diabetes; by 2040, this is expected to increase to 71.1 million. Of the 57 million global deaths in 2008, 36 million (63%) were due to noncommunicable diseases (NCDs) and 17.3 million (30%) were due to CVDs. Almost 80% of NCD deaths occur in low and middle income countries and it is the most frequent cause of death in most countries, except in Africa [2].

Careful glucose control, effective control of blood pressure, and effective management of risks in the presymptomatic phases of CVDs have been shown to reduce complications [3–6]. Prevention of complications of diabetes is about ensuring that patients have a good quality of life and includes lifestyle management such as diet and physical activity [7]. Controlling hypertension can decrease CV events such as coronary heart disease, congestive heart failure, stroke, and renal failure [3, 6].

Telehealth applications have shown positive effects for people with hypertension [8], CVD risks [9], and congestive heart failure [10, 11]. Furthermore, such applications influence patients' awareness about their own health [12, 13]. A review study found that technology intervention treatments result in positive behavioural changes among patients and are potentially highly beneficial for the management of chronic illnesses such as type 2 diabetes [14]. Another review supports the use of a self-management health information technology approach to improve glycaemic control. The effect of this approach was significantly greater when the technology used a web-based application, when a mechanism was provided for patients to enter their health data (manually or automatically), and when the technology was operated in the home or with no restrictions regarding location [15]. Furthermore, it was shown that telehealth was an effective model for the provision of diabetes care to rural patients compared to face-to-face visits [16]. Research on home health telemonitoring has also shown contradictory results; for example, Wakefield et al. [17] found that the addition of technology alone did not improve outcomes related to haemoglobin A1c.

When implementing technology in health care, there is a need for effective and responsive clinical processes to optimize the use of the additional data. In a study about implementing blood glucose and blood pressure in home health telemonitoring in primary care practices for patients with diabetes, stakeholder groups (patients, nurse care coordinators, and physicians) expressed that the careful consideration of workflow and information flow would help enable effective implementations [18]. It was also considered that practices need to understand the capabilities and limitations of the technology, the involvement of the patients and stakeholders, and their willingness to use it. In order to have successful implementation of different self-management applications, several perspectives must be considered. This study intends to add knowledge based on the views of both patients and healthcare personnel in regard to the online self-management of patients with chronic conditions. Thus, the aim of this study was to describe patients' and healthcare personnel's experiences of using health coaching with online self-management in primary health care.

2. Method

2.1. Context. The study was conducted in four healthcare centres in the county of Norrbotten in the northern part of Sweden. It comprises 25 percent of Sweden's land area and a population of 250,000 inhabitants. The study is a part of the Renewing Health project; the project included nine regions in Europe aiming to implement large-scale, real-life test beds for the validation and subsequent evaluation of innovative telemedicine services using a patient-centred approach and a common rigorous assessment methodology [19].

2.2. The Intervention. The Swedish field trial in the Renewing Health project developed a method that combined health coaching with the online management of patients' data, where the patient becomes more actively involved by self-monitoring his or her own health and health care via a national patient portal. The portal provides secure access to their health information for all Swedish citizens and supports electronic interaction with healthcare professionals. During the field trial, patients used their own computers; patients without access to a computer were provided with an iPad. The preventive health and diagnostic measurement equipment for self-monitoring were also provided to patients during the field trial.

The intervention was initiated with group sessions that aimed to educate and motivate patients to undertake lifestyle changes. The patients were trained to manage their health information and interact with the healthcare professionals through the application. A health activity plan was developed for each patient, and during the time frame established for the study, patients performed health-promoting activities and reported parameters such as the number of steps taken in a day, pulse, and the duration of physical activity. Based on their diagnoses, the patients measured and reported medical parameters such as blood pressure, blood glucose, prothrombin complex (PK) values, and 2-channel ECG. Approximately every second month, the results were reviewed and the health activity plan for each patient was revised if necessary. The patients then received feedback from the healthcare professional via either email or video. Feedback could be about reported medical parameters, changes in drug treatment, and physical activities. General practitioners, diabetes nurses, physiotherapists, and nutritionists cooperated to manage patient interactions.

2.3. Study Design. In this study, a pragmatic randomised controlled trial was conducted. The methodology used was in accordance with the model for assessment of telemedicine applications (MAST) [20]. This ensured that the outcomes with regard to safety, clinical impact, patient perception, economic aspects, and organisational aspects were assessed in accordance with scientific guidelines.

2.4. Participants and Procedure

2.4.1. The Quantitative Study. In May 2011, 4796 eligible patients who met the inclusion criteria (Table 1) were contacted through an informational letter sent from their healthcare centres. Of these, 4057 were excluded due to their decisions to decline to participate or because they did not meet the inclusion criteria, leaving 739 participants. After the participants had signed an informed consent form, randomisation was performed following standard procedures (PC-based generation of random integer sequences and allocation based on consecutive assignment). Randomisation was performed by a statistician at the Research and Development Unit of the Norrbotten County Council. During the intervention period, 180 participants in the intervention group and 54 participants in the control group were lost to follow-up due to reasons that included being too ill, finding the technology too difficult to manage, changing healthcare centres, and death. At the end of the trial, 15 March 2013, all 253 participants in the intervention group were approached by the contact person at each primary healthcare centre, where they completed the questionnaire, which took about 15 minutes. Of the remaining 253 participants, 245 completed the questionnaire. The response rate was 96 percent.

2.4.2. The Qualitative Study. A total of 33 patients (16 women and 17 men) from the four healthcare centres included in the Renewing Health project participated. The patients were between 45 and 89 years old (md = 66) and were diagnosed with either type 2 diabetes, heart disease, or hypertension. During spring of 2013, the contact person at each primary healthcare centre distributed an invitation letter to patients in the intervention group to participate in an interview study about their experiences of the intervention. Invitations

Table 1: Inclusion criteria.

Diabetes type 2	CVD	Hypertension
Diagnosed > three months prior to the enrolment	Diagnosis of ischemic heart disease	Diagnosis of hypertension
HbA1c > 6.5%		
Age > 18 years	Age > 18 years	Age > 18 years
Capability to fill in questionnaires in their own language	Capability to fill in questionnaires in their own language	Capability to fill in questionnaires in their own language
Capability to use the devices provided	Capability to use the devices provided	Capability to use the devices provided
Being cognitively able to participate	Being cognitively able to participate	Being cognitively able to participate

were based on the participants having participated in or withdrawn from the study. Of 39 patients who were invited and 35 accepted, 2 declined later due to personal reasons. The researchers contacted the patients to schedule appointments to be interviewed at their convenience.

Four focus group discussions were held with the healthcare staff ($n = 22$) at the participating primary healthcare centres involved in the project. The participants were between 39 and 65 years old (md = 54) and had worked between 13 and 43 years (md = 24.5). The participants' professions included a biomedical scientist, diabetes nurses, district nurses/nurses, an occupational therapist, physicians, physiotherapists, a medical secretary, and enrolled nurses.

2.5. Data Collection

2.5.1. Questionnaire, Service User Technology Acceptability Questionnaire (SUTAQ). The questionnaire was developed by NHS England Whole System Demonstrator Programme [21] and was translated into Swedish and then back-translated to English. A pilot trial, which resulted in one change, was conducted with 10 people from an earlier e-health study. The questionnaire consists of 22 items (statements) in a Likert-type scale that includes both positive and negative statements in order to reduce the risk of bias. The topics include questions about the following: (1) enhanced care: did patients believe telemedicine enhanced the care they received? (2) Increased accessibility: did they think that it increased accessibility to healthcare services? (3) Privacy and discomfort: did they believe that it created problems related to their privacy and/or made them feel uncomfortable? (4) Care personnel concerns: did they have concerns about the personnel involved in the process of telemedicine? (5) Kit (here in this study; PC, iPad, blood pressure, pulse, step, and PK meters) as substitution: did they see it as a substitute to their usual care? (6) Satisfaction: were they satisfied with it overall? The answers to all items (questions) in the questionnaire were coded as follows: 1 = strongly agree, 2 = moderately agree, 3 = mildly agree, 4 = mildly disagree, 5 = moderately disagree, and 6 = strongly disagree.

2.5.2. Interviews with the Patients. Personal interviews were conducted with 33 patients from the intervention group, both those who participated throughout the duration of the project ($n = 27$) and those who withdrew from participation ($n = 6$). The interviews were semistructured, and the participants were asked to talk about their experiences of communicating with the physician and/or diabetes nurse via a web application, their thoughts about getting care through computers or mobile phone, how they experienced the function of technology, and how they believed the application supported their self-care abilities. The interviews were digitally recorded; they lasted approximately 15 to 20 minutes and were later transcribed verbatim.

2.5.3. Focus Group Discussions with Healthcare Personnel. The focus group discussions focused on how the healthcare staff experienced communicating with patients through the web application. The healthcare staff was asked to talk about their experiences of care through computers or mobile phones, how they experienced the technology, and whether or not the application supported patient self-care. The discussions were digitally recorded, lasted approximately 30 to 60 minutes, and were later transcribed verbatim.

2.6. Data Analysis

2.6.1. Quantitative Method

Questionnaire. Based on the answers to the items, six subscales were identified as follows: enhanced care (based on items 17, 15, 10, 11, and 13); increased accessibility (based on items 1, 3, 4, and 19); privacy and discomfort scale (based on items 5, 2, 8, and 12); care personnel concerns (based on items 9, 21, and 20); kit as substitution (based on items 18, 22, and 16); and satisfaction (based on items 7, 6, and 14). The calculation of the scales was performed by subtracting the mean value of the items from 7.

For all subscales, the interpretation is that a higher value reflects a higher degree of agreement with the subscale. A high value on the subscale "satisfaction," for example, 5.5, reflects a high degree of agreement and, therefore, a high degree of satisfaction. The two subscales "privacy and discomfort" and "care personnel concerns" are based on negative statements in the items. Therefore, a high value on these subscales reflects a high degree of agreement with this negative aspect of the kit. For example, a high value of, for example, 5.5, on the subscale "care personnel concerns" reflects that the patients are, to a high degree, concerned with regard to the personnel taking care of them by using the kit.

2.6.2. Qualitative Method

Interviews and Focus Group Discussions. Both the interviews with the patients and the focus group discussions with the healthcare personnel were analysed with a qualitative content analysis [22]. The method can be described as a process of identifying, coding, and categorising the primary pattern of the data (i.e., the content). The data analysis started with reading each interview several times to get a sense of the content. After that, guided by the aim of the study, a reading followed to identify textual units. The textual units were then condensed and sorted into categories based on similarities in content. The categories were then related to each other and subsumed into final categories.

3. Ethical Approval

Informed consent was collected after the participants were informed orally and in writing about the study's purposes. Participants were assured that they could withdraw from the study without giving any explanation; that the results would not be linked to individuals; and that all study results would maintain confidentiality. The study was conducted according to the Ethical Review Act (The Ministry of Education and Cultural Affairs, 2003:460) and approved by the Regional Ethical Review Board (Dnr 2010/386-31M).

4. Results

The results are presented in two parts. In the first part, results from the questionnaire are presented (Table 2), and in the second part, the results from the interviews with the patients and the focus group discussions with the healthcare personnel are presented.

4.1. Part I: Results of the Quantitative Analysis. In the subscale "enhanced care," participants moderately agreed that the intervention would enhance their ability to take care of their own health or would be a good addition to their regular health care. The kit allowed them to be less concerned about their health, and they would recommend it to people with similar conditions. They also mildly to moderately agreed that the intervention increased accessibility to care and healthcare professionals. By using the kit, the participants saved time because they did not have to visit the GP clinic as often as before. The kit was perceived to increase access to care and made it easier to improve their health. Participants strongly disagreed about being concerned about their privacy and worrying about their private information being compromised by using the kit, and they expressed that they were comfortable using it. They did not perceive that the kit interfered with their everyday routines. They also moderately disagreed about being concerned about staff being competent enough or risking lack of continuity of care. They were not concerned that the healthcare personnel had access to their healthcare history. Participants mildly agreed that the kit was a positive addition to their regular health care and allowed them to be less concerned about their health status. They had concerns about the kit being suitable as a replacement for regular to face-to-face consultations. Overall, the participants strongly agreed that they were satisfied with the service with regard to the kit and that it was easy to understand and reliable.

4.2. Part II: Results of the Qualitative Analysis with Patients and Healthcare Personnel

4.2.1. The Patients. The analysis of the interviews with the patients resulted in four categories as follows: experiencing the technology, the importance of feedback, self-care, and privacy. The results are illustrated with quotations from the interviews.

Experiencing the Technology. Participants described that using the technology was, overall, a positive experience and that it was both exciting and interesting. They considered the technology to be user friendly, and the general opinion was that it worked well. Several participants described that the technology was a bit difficult the first time they used it. One participant expressed, "The technology works well and the equipment works well and it was easy to use." This was also described by patients with limited experience using computers. One participant said, "What surprised me was that there were many elderly people not skilled with computers, but it works well for them too." Some participants even said that it had made them more interested in wanting to learn more about technology.

The Importance of Feedback. Participants highlighted the importance of receiving feedback from healthcare staff when they had reported data. One participant said, "I don't believe that technology can be good if you do not have individual follow-up or feedback, but I think that the feedback can be handled by phone or mail; it's not necessary to have personal meetings." The participants described varying experiences regarding how the feedback had worked, but many said they wished that the feedback had been better. One participant expressed, "No feedback at all. You could see if someone [the healthcare staff] had been checking it, but there was never anyone who had been checking it. It felt like sending [data] into a black hole." There were also participants who had the opposite opinion, as one participant said, "I always got feedback on reported measurements, so they [the healthcare staff] had control."

Self-Care. Participants expressed varying opinions regarding self-care; some patients said that their health had improved, and others said that there was no difference. One participant said, "My health has definitely improved because I understand the importance of exercise." Another said, "I don't feel that my health has improved." The participants agreed that using the technology gave them increased control and insight about the importance of how exercise affects their health. They stated that reporting their physical activities motivated them to exercise more often than before. One participant expressed, "It engages yourself in a different way and makes you feel confident when you have control. This is two very positive things." The participants also stated that having control of their own health and measurements gave them

TABLE 2: Results questionnaire, Service User Technology Acceptability Questionnaire (SUTAQ).

Subscales	Diabetes $n = 51$	CVD $n = 48$	Hypertension $n = 154$
Enhanced care	5.10 (0,63), 5.2 $n = 48$	4.78 (1,01), 4.8 $n = 45$	5.04 (0,85), 5.2 $n = 149$
Missing	3	3	5
Increased accessibility	4.55 (1,07), 4.8 $n = 48$	4.15 (1,34), 4.5 $n = 45$	4.49 (1,10), 4.8 $n = 149$
Missing	3	3	5
Privacy and discomfort	1.53 (0,66), 1.3 $n = 48$	1.43 (0,51), 1.3 $n = 46$	1.51 (0,60), 1.3 $n = 151$
Missing	3	2	3
Care personnel concerns	1.97 (0,85), 2.0 $n = 48$	1.93 (1,01), 1.7 $n = 44$	2.01 (0,99), 1.7 $n = 151$
Missing	3	4	3
Kit as substitution	3.96 (0,83), 4.0 $n = 47$	3.45 (1,01), 3.7 $n = 45$	3.82 (0,88), 4.0 $n = 150$
Missing	4	3	4
Satisfaction	5.68 (0,52), 6.0 $n = 47$	5.41 (0,94), 5.7 $n = 46$	5.57 (0,70), 6.0 $n = 149$
Missing	4	2	5

a sense of security or safety. The participants expressed that health care provided this way will be part of the future and that it will expand. One participant expressed, "In the future, it will become even more of this. Yes, especially for those who live at some distance from the healthcare centre."

Privacy. The participants were consistent in regard to not being worried about their privacy being threatened. One participant said, "No. no, no, I don't feel that my privacy has been threatened. If there is anyone who wants to read, let them." Another said, "I've never even had a thought about it being an intrusive invasion of privacy." They also expressed that the reported measurements were not a secret or something they needed to hide from others. As one participant said, "It's not a secret; there is nothing to be ashamed of."

Experiences of People Who Withdrew from Participation. The interviews with those who withdrew from participation in the intervention showed similar experiences to those who participated throughout the duration of the project. Some reasons for withdrawing are shown in the quotations. As one participant said, "I changed healthcare centres so I could not continue my participation. I wanted to continue." Another participant expressed, "I had problems with my e-ID so I chose to leave, but I think it was due to my own lack of knowledge."

4.2.2. The Healthcare Personnel. The analysis of the focus group discussions with the healthcare personnel resulted in five categories as follows: reluctance to change the way they have been working, strengthening self-care, opinions about the application, and something for the future. The categories are presented below supported by quotations from the discussions.

Reluctance to Change the Way They Have Been Working. Healthcare personnel emphasized that they were forced to change their working methods and found it difficult to work in this new way. One participant said, "One has always a certain resistance to do something new." Another participant said, "It's a tradition hard to change...you're used that the patient visits the health centre." Healthcare staff described that they used the application when the patient visited the healthcare centre, which means that the staff used the application in the conventional care mode. They did not follow up on the data the patient registered in the application that was available on the national patient portal. As one participants expressed, "...have commented on it occasionally, ... I've used it when I met a patient and used it as their own control."

Strengthening Self-Care. Strengthening self-care was something that the healthcare personnel thought of as beneficial for the patients. One participant said, "Now the patients can use the system ... and it's for their own benefit and care." The healthcare personnel expressed that the advantage with the application was that it made the patient more aware of his or her own health and self-care. It was a possibility for the patients to notice when they exercised and to follow their blood pressure or their blood sugar. As one participant stated, "It's for them."

Opinions about the Application. The healthcare personnel had many opinions about the application. They expressed that in the beginning it was difficult to use because it did not function properly all the time. The healthcare personnel considered that there were too many steps they had to take before they could enter and start to work with the application. Some of the healthcare personnel expressed that to use the application in their daily work was a generational issue. As one participant said, "I think it's a generational issue. Should I be able to use it, it must be very easy to follow. Basically self-explanatory."

Something for the Future. The healthcare personnel highlighted that this method of working was something for the future. They believed that in several years the patients would be ready to master the technology. The healthcare personnel said, "you just have to look at your grandchildren and how they handle the computer and iPad and whatever it is called." They also expressed that support from the physicians was essential for the implementation of this method of working. Several participants expressed the importance of support from doctors.

5. Discussion

The main finding in the study is that both healthcare personnel and patients experienced the intervention to be valuable and to function well, but it is evident that there were different expectations about the fulfilment of the intervention. Patients expected feedback and support, while healthcare staff expected patients to perform self-management tasks mostly without staff support.

Thus, healthcare personnel regarded the intervention as valuable for patients to perform self-management but preferably without them supporting the patients. They meant that the intervention enabled them to save time and focus on more severely ill patients. According to a review study, relatively little research attention has been given to the effects of e-health on roles and responsibilities, risk management, ways to engage with professionals, and ensuring that the potential benefits of new technologies are made transparent through the interventions' evaluations and feedback [23]. Greater focus should be directed to empirical investigations in order to identify and anticipate how e-health services will impact everyday clinical practices and to examine how new e-health services will affect clinical interactions and activities and the allocation and performance of clinical work, as well as different methods of engaging with professionals before and during the implementation of e-health services [18, 23, 24]. The results of a study comparing the Agile Process and the Incremental Process indicate that development performance and product quality achieved by following the Agile Process were superior to those achieved by following the Incremental Process in the projects compared [25]. Agile models offer a smooth and flexible approach aiming to respond to changing requirements; adjustments to supportive tools under development can be adjusted during the process as needed. It is beneficial when requirements are instable and constantly changing. The Incremental model is a modified version of the Waterfall model, where the product is developed incrementally in parts as a response to increasing product sizes and are delivered in sequences, each with a wider functionality. It is beneficial when requirements are incomplete at the start of the project and elicited in time. [26].

Patients in the intervention group were highly satisfied, believing that the intervention enhanced their care and increased accessibility without causing concerns about privacy, discomfort, or the involvement of personnel. In general, however, it was not seen as a substitute for their usual care, although it was regarded as comparable to an "in room meeting." This is in line with the results of a literature review [27] showing that patients prefer a combination of telecare and traditional healthcare delivery. Therefore, telemedicine must be used as a complement and not a replacement for standard health care. According to Bardram et al. [28], information and communication technology (ICT) used in home health care must take into consideration the role technology should play in its use by patients and healthcare professionals. Home monitoring devices or systems can help support patients to have greater flexibility in their lives and to be more independent when managing their medical conditions. If patients feel that home-based self-care benefits and empowers them, they are more likely to continue to use it [29].

Although generally positive about handling the technical application and performing self-management care, the patients in the study commented strongly that they lacked support and feedback about the registered data from the healthcare personnel, and they felt that this left them in limbo. For telehealth to be a successful tool, it is necessary to ensure adequate follow-up and feedback to the patient [29, 30]. Without adequate participant education or with low health-literacy levels, the result tends to be lower compliance, while active participation with human support from a healthcare service provider reinforces good compliance behaviour [29]. The results in one study showed that elderly and/or chronically ill persons who have home telecare contacts at fixed times every day perceive greater advantages of home telecare; they also perceive the technology as more compatible and less complex, and they perceive more observability compared to clients who have home telecare contacts based only on their own initiative [31].

Healthcare personnel in the study thought that the intervention was something for the future and did not change their way of organising care work in order to support patients using the application. If they used the application, it was used in conventional care. According to Miller, healthcare personnel have to see the benefits of ICT; otherwise, they might have difficulty seeing the technology as part of their daily work routine [32]. Another study demonstrated that when barriers to successful implementation exist, healthcare personnel can lose their faith in using technology, for example, telemonitoring for patients with chronic illnesses, and instead perform tasks traditionally delivered face-to-face [33]. Addressing such barriers is of critical importance for the successful implementation of telehealth in routine healthcare practices. In an evaluation of a telehealth service for patients with chronic obstructive pulmonary disease and heart failure, several barriers were identified to affect the level of telehealth adoption by patients, including a preference for face-to-face physical contact with their healthcare personnel, technology anxiety, technical problems, and the belief that telehealth is unnecessary [34].

There were a considerable number of dropouts in the intervention group. Reasons included becoming too ill, finding the technology too difficult to handle, changing healthcare centres, and death. In a meta-analysis, the reasons for patients dropping out or withdrawing are important to recognise, as they can significantly inform the future development and design of information technology used for healthcare treatments [14]. Furthermore high amount of dropouts can compromise the validity of the results. Improvements in telemedicine require knowledge and understanding of how users (patients) physically and emotionally interact with and react to the technologies [18]. In our study, the information about the reasons for dropouts and withdrawals shows that more careful consideration is required before offering this kind of electronic healthcare service.

6. Conclusion

The main conclusion remains that telemedicine, for example, the use of ICT in healthcare services, is associated with high user satisfaction and acceptability by patients, a very significant result in an era of indisputable consumer sovereignty and patient-centred healthcare systems. It seems that healthcare personnel are convinced about ICT's benefits for patients and that this is something for the future. However, they are not convinced about its benefits for healthcare organisations. For the successful implementation of telemedicine, organisational changes are necessary.

Acknowledgments

This project was funded by the EU through the ICT Policy Support Programme, as part of the Competitiveness and Innovation Framework Programme (CIP), and by the Norrbotten County Council and Luleå University of Technology. The authors particularly thank the patients, healthcare staff, and the members of the project staff who participated.

References

[1] "Federation," in *Proceedings of the Federation*, Brussels, Belgium, 2015, http://www.diabetesatlas.org.

[2] S. Mendis, P. Puska, and B. Norrving, *Global atlas on cardiovascular disease prevention and control*, World Health Organization, 2011, http://www.who.int/cardiovascular_diseases/publications/atlas_cvd/en/index.html.

[3] F. J. He and G. A. MacGregor, "Cost of poor blood pressure control in the UK: 62 000 unnecessary deaths per year," *Journal of Human Hypertension*, vol. 17, no. 7, pp. 455–457, 2003.

[4] F. Ismail-Beigi, T. Craven, M. A. Banerji et al., "Effect of intensive treatment of hyperglycaemia on microvascular outcomes in type 2 diabetes: an analysis of the ACCORD randomised trial," *The Lancet*, vol. 376, no. 9739, pp. 419–430, 2010.

[5] I. M. Stratton, A. I. Adler, H. A. W. Neil et al., "Association of glycaemia with macrovascular and microvascular complications of type 2 diabetes (UKPDS 35): prospective observational study," *British Medical Journal*, vol. 321, no. 7258, pp. 405–412, 2000.

[6] WHO, "A global brief on hypertension: silent killer global public health crisis," 2013, http://apps.who.int/iris/bitstream/10665/79059/1/WHO_DCO_WHD_2013.2_eng.pdf.

[7] S. E. Inzucchi, R. M. Bergenstal, J. B. Buse et al., "Management of hyperglycemia in type 2 diabetes: a patient-centered approach: position statement of the American Diabetes Association (ADA) and the European Association for the Study of Diabetes (EASD)," *Diabetes Care*, vol. 35, no. 6, pp. 1364–1379, 2012.

[8] B. J. Wakefield, J. E. Holman, A. Ray et al., "Effectiveness of home telehealth in comorbid diabetes and hypertension: A randomized, controlled trial," *Telemedicine and e-Health*, vol. 17, no. 4, pp. 254–261, 2011.

[9] P. Kothapalli, A. A. Bove, W. P. Santamore, C. Homko, and A. Kashem, "Factors affecting frequency of patient use of internet-based telemedicine to manage cardiovascular disease risk," *Journal of Telemedicine and Telecare*, vol. 19, no. 4, pp. 205–208, 2013.

[10] S. Dang, S. Dimmick, and G. Kelkar, "Evaluating the evidence base for the use of home telehealth remote monitoring in elderly with heart failure," *Telemedicine Journal and E-Health : The Official Journal of the American Telemedicine Association*, vol. 15, no. 8, pp. 783–796, 2009.

[11] J. Polisena, K. Tran, K. Cimon et al., "Home telemonitoring for congestive heart failure: A systematic review and meta-analysis," *Journal of Telemedicine and Telecare*, vol. 16, no. 2, pp. 68–76, 2010.

[12] C. R. Lyles, L. T. Harris, T. Le et al., "Qualitative evaluation of a mobile phone and web-based collaborative care intervention for patients with type 2 diabetes," *Diabetes Technology & Therapeutics*, vol. 13, no. 5, pp. 563–569, 2011.

[13] J. L. Pecina, K. S. Vickers, D. M. Finnie, J. C. Hathaway, G. J. Hanson, and P. Y. Takahashi, "Telemonitoring increases patient awareness of health and prompts health-related action: Initial evaluation of the TELE-ERA study," *Telemedicine and e-Health*, vol. 17, no. 6, pp. 461–466, 2011.

[14] S. Jalil, T. Myers, and I. Atkinson, "A Meta-Synthesis of Behavioral Outcomes from Telemedicine Clinical Trials for Type 2 Diabetes and the Clinical User-Experience Evaluation (CUE)," *Journal of Medical Systems*, vol. 39, no. 3, 2015.

[15] D. Tao and C. K. L. Or, "Effects of self-management health information technology on glycaemic control for patients with diabetes: A meta-analysis of randomized controlled trials," *Journal of Telemedicine and Telecare*, vol. 19, no. 3, pp. 133–143, 2013.

[16] E. Ciemins, P. Coon, R. Peck, B. Holloway, and S.-J. Min, "Using telehealth to provide diabetes care to patients in rural Montana: Findings from the promoting realistic individual self-management program," *Telemedicine and e-Health*, vol. 17, no. 8, pp. 596–602, 2011.

[17] B. J. Wakefield, R. J. Koopman, L. E. Keplinger et al., "Effect of home telemonitoring on glycemic and blood pressure control in primary care clinic patients with diabetes," *Telemedicine and e-Health*, vol. 20, no. 3, pp. 199–205, 2014.

[18] R. J. Koopman, B. J. Wakefield, J. L. Johanning et al., "Implementing home blood glucose and blood pressure telemonitoring in primary care practices for patients with diabetes: Lessons learned," *Telemedicine and e-Health*, vol. 20, no. 3, pp. 253–260, 2014.

[19] Renewing Health, "REgioNs of Europe WorkINg toGether for HEALTH," http://www.renewinghealth.eu/.

[20] K. Kidholm, A. G. Ekeland, L. K. Jensen et al., "A model for assessment of telemedicine applications: Mast," *International Journal of Technology Assessment in Health Care*, vol. 28, no. 1, pp. 44–51, 2012.

[21] A. Steventon, M. Bardsley, J. Billings et al., "Effect of telehealth on use of secondary care and mortality: Findings from the Whole System Demonstrator cluster randomised trial," *BMJ*, vol. 344, no. 7865, Article ID e3874, 2012.

[22] B. Downe-Wamboldt, "Content analysis: Method, applications, and issues," *Health Care for Women International*, vol. 13, no. 3, pp. 313–321, 1992.

[23] F. S. Mair, C. May, C. O'Donnell, T. Finch, F. Sullivand, and E. Murray, "Factors that promote or inhibit the implementation of e-health systems: An explanatory systematic review," *Bulletin of the World Health Organization*, vol. 90, no. 5, pp. 357–364, 2012.

[24] A. Barakat, R. D. Woolrych, A. Sixsmith, W. D. Kearns, and H. S. M. Kort, "Ehealth technology competencies for health professionals working in home care to support older adults to age in place: Outcomes of a two-day collaborative workshop," *Journal of Medical Internet Research*, vol. 15, no. 9, article no. e10, 2013.

[25] A. Tarhan and S. G. Yilmaz, "Systematic analyses and comparison of development performance and product quality of Incremental Process and Agile Process," *Information and Software Technology*, vol. 56, no. 5, pp. 477–494, 2014.

[26] Alliance Agile, "Manifesto for Agile software development," 2001 http://agilemanifesto.org/.

[27] T. L. Williams, C. R. May, and A. Esmail, "Limitations of patient satisfaction studies in telehealthcare: A systematic review of the literature," *Telemedicine and e-Health*, vol. 7, no. 4, pp. 293–316, 2001.

[28] J. E. Bardram, C. Bossen, and A. Thomsen, "Designing for transformations in collaboration: A study of the deployment of homecare technology," in *Proceedings of the 2005 International ACM SIGGROUP Conference on Supporting Group Work, GROUP'05*, pp. 294–303, USA, November 2005.

[29] A. Maeder, N. Poultney, G. Morgan, and R. Lippiatt, "Patient Compliance in Home-Based Self-Care Telehealth Projects," *Journal of Telemedicine and Telecare*, vol. 21, no. 8, pp. 439–442, 2015.

[30] A. L. Bui and G. C. Fonarow, "Home monitoring for heart failure management," *Journal of the American College of Cardiology*, vol. 59, no. 2, pp. 97–104, 2012.

[31] J. M. Peeters, A. J. E. De Veer, L. Van der Hoek, and A. L. Francke, "Factors influencing the adoption of home telecare by elderly or chronically ill people: a national survey," *Journal of Clinical Nursing*, vol. 21, no. 21-22, pp. 3183–3193, 2012.

[32] E. A. Miller, "The continuing need to investigate the nature and content of teleconsultation communication using interaction analysis techniques," *Journal of Telemedicine and Telecare*, vol. 17, no. 2, pp. 55–64, 2011.

[33] J. Taylor, E. Coates, L. Brewster, G. Mountain, B. Wessels, and M. S. Hawley, "Examining the use of telehealth in community nursing: Identifying the factors affecting frontline staff acceptance and telehealth adoption," *Journal of Advanced Nursing*, vol. 71, no. 2, pp. 326–337, 2015.

[34] B. Odeh, R. Kayyali, S. Nabhani-Gebara, N. Philip, P. Robinson, and C. R. Wallace, "Evaluation of a Telehealth Service for COPD and HF patients: Clinical outcome and patients' perceptions," *Journal of Telemedicine and Telecare*, vol. 21, no. 5, pp. 292–297, 2015.

26

What Kind of Information and Communication Technologies Do Patients with Type 2 Diabetes Mellitus Prefer?

Iván Chérrez-Ojeda,[1,2] Emanuel Vanegas,[1,2] Erick Calero,[2] Karin Plaza,[2] Jose A. Cano,[1,2] Juan Carlos Calderon,[1,2] Jorge Valdano,[1] Jorge Oswaldo Gutierrez,[1] and Jose Guevara[2]

[1] *Universidad Espíritu Santo, Samborondón, Ecuador*
[2] *Respiralab Research Group, Respiralab, Guayaquil, Ecuador*

Correspondence should be addressed to Iván Chérrez-Ojeda; ivancherrez@gmail.com

Academic Editor: Carlos De Las Cuevas

Purpose. The purpose of this study is to assess the frequency of use of information and communication technologies and patterns of preference among Ecuadorian patients with diabetes. *Methods.* We conducted an anonymous cross-sectional survey on type 2 diabetes mellitus. A chi-square test for association and adjusted regression analyses were performed. *Results.* 248 patients were enrolled, with a mean sample age of 57.7 years. SMS was the most used ICT (66.0%). The Internet was used by 45.2% of patients to obtain information about diabetes. SMS and email were rated as the most useful ICTs for receiving information (64.5% and 28.1%, resp.) and asking physicians about diabetes (63.8% and 26.1%, resp.). Patients were also interested in receiving disease information (82.4%) and asking physicians about diabetes (84.7%) through WhatsApp. Adjusted logistic regressions revealed that individuals aged 55 years or younger, those with superior degree level, and those with long diabetes history preferred email for receiving information and asking physicians about diabetes compared to those above 55 years, those with low education level, and those with short diabetes history, respectively. *Conclusion.* Understanding preferences of ICTs among patients with diabetes could facilitate application development targeted towards specific requirements from patients.

1. Introduction

Diabetes mellitus (DM) is one of the most prevalent chronic diseases worldwide, representing an important cause of mortality and morbidity. In 2014, the NCD Risk Factor Collaboration estimated that 422 million adults were living with diabetes [1]. Latin Americans are an example of the most affected groups by this disease [2]. The prevalence of diabetes in this population is up to 14.3%. Furthermore, 12.4% of adolescents in Ecuador met the criteria for prediabetes [3, 4].

The increase in rates of nonadherence to medication, especially in low socioeconomic populations, has raised concerns about the considerable burden—both societal and individual—of this disease. Therefore, new strategies to improve clinical outcomes involving better communication between healthcare providers and patients are now being explored, giving rise to a heightened interest in the use of information and communication technologies (ICTs) for medical purposes [5–7].

ICTs are broadly defined as technologies used to communicate, manipulate, and store data by electronic means. This concept includes email, SMS text messaging, video chat (i.e., Skype or Hangouts), and online social media (i.e., Facebook or Twitter) as well as all the different computing and mobile-type devices (smartphones and tablets) that perform a wide range of communication and information functions [8, 9]. Recent studies have suggested that the use of ICTs in general may have a positive effect on patients with diabetes by facilitating communication between healthcare professionals and patients, as well as by helping patients learn more about their day-to-day care [10–12].

A recent systematic review and a meta-analysis demonstrated that the use of mHealth significantly improved self-management and glycemic levels measured with HbA1c. Interventions included text messaging, web interfaces, apps, phone calls, computer-based interventions, and social media [10–13]. However, many people stop using a healthcare app shortly after downloading it, suggesting that developers need to address consumer concerns better and that clinical trials are required to test the efficacy of health apps to broaden their appeal and wider use [14–16]. The same concern applies to social media, such as Facebook, where there are profiles that promote therapeutic modalities that are not approved by the FDA and could not be beneficial for a patient with diabetes [17].

Still, little is known about Hispanic population [18]. The aim of this study is to assess the frequency of use of information and communication technologies and patterns of preference among Ecuadorian patients with diabetes. These results might aid in developing new ICTs to promote self-management and improve diabetes outcomes.

2. Materials and Methods

We conducted an anonymous cross-sectional survey in which 248 patients with type 2 diabetes from Ecuador rated their typical frequency of ICT usage. Eligible outpatients from either public or private practices in Guayaquil (Ecuador) were surveyed using the Spanish version of the Michigan asthma questionnaire [19]. The survey included 22 items and collected information about demographics, use of cell phones, the interest of patients in using ICTs to receive information about diabetes, and the interest of patients in using ICTs to communicate with healthcare providers about diabetes.

The inclusion criteria employed in this survey were patients older than 18 years who have a diabetes diagnosis of at least 1 year. We excluded patients with psychiatric diseases or language impairment and those who found it difficult to visualize the survey.

2.1. Ethical Considerations. The study was reviewed by the ethics committee of Kennedy Hospital in Guayaquil, Ecuador. We obtained informed consent before participation in the survey. We guaranteed that the identities of the patients would not be revealed.

2.2. Statistical Analysis. For each ICT, responses to frequency of use were dichotomized into categories of “at least once a week” and “less than once a week.” Age, gender, education level, and years since diabetes diagnosis were used as independent variables on each analysis. Age was categorized into adults (≤55 years of age) and old adults (>55 years of age). Education level was categorized into none/pretertiary and undergraduate/postgraduate. Time since diabetes diagnosis was categorized as ≤8 years and >8 years.

We performed a chi-square test to assess the association among Internet access or owning a cellphone or smartphone and age, gender, education level, and years since diagnosis. We employed the same test to determine the association between same independent variables and the frequency of use of each ICT type and using each ICT to obtain information about their disease.

We performed similar analyses on the associations between the independent variables described and the degree of interest (dichotomized into “high or some interest” and “little or no interest”) in receiving information through each ICT type and interest in communicating (seeking physician) through ICT media type.

We performed adjusted regression analyses between the set of independent variables and use (“at least once a week” and “less than once a week”) and interest in receiving information and communicating through each ICT. Analysis was adjusted for age, gender, education level, and years since diagnosis. Reference categories were >55 years old, male, no education/pretertiary education, and ≤8 years since diagnosis, respectively. Finally, we performed separated nonadjusted analysis between frequency of use of an ICT and interest in receiving information and communicating with physician through that same ICT.

All the data were analyzed using SPSS software, version 24.0 (SPSS Inc., Chicago, IL, USA). We performed Fisher’s exact test where necessary. A p value of less than 0.05 was considered statistically significant.

3. Results

Of the 290 surveys delivered to patients with diabetes, 248 patients filled the survey and were included in this study (nonresponse rate of 14.48%). Mean sample age was 57.7 years (standard deviation [SD]: 10.4). Mean ages of patients ≤55 years and >55 years were 47.75 (SD: 6.02) and 64.38 (SD: 6.65), respectively. Average time with diabetes was 9.4 years (SD: 6.5) and the mean years of diabetes for the ≤8 and >8 years groups were 4.53 (SD: 2.42) and 14.66 (SD: 5.26), respectively. Most patients were female (62.1%) and reported having secondary education (38.7%) (Table 1).

3.1. Internet Access and Owning Cellphone or Smartphone. From all, 69.4% reported that they owned a cellphone, of which 46.8% were smartphones and 22.6% were regular mobile phones (Table 2). Internet access was reported by only 27.2% (Table 2). Individuals aged ≤55 were associated with a higher proportion of owning a cellphone and smartphone, as well as having access to Internet (Table 2).

3.2. Use of ICTs at Least Once a Week. SMS was the most used ICT (66.0%), followed by the Internet (36.3%), Facebook (31.5%), and email (27.9%). Overall, being 55 years old or younger was associated with a higher proportion of respondents for using every ICT at least once a week compared to patients aged above 55 years (Table 2). Regarding education level, the highest educated patients reported the highest use of ICTs (Supplemental Appendix, Table S2).

3.3. Use of ICTs for Seeking Diabetes Information. The Internet was used by 45.2% of patients to obtain information about diabetes. Other ICTs were not used frequently for this purpose (Table 2). Patients with the highest education degree

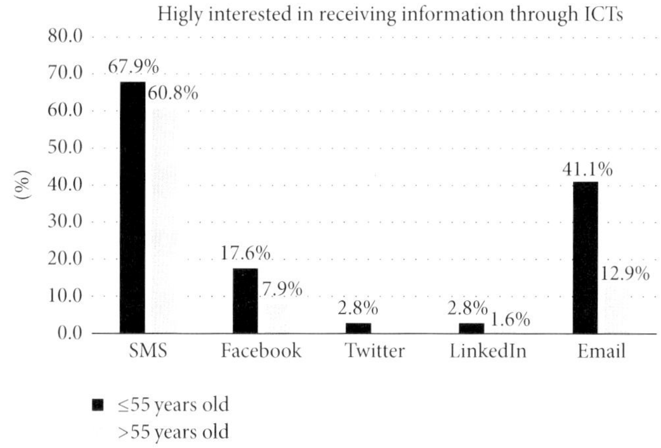

Figure 1: Proportion of patients who are highly interested in receiving information about diabetes through each ICT type.

Table 1: Demographic information of surveyed population.

Characteristics	Patients (n = 248) n (%)
Age (years)	
≤55 years old	100 (40.3)
>55 years old	148 (59.7)
Gender	
Male	89 (35.9)
Female	154 (62.1)
Race	
White	14 (5.6)
Native	0 (0)
Hispanic/mestizo	220 (88.7)
Black	7 (2.8)
Other	0 (0)
Education level	
None	30 (12.1)
Primary school	86 (34.7)
Secondary school	96 (38.7)
Undergraduate	32 (12.9)
Postgraduate	1 (0.4)
Years with diabetes	
≤8	127 (51.2)
>8	116 (46.8)

(68.0%) presented a higher proportion of individuals using Internet to seek information than those with no education/pretertiary education (39.0%) (Supplemental Appendix, Table S2). Analysis by years with disease reveals that patients with more than 8 years with diabetes represented the highest frequency of using Internet for this purpose (Supplemental Appendix, Table S3).

3.4. High Interest in Receiving Disease Information Using ICTs. SMS (64.5%) was the most rated ICT for patients to receive information about their disease, followed by email (28.1%) (Table 2). Regarding gender, males presented the highest proportion of being interested in receiving information through SMS (73.3%) and Facebook (21.4%) (Supplemental Appendix, Table S1). On the other hand, analysis by age and education shows that younger responders with the highest education degree had the highest number of patients interested in receiving information by email (Figure 1) (Table 2; Supplemental Appendix, Table S2).

3.5. High Interest in Asking for Physician's Information Using ICT. SMS and email were rated as useful when it came to asking physicians for information about diabetes (63.8% and 26.1%, resp.) (Table 2). Analysis by age shows that patients with 55 years of age or younger presented the highest rate of being highly interested in communicating with physicians through email (37.1%) (Figure 2 and Table 2). Also males (75.0%) presented a higher percentage of patients with high interest in same subject through SMS than females (54.1%) (Supplemental Appendix, Table S1).

Regarding education level, the highest degree was associated with the greatest proportion of patients being highly interested in requesting information from a physician through SMS and email (81.5 and 45.8%, resp.) (Supplemental Appendix, Table S2).

3.6. Interest in Receiving Disease Information and Communicating with Physicians through WhatsApp. A great proportion of patients were interested in receiving disease information (82.4%) and asking physicians about diabetes (84.7%) through WhatsApp. A superior number of patients with 55 years of age or younger (88.6%) were associated with interest in receiving information about diabetes through WhatsApp. Differences between the other variables' categories were not statistically significant.

3.7. Logistic Regression Analysis. Adjusted analysis reveals that patients with 55 years of age or younger are more likely to be interested in receiving information about diabetes (OR: 8.77) and communicating with physicians (5.96) through email than those above 55 years of age (reference category)

Table 2: Use, obtaining information, interest in receiving information, and interest in asking a physician through ICT types by age.

	≤55 years old (*n* = 100)	>55 years old (*n* = 148)	Chi-square *p* value	Total (*n* = 248)
Internet access	48.0	13.0	.000	27.2
Owning				
Cellphone	90.0	55.4	.000	69.4
Smartphone	64.3	27.0	.000	46.8
Use of ICT type (at least once a week)				
SMS	75.6	55.8	.009	66.0
Facebook	45.9	15.9	.000	31.5
Twitter	20.8	4.4	.004	12.9
YouTube	38.4	8.8	.000	24.1
Email	41.7	13.2	.000	27.9
Internet	52.0	19.7	.000	36.3
LinkedIn	5.6	0.0	.120[a]	2.9
Skype	6.9	1.5	.211[a]	4.3
Uses ICT to obtain information about disease				
Internet	54.7	35.2	.018	45.2
Facebook	8.3	2.9	.275[a]	5.6
Twitter	4.2	1.4	.620[a]	2.8
YouTube	4.2	1.4	.620[a]	2.8
Email	15.3	4.3	.028	9.9
Interest in receiving information through ICT type (high/some interest)				
SMS	67.9	60.8	.358	64.5
Facebook	17.6	7.9	.096	13.1
Twitter	2.8	0.0	.499[a]	1.5
LinkedIn	2.8	1.6	1.000[a]	2.2
Email	41.1	12.9	.000	28.1
Interest in asking physician through ICT type (high/some interest)				
SMS	69.3	58.1	.154	63.8
Facebook	13.9	4.6	.064	9.5
Twitter	0.0	1.6	.478[a]	0.7
LinkedIn	1.4	1.6	1.000[a]	1.5
Email	37.1	14.1	.002	26.1
Interest in receiving information through WhatsApp (yes/no)				
Interested	88.9	65.0	.034[a]	82.4
Interest in asking physician about disease through WhatsApp (yes/no)				
Interested	90.6	68.4	.056[a]	84.7

Notes. All data are presented as percentages. Differences in values between the two age groups are significant at .05 significance level. [a]Fisher's exact test performed.

(Table 3). Also responders aged 55 years or younger were more interested in both receiving information (OR: 5.49) and communicating with their physicians (OR: 4.96) using WhatsApp than patients above 55 years of age (Table 3).

Furthermore, females were associated with a lesser chance of being highly interested in receiving information through Facebook (OR: 0.21) and communicating with physicians through SMS (OR: 0.42) than males (reference category) (Table 3). Moreover, patients with superior degree presented greater odds of being interested in receiving information about their disease through email (OR: 4.32) than those with no schooling or pretertiary education (reference category) (Table 3).

In addition, a greater likelihood of being highly interested in receiving information about disease (OR: 2.70) and communicating with physicians (OR: 2.92) through email was associated with patients diagnosed with diabetes for more than 8 years when compared to those having the disease

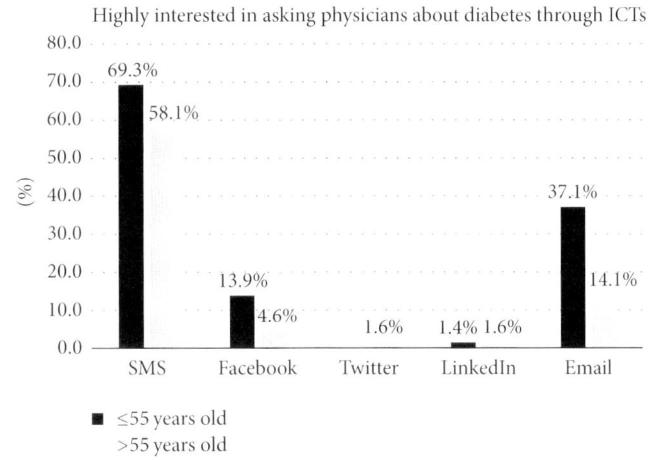

FIGURE 2: Proportion of patients who are highly interested in asking physicians about diabetes through each ICT type.

TABLE 3: Characteristics of frequent users of selected ICT types (≥1 X/week) showing high/some interest in receiving information and asking physicians about diabetes.

Variable	Interest in receiving information through ICT type OR (95% CI)	Interest in asking physicians through ICT type OR (95% CI)
SMS (n = 159)		
Gender[a]		
Female	0.49 (0.24–1.01)	**0.42 (0.20–0.89)**
Weekly SMS use[b]	**7.52 (3.49–16.24)**	**7.33 (3.37–15.94)**
Facebook (n = 143)		
Gender		
Female	**0.21 (0.07–0.69)**	0.77 (0.23–2.55)
Years with diabetes[c]		
>8 years	**0.25 (0.07–0.90)**	0.33 (0.08–1.30)
Weekly Facebook use	**14.50 (3.92–53.59)**	**8.89 (2.30–34.32)**
Email (n = 140)		
Age[d]		
≤55 years old	**8.77 (2.73–28.20)**	**5.96 (1.96–18.16)**
Education level[e]		
Undergraduate/postgraduate	**4.32 (1.39–13.39)**	2.75 (0.91–8.31)
Years with diabetes		
>8 years	**2.70 (1.02–7.17)**	**2.92 (1.07–7.94)**
Weekly email use	**47.05 (15.75–140.59)**	**25.47 (9.29–69.85)**
WhatsApp		
Age[a]		
≤55 years old	**5.49 (1.42–21.20)**	**4.96 (1.16–21.30)**

Notes. Regression analysis was adjusted for variables such as age, gender, education level, and years with diabetes. Regression analysis using weekly ICT type was performed separately (nonadjusted). Bolded values are significant at 0.05 significance level. OR, odds ratio; CI, confidence interval. [a]Reference "gender" category is male. [b]Reference "ICT use" category is "less than once a week." [c]Reference "years with diabetes" category is ≤8 years. [d]Reference "age" category is >55 years old. [e]Reference "educational level" category is no education/pretertiary.

for 8 years or less (reference category) (Table 3). However, these patients were also less likely to be highly interested in receiving information through Facebook (OR: 0.25) than the reference.

Finally, nonadjusted regressions found that responders that used SMS, Facebook, and email at least once a week were more likely to be highly interested in receiving disease information and communicating with physicians through these same ICTs when compared to responders using the ICT less than once a week (reference category) (Table 3).

If an individual indicated no interest in using an ICT to receive information or communicate with their physician, we included open-ended questions to explain why. However, only 0.40% ($n = 1$) was not interested in receiving information through any type of ICT, while all patients were interested in at least one ICT for asking physicians about diabetes. The patient that was not interested in receiving information through any ICT type explained that she preferred to communicate directly with her physician through phone calls or personally.

4. Discussion

Essential DM self-management is generally divided into different domains: nutritional management, exercise and physical activity, blood glucose monitoring and medication utilization, risk reduction, problem solving, and healthy coping [20, 21].

However, DM patients who do not receive education may suffer from many complications because of poor self-management [22, 23]. This is where information and communication technologies may play a major role to improve the clinical condition of patients. The rapid diffusion, low cost, and general availability of ICTs make them an attractive platform for managing care, communication, and interventions in chronic diseases as part of Self-Management Education (SME). For instance, telehealth interventions have shown positive effects on improving the DM control self-management in primary healthcare settings [24]. Anyway, in the present study, we found that 72.8% of patients have no access to Internet, and less than half have a smartphone. These results highlight the fact that access to technology in Latin America is restricted to a small group, which represents a limitation for health interventions through ICTs.

It has been reported that Latinos living in California make greater use of SMS, email, and Facebook than any other ICT [25, 26]. The present study suggests that SMS and email were the most useful tools for all patients for receiving DBT information and communicating with physicians, regardless of age, gender, education, or years with disease. There are several practical reasons for using SMS. It costs less than voice messaging, and it can reach people whose phones are switched off. Furthermore, SMS messaging is silent, which means that it can be used in places where it may be impractical to hold a conversation [27].

Regarding email, we found that patients with a diagnosis of DM of more than 8 years were approximately 3 times more likely to be interested in receiving information and communicating with physicians through email. Our findings are similar to those reported by Giménez-Pérez et al., where patients with a type I DM diagnosis of 18.4 years prefer communicating with healthcare professionals through email instead of Facebook [28]. In both studies, the population subject to analysis was above the second half of adulthood. Even though we found that patients above 55 years of age were less likely to use ICTs for these purposes, the preference of using only email in this group could be due to aging and chronicity of the disease, which predispose patients to become isolated from society, and feeling of loneliness [29]. Likewise, in Giménez-Pérez et al.'s study, patients in the fourth quartile of age (52 y–75 y) presented the lowest proportion of willingness to share information online with professionals. These data support the fact that a long history of chronic disease in the setting of advanced age favors the development of loneliness. A systematic review of loneliness and common chronic physical conditions in adults establishes how such behavior can be a significant biopsychosocial stressor that can complicate the course of the disease through reciprocal relationship with outcomes of diabetes [30].

WhatsApp is a cross-platform instant messaging application that allows smartphone users to exchange text, image, video, and audio messages for free. In Latin America, around two-thirds of Internet users are now "WhatsApping" in contrast with North Americans who have a somewhat lesser frequency of use of WhatsApp [31]. Our results suggest that WhatsApp could be appropriate for patients aged 55 or younger since they are five times more likely to receive information and communicate with physician through this ICT than others. Owing to the different categories of interest used in analysis for WhatsApp and other electronic networks, they cannot be directly compared.

Currently, in Latin America, some mobile operators offer different plans that include unlimited data usage exclusively for WhatsApp and Facebook services. This is probably one of the reasons why Latin America has a high social media penetration rate compared with other global regions [31]. We found among participants that Facebook was used as the third option for receiving and communicating with physicians, though it was a small proportion of patients.

There are different Facebook support groups, where patients can share their stories, learn from others, increase their knowledge, and build up hope. In a systematic review, examining the benefits of social media in chronic diseases, 45% of studies identified a positive impact with respect to support (via blogs) and disease modification (via Facebook) [9]. Furthermore, two qualitative studies about diabetes-related Facebook groups conducted by Greene et al. reported that more than 60% of wall-post topics were based on sharing information about diabetes [17, 32].

Level of education and income might influence ICT use in Hispanics. Hispanics with more education and with higher household incomes are more likely to report using the Internet. As a matter of fact, in 2015, only two-thirds of Hispanics (67%) with an education degree lower than high school reported being online, while 95% of those with at least some college experience were online during the year [33]. Our results show a similar pattern, where patients with higher education levels presented a higher proportion of using every

ICT more frequently, looking for information through such ICTs, and being interested in receiving and communicating with physicians than those with the lowest education degree.

Our results have important implications for designing interventions using ICTs to improve patient education and communication between healthcare professionals and patients. Given the fact that most of the population in Latin America belongs to a low socioeconomic status and public healthcare is not equally accessible to all individuals, it is imperative to find methods to diffuse medical advice efficiently. In developing nations, people living in urban areas have a reasonable chance of access to medical care, while those in semiurban or rural areas do not have such chance. If available, the former group may have access to very limited, if not deficient, healthcare. Our results suggest that email and SMS were used by patients in every age group. Also other social media channels, such as WhatsApp and Facebook, are becoming increasingly popular among patients. Even though it has been reported that there is a significant difference in preferences of health information technology tools used between rural and urban citizens in the United States, there is no current information on whether such observation replicates in Latin America [34].

Our study has some limitations. First, it was not conducted in all Latin American countries, and the preferred use of ICTs in other countries could differ. Our participants knew the purpose of the study, which may have affected the answers some of them gave. Our survey has not been validated, and our results could lead to biased or inaccurate conclusions. Finally, due to missing data in the surveys that were left blank by patients who did not want to fill the study survey, our group could not establish whether any significant differences existed between the respondent and nonrespondent groups.

However, one strength point of this study is that it covered a reasonably large sample size of DM patients. The sample included participants of different age, gender, and education level and, to the best of our knowledge, our study is the first to explore the use and preference of ICTs in Latin American DM patients.

Future research is needed to confirm our findings and assess the real use of ICTs tools as an appropriate development of mobile health applications. Any programmatic solution must be accompanied by a distribution strategy to increase patient acceptance and use of health care-related applications. Physicians should be enrolled with app developers to evaluate the design and development of such tools.

5. Conclusion

There are different preferences of ICTs in type 2 DM patients. SMS and email were the most useful tools for all patients for receiving DBT information and communicating with physicians. A higher education degree is associated with a higher interest of using ICTs for health-related purposes. The widespread use of ICTs opens new possibilities to the relationship between physicians and patients, improving channels of communication that go in both directions.

Acknowledgments

The authors acknowledge the guidance and knowledge imparted by the MECOR Program for this study, especially from Sonia Buist, M.D., and Ana Menezes, M.D. The authors are grateful for the support provided by Michell Torres, as well as all members of the Respiralab team.

References

[1] NCD Risk Factor Collaboration (NCD-RisC), "Worldwide trends in diabetes since 1980: a pooled analysis of 751 population-based studies with 4.4 million participants," *The Lancet*, vol. 387, no. 10027, pp. 1513–1530, 2016.

[2] American Diabetes Association, "Standards of Medical Care in Diabetes—2017," *Diabetes Care*, vol. 40, pp. S4–S135, 2017.

[3] V. Irazola, A. Rubinstein, L. Bazzano et al., "Prevalence, awareness, treatment and control of diabetes and impaired fasting glucose in the Southern Cone of Latin America," *PLoS ONE*, vol. 12, no. 9, Article ID e0183953, 2017.

[4] S. L. Casapulla, C. A. Howe, G. R. Mora et al., "Cardiometabolic risk factors, metabolic syndrome and pre-diabetes in adolescents in the Sierra region of Ecuador," *Diabetology & Metabolic Syndrome*, vol. 9, no. 1, article 24, 2017.

[5] D. C. Buse and R. B. Lipton, "Facilitating communication with patients for improved migraine outcomes," *Current Pain and Headache Reports*, vol. 12, no. 3, pp. 230–236, 2008.

[6] B. Bender, "Physician-patient communication as a tool that can change adherence," *Annals of Allergy, Asthma & Immunology*, vol. 103, pp. 1-2, 2009.

[7] P. A. Newcomb, K. W. McGrath, J. K. Covington, S. C. Lazarus, and S. L. Janson, "Barriers to patient-clinician collaboration in asthma management: the patient experience," *Journal of Asthma*, vol. 47, no. 2, pp. 192–197, 2010.

[8] B. E. Perron, H. O. Taylor, J. E. Glass et al., "Information and communication technologies in social work," *Advances in Social Work*, vol. 11, pp. 67–81, 2010.

[9] R. Patel, T. Chang, S. R. Greysen, and V. Chopra, "Social media use in chronic disease: A systematic review and novel taxonomy," *American Journal of Medicine*, vol. 128, no. 12, pp. 1335–1350, 2015.

[10] L. I. Faruque, N. Wiebe, A. Ehteshami-Afshar et al., "Effect of telemedicine on glycated hemoglobin in diabetes: A systematic review and meta-analysis of randomized trials," *Canadian Medical Association Journal*, vol. 189, no. 9, pp. E341–E364, 2017.

[11] M. Cui, X. Wu, J. Mao, X. Wang, M. Nie, and N. C. Barengo, "T2DM self-management via smartphone applications: a systematic review and meta-analysis," *PLoS ONE*, vol. 11, no. 11, Article ID e0166718, 2016.

[12] G. Petrovski, M. Zivkovic, and S. S. Stratrova, "Social media and diabetes: can Facebook and Skype improve glucose control in patients with type 1 diabetes on pump therapy? One-year experience," *Diabetes Care*, vol. 38, no. 4, pp. e51–e52, 2015.

[13] D. A. Greenwood, P. M. Gee, K. J. Fatkin, and M. Peeples, "A systematic review of reviews evaluating technology-enabled diabetes self-management education and support," *Journal of Diabetes Science and Technology*, vol. 11, no. 5, pp. 1015–1027, 2017.

[14] P. Krebs and D. T. Duncan, "Health app use among US mobile phone owners: a national survey," *JMIR mHealth and uHealth*, vol. 3, no. 4, article e101, 2015.

[15] A. C. Wu, J. F. Carpenter, and B. E. Himes, "Mobile health applications for asthma," *Journal of Allergy and Clinical Immunology: In Practice*, vol. 3, no. 3, pp. 446–448.e16, 2015.

[16] K. Huckvale, C. Morrison, J. Ouyang, A. Ghaghda, and J. Car, "The evolution of mobile apps for asthma: An updated systematic assessment of content and tools," *BMC Medicine*, vol. 13, no. 1, article 58, 2015.

[17] J. A. Greene, N. K. Choudhry, E. Kilabuk, and W. H. Shrank, "Online social networking by patients with diabetes: A qualitative evaluation of communication with Facebook," *Journal of General Internal Medicine*, vol. 26, no. 3, pp. 287–292, 2011.

[18] J. Hudnut-Beumler, E. Po'e, and S. Barkin, "The use of social media for health promotion in hispanic populations: a scoping systematic review," *JMIR Public Health and Surveillance*, vol. 2, no. 2, article e32, 2016.

[19] A. P. Baptist, M. Thompson, K. S. Grossman, L. Mohammed, A. Sy, and G. M. Sanders, "Social media, text messaging, and emailpreferences of asthma patients between 12 and 40 years old," *Journal of Asthma & Allergy Educators*, vol. 48, no. 8, pp. 824–830, 2011.

[20] B. Stetson, D. Schlundt, M. Peyrot et al., "Monitoring in diabetes self-management: Issues and recommendations for improvement," *Population Health Management*, vol. 14, no. 4, pp. 189–197, 2011.

[21] D. Tomky, M. Cypress, D. Dang et al., "Aade position statement," *The Diabetes Educator*, vol. 34, pp. 445–449, 2008.

[22] J. Barlow, C. Wright, J. Sheasby, A. Turner, and J. Hainsworth, "Self-management approaches for people with chronic conditions: a review," *Patient Education and Counseling*, vol. 48, no. 2, pp. 177–187, 2002.

[23] S. R. Shrivastava, P. S. Shrivastava, and J. Ramasamy, "Role of self-care in management of diabetes mellitus," *Journal of Diabetes and Metabolic Disorders*, vol. 12, no. 1, article 14, 2013.

[24] C. So and J. Chung, "Telehealth for diabetes self-management in primary healthcare—a systematic review and meta-analysis," *Journal of Telemedicine and Telecare*, Article ID 1357633X1770055, 2017.

[25] M. S. Bender, J. Choi, S. Arai, S. M. Paul, P. Gonzalez, and Y. Fukuoka, "Digital technology ownership, usage, and factors predicting downloading health apps among Caucasian, Filipino, Korean, and Latino Americans: the digital link to health survey," *JMIR mHealth and uHealth*, vol. 16, no. 10, article e43, 2014.

[26] Nielsen, Multiplying Mobile: How Multicultural Consumers are Leading Smartphone Adoption, http://www.nielsen.com/us/en/insights/news/2014/multiplying-mobile-how-multicultural-consumers-are-leading-smartphone-adoption.html.

[27] W. A. Kaplan, "Can the ubiquitous power of mobile phones be used to improve health outcomes in developing countries?" *Globalization and Health*, vol. 2, no. 1, article 9, 2006.

[28] G. Giménez-Pérez, A. Recasens, O. Simó et al., "Use of communication technologies by people with type 1 diabetes in the social networking era. A chance for improvement," *Primary Care Diabetes*, vol. 10, no. 2, pp. 121–128, 2016.

[29] M. A. Barlow, S. Y. Liu, and C. Wrosch, "Chronic illness and loneliness in older adulthood: The role of self-protective control strategies," *Health Psychology*, vol. 34, no. 8, pp. 870–879, 2015.

[30] T. Petitte, J. Mallow, E. Barnes, A. Petrone, T. Barr, and L. Theeke, "A systematic review of loneliness and common chronic physical conditions in adults," *The Open Psychology Journal*, vol. 8, no. 1, pp. 113–132, 2015.

[31] K. Young, "WhatsApp usage highest in LatAm," GlobalWebIndex, The trends to watch in 2017 ed, United Kingdom, 2016.

[32] Y. Zhang, D. He, and Y. Sang, "Facebook as a platform for health information and communication: a case study of a diabetes group," *Journal of Medical Systems*, vol. 37, no. 3, article 9942, 2013.

[33] A. Brown, G. López, and M. H. Lopez, Digital Divide Narrows for Latinos as More Spanish Speakers and Immigrants Go Online, 2016, http://www.pewhispanic.org/2016/07/20/1-internet-use-among-hispanics/.

[34] A. J. Greenberg, D. Haney, K. D. Blake, R. P. Moser, and B. W. Hesse, "Differences in access to and use of electronic personal health information between rural and urban residents in the United States," *The Journal of Rural Health*, 2016.

Permissions

All chapters in this book were first published in IJTA, by Hindawi Publishing Corporation; hereby published with permission under the Creative Commons Attribution License or equivalent. Every chapter published in this book has been scrutinized by our experts. Their significance has been extensively debated. The topics covered herein carry significant findings which will fuel the growth of the discipline. They may even be implemented as practical applications or may be referred to as a beginning point for another development.

The contributors of this book come from diverse backgrounds, making this book a truly international effort. This book will bring forth new frontiers with its revolutionizing research information and detailed analysis of the nascent developments around the world.

We would like to thank all the contributing authors for lending their expertise to make the book truly unique. They have played a crucial role in the development of this book. Without their invaluable contributions this book wouldn't have been possible. They have made vital efforts to compile up to date information on the varied aspects of this subject to make this book a valuable addition to the collection of many professionals and students.

This book was conceptualized with the vision of imparting up-to-date information and advanced data in this field. To ensure the same, a matchless editorial board was set up. Every individual on the board went through rigorous rounds of assessment to prove their worth. After which they invested a large part of their time researching and compiling the most relevant data for our readers.

The editorial board has been involved in producing this book since its inception. They have spent rigorous hours researching and exploring the diverse topics which have resulted in the successful publishing of this book. They have passed on their knowledge of decades through this book. To expedite this challenging task, the publisher supported the team at every step. A small team of assistant editors was also appointed to further simplify the editing procedure and attain best results for the readers.

Apart from the editorial board, the designing team has also invested a significant amount of their time in understanding the subject and creating the most relevant covers. They scrutinized every image to scout for the most suitable representation of the subject and create an appropriate cover for the book.

The publishing team has been an ardent support to the editorial, designing and production team. Their endless efforts to recruit the best for this project, has resulted in the accomplishment of this book. They are a veteran in the field of academics and their pool of knowledge is as vast as their experience in printing. Their expertise and guidance has proved useful at every step. Their uncompromising quality standards have made this book an exceptional effort. Their encouragement from time to time has been an inspiration for everyone.

The publisher and the editorial board hope that this book will prove to be a valuable piece of knowledge for researchers, students, practitioners and scholars across the globe.

List of Contributors

Mohd Khanapi Abd Ghani and Mustafa Musa Jaber
Biomedical Computing and Engineering Technologies (BIOCORE) Applied Research Group, Faculty of Information and Communication Technology, Universiti Teknikal Malaysia Melaka, Durian Tunggal, 75450 Ayer Keroh, Malacca, Malaysia

DavidMaunder, Julien Epps, Eliathamby Ambikairajah and Branko Celler
School of Electrical Engineering and Telecommunications, The University of New SouthWales, Sydney, NSW2052, Australia

Catherine McCabe, John Dinsmore, Anne Marie Brady, Gabrielle Mckee and Sharon O'Donnell
School of Nursing & Midwifery, Trinity College Dublin, 24 D'Olier Street, Dublin 2, Ireland

David Prendergast
Intel Ireland Ltd., Collinstown Industrial Park, Leixlip, County Kildare, Ireland

AyaWilliams, Rachel LaRocca, Trina Chang, Nhi-Ha Trinh, Maurizio Fava and Albert Yeung
Massachusetts General Hospital Depression Clinical and Research Program, One Bowdoin Square 6th floor, Boston, MA 02114, USA

Joseph Kvedar
Massachusetts General Hospital Center for Connected Health, 25 New Chardon Street, Suite 300, Boston, MA 02114, USA

Paola Pierleoni, Luca Pernini, Alberto Belli and Lorenzo Palma
Dipartimento di Ingegneria dell'Informazione, Universit´a Politecnica delle Marche, Via Brecce Bianche, 60131 Ancona, Italy

Tiziana Volpe
Community Health Systems Resource Group,The Hospital for Sick Children, 555 University Avenue, Toronto, ON, Canada M5G 1X8

Katherine M. Boydell
Community Health Systems Resource Group,The Hospital for Sick Children, 555 University Avenue, Toronto, ON, Canada M5G 1X8
Child Health Evaluative Sciences, Research Institute,The Hospital for Sick Children, 555 University Avenue, Toronto, ON, Canada M5G 1X8
Dalla Lana School of Public Health,University of Toronto, 155 College Street, 6th Floor, Toronto,ON, Canada M5T 3M7
Department of Psychiatry, Faculty of Medicine, University of Toronto, 250 College Street, 8th Floor, Toronto, ON, Canada M5T 1R8

Antonio Pignatiello
Department of Psychiatry, Faculty of Medicine, University of Toronto, 250 College Street, 8th Floor, Toronto, ON, Canada M5T 1R8
Department of Telepsychiatry, TeleLink Mental Health Program,The Hospital for Sick Children, 555 University Avenue, Toronto, ON, Canada M5G 1X8

Kjærsti Thorsteinsen
Tromsø Telemedicine Laboratory, Department of Psychology, University of Tromsø, 9037 Tromsø, Norway

Joar Vittersø
Department of Psychology, University of Tromsø, 9037 Tromsø, Norway

Gunnvald Bendix Svendsen
Brand Management, Telenor ASA, Snarøyveien 30, 1331 Fornebu, Norway

T. Vigneswari
Kings College of Engineering, Punalkulam, Tamilnadu 613303, India
System Software Group, M.A.M College of Engineering, Tiruchirappalli, Tamilnadu 621105, India

M. A. Maluk Mohamed
System Software Group, M.A.M College of Engineering, Tiruchirappalli, Tamilnadu 621105, India

Emma Derbyshire and Darren Dancey
School of Healthcare Science, John Dalton East Building, Oxford Road, Manchester M1 5GD, UK

Claude Takenga and Rolf-Dietrich Berndt
Infokom GmbH, 17034 Neubrandenburg, Germany

Olivier Musongya, Joël Kitero, Remi Katoke and Kakule Molo
Health Department, Baptist Church in Central Africa (CBCA), Goma, Democratic Republic of Congo

Basile Kazingufu, Malikwisha Meni and Mambo Vikandy
Ruwenzori State University (UOR), Butembo, Democratic Republic of Congo

Henri Takenga
Provincial Health Division (DPS), Ministry of Health, North Kivu, Goma, Democratic Republic of Congo

Annette M. Johansson, Inger Lindberg and Siv Söderberg
Division of Nursing, Department of Health Science, Luleå University of Technology, 971 87 Luleå, Sweden

Roberto Tapia-Conyer, Rodrigo Saucedo, Hector Gallardo and Ricardo Mujica
Instituto Carlos Slim de la Salud, Insurgentes Sur 3500, 14060 Ciudad de México, DF, Mexico

Carlos Meier, Joseph Smith, Daniel Estrada, Karen Becerra, Jonathan Mack, Michael Casale and Shelley Lyford
Gary and Mary West Health Institute, 10350 N Torrey Pines Road, La Jolla, CA 92037, USA

Antonio Sanchez and Ramon Sabido
Servicios de Salud de Yucatán, Calle 72, No. 463 Entre 53 y 55, Centro, 97000Merida, YUC, Mexico

Falin Wu, Hengyang Zhao and Yan Zhao
School of Instrumentation Science and Optoelectronics Engineering, Beihang University, Beijing 100191, China

Haibo Zhong
Space Star Technology Co., Ltd., Beijing 100086, China

Kevin R. Tarlow, Timothy R. Elliott and Daniel F. Brossart
Educational Psychology, Texas A & M University, College Station, TX 77843, USA

Carly E. McCord
School of Public Health, Texas A & M Health Science Center, 8441 Highway 47, Clinical Building 1, Suite 1300, Bryan, TX 77807, USA

Selma Limam Mansar, Shashank Jariwala, Nawal Behih, Maahd Shahzad and Aysha Anggraini
Information Systems Program, Carnegie Mellon University, Doha, Qatar

Priyanka Kakria and N. K. Tripathi
School of Engineering and Technology, Asian Institute of Technology, Phaholyothin Highway, Klong Luang, Pathumthani 12120,Thailand

Peerapong Kitipawang
International College of Medicine, Thammasat University, Rangsit Campus, Phaholyothin Highway, Klong Luang, Pathumthani 12120, Thailand

Juan Pablo Sáenz
Dipartimento di Automatica e Informatica, Politecnico di Torino, Turin, Italy

Mónica Paola Novoa
Fundacíon Universitaria de Ciencias de la Salud, Hospital de San José, Bogotá, Colombia

Darío Correal
Departamento de Ingeniería de Sistemas y Computaci´on, Universidad de los Andes, Bogotá, Colombia

Bell Raj Eapen
McMaster University, Hamilton, ON, Canada

Natthaporn Sudas Na Ayutthaya
Department of Pharmacy, Kamphaeng Phet Hospital, Mueang Kamphaeng Phet,Thailand
Faculty of Pharmaceutical Sciences, Naresuan University, Phitsanulok,Thailand

Itsarawan Sakunrak and Teerapon Dhippayom
Faculty of Pharmaceutical Sciences, Naresuan University, Phitsanulok,Thailand

Fan Yang and Lisa Gee
Department of International Health, Johns Hopkins Bloomberg School of Public Health, 615 N.Wolfe Street, Room E5030, Baltimore, MD 21205, USA

Jessica D. Rothstein, Larissa Jennings, Alain B. Labrique and Amnesty E. LeFevre
Department of International Health, Johns Hopkins Bloomberg School of Public Health, 615 N.Wolfe Street, Room E5030, Baltimore, MD 21205, USA
Johns Hopkins University Global mHealth Initiative, 615 N.Wolfe Street, Room 5635, Baltimore, MD 21205, USA

Karen Romano, David Hutchful and Anitha Moorthy
Grameen Foundation, No. 25 Labone Crescent, Accra, Ghana

Karin Halje
Young Adults Centre, Region Östergötland, 58185 Linköping, Sweden

Joakim Ekberg
Department of Medical and Health Sciences, Linköping University, 58183 Linköping, Sweden

Unit for Health Analysis, Centre for Healthcare Development, Region Östergötland, 58185 Linko¨ping, Sweden

Toomas Timpka
Department of Medical and Health Sciences, Linköping University, 58183 Linköping, Sweden
Unit for Health Analysis, Centre for Healthcare Development, Region Östergötland, 58185 Linköping, Sweden
Department of Computer and Information Science, Linköping University, 58183 Linköping, Sweden

Magnus Bång, Anders Fröberg and Henrik Eriksson
Department of Computer and Information Science, Linköping University, 58183 Linköping, Sweden

Antonio J. Salazar
Electrophysiology and Telemedicine Laboratory, University of Los Andes, Carrera 1 Este No. 19A-40, Bogotá, Colombia

Nicolás Useche, Aníbal J. Morillo and Sonia Bermúdez
Primary Stroke Center, University Hospital of Fundaci´on Santa Fe de Bogotá, Calle 119 No. 7-75, Bogotá, Colombia
School of Medicine, Universidad El Bosque, Av. Cra 9 No. 131A-02, Bogotá, Colombia

Manuel Granja
Baptist Health, Lyerly Neurosurgery, 800 Prudential Drive, Jacksonville, FL 32207, USA

Aihua Fan
Xían PolytechnicUniversity, Shaanxi, China

Di Lin and Yu Tang
University of Electronic Science and Technology of China, Sichuan, China

Tarsh Pandit and Robin A. Ray
College of Medicine and Dentistry, James Cook University, Townsville, QLD, Australia

Sabe Sabesan
College of Medicine and Dentistry, James Cook University, Townsville, QLD, Australia
Tropical Centre for Telehealth Practice and Research, Townsville Hospital and Health Services, Townsville, QLD, Australia

Mahnaz Behroozi and Ashkan Sami
Department of CSE and IT, School of Electrical Engineering and Computer Science, Shiraz University, Shiraz 71348-51154, Iran

Inger Lindberg and Birgitta Lindberg
Division of Nursing, Department of Health Science, Luleå University of Technology, 971 87 Luleå, Sweden

Siv Söderberg
Department of Nursing Sciences, Mid Sweden University, 83125 Östersund, Sweden

Jorge Valdano and Jorge Oswaldo Gutierrez
Universidad Espíritu Santo, Samborond´on, Ecuador

Iván Chérrez-Ojeda, Emanuel Vanegas, Jose A. Cano and Juan Carlos Calderon
Universidad Espíritu Santo, Samborond´on, Ecuador
Respiralab Research Group, Respiralab, Guayaquil, Ecuador

Erick Calero, Karin Plaza and Jose Guevara
Respiralab Research Group, Respiralab, Guayaquil, Ecuador

Index